BRAINPOWER
COOKBOOK

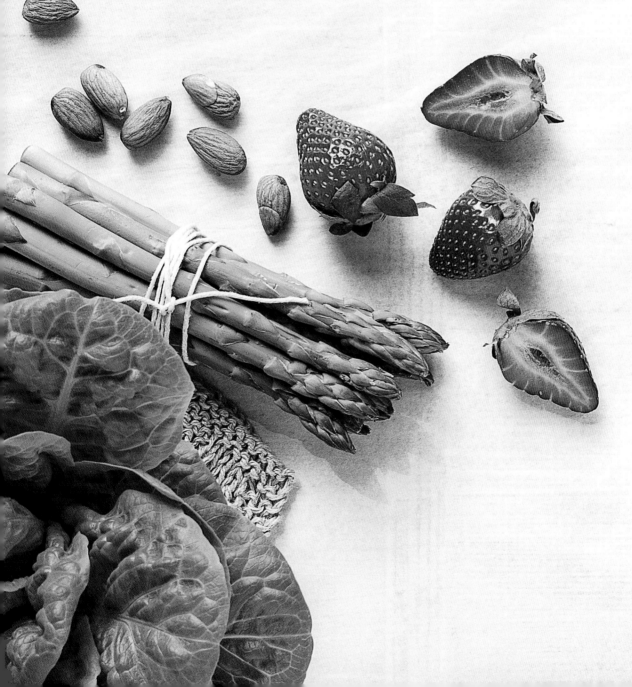

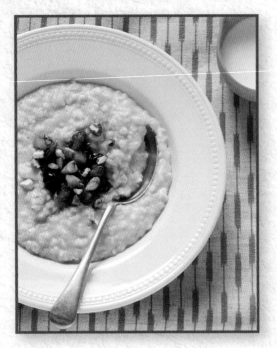
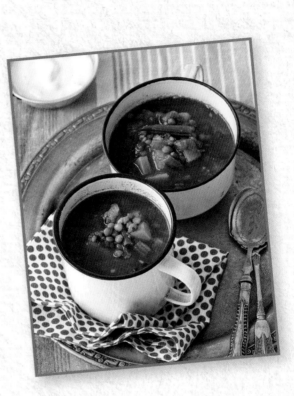
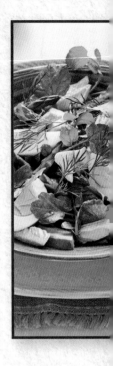
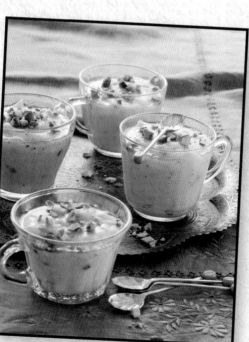
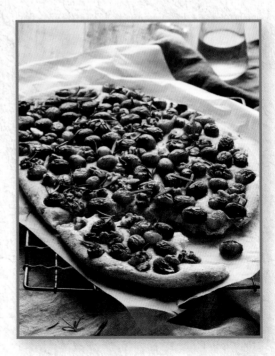

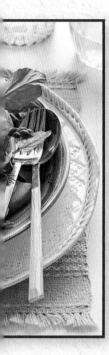
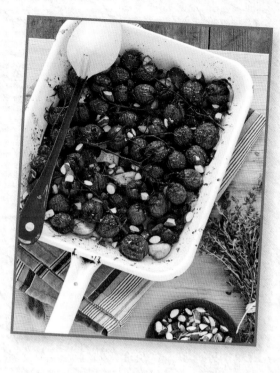
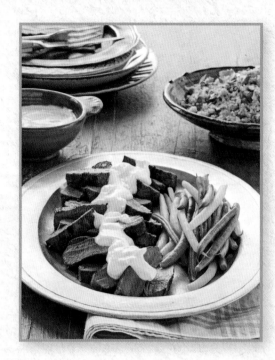

BRAINPOWER
COOKBOOK

175 GREAT RECIPES
to Think Fast, Keep Calm Under Stress,
and Boost Your Mental Performance

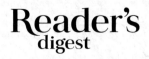

Reader's
digest

New York/Montreal

Foreword

The human brain is a complex and intriguing organ that we are only just beginning to understand. Not only is it the seat of our consciousness and individuality, it enables our thoughts, emotions, movements, sleep and vital functions. Our brains require a lot of energy to function well, and a healthy diet is essential for providing our brains with power. As a clinician and a researcher, it is an exciting time to be working in the field of neuroscience, since we now know that the brain is capable of changing in response to the environment, and that we can influence the health and well-being of our brain throughout our lifespan.

In my clinical role, I have for many years faced the unfortunate task of informing people of irreparable brain damage. It is imperative that we take whatever steps we can to prevent damage and to bolster the resilience of our brains against disease. We need to take a multifactorial approach to keeping our brain healthy, and we must implement these strategies as early as possible, preferably no later than midlife. Nutrition is just one aspect of a healthy lifestyle preventative approach. It is also important that we exercise regularly, get adequate sleep, reduce stress and tackle depression, keep our brain active and maintain a balanced social and working life. In addition, the role of vascular risk factors in terms of maintaining brain health cannot be understated. In general, 'what is good for your heart is good for your brain'.

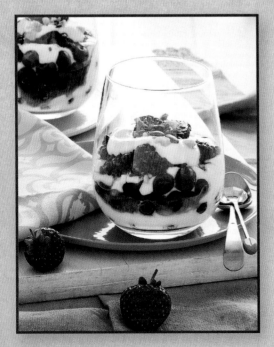

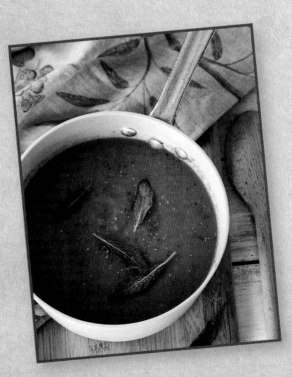

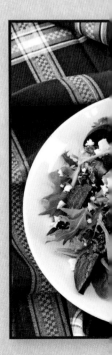

This means that we must strive to keep our blood pressure in check, keep our cholesterol and blood glucose levels down, and maintain a healthy weight. A healthy, balanced diet can help to tackle all of these factors, while also providing protection against free radicals and other harmful substances.

The *Brainpower Cookbook* will provide you with the inspiration you need to take control of your diet, your lifestyle and your brain. It not only covers the essentials behind the science of healthy nutrition, but provides recipes that are thoughtful, tasty and practical. It may even provide you with some interesting brain trivia to discuss at your next dinner party. The vast range of recipes incorporates a wide variety of fresh ingredients that will promote optimal vascular health, boost antioxidants, reduce levels of brain inflammation and, most importantly, promote a sense of well-being. This book is a must-have for any person, at any life stage, who values a healthy brain as much as indulging in culinary delights.

Associate Professor Sharon Naismith

Clinical Neuropsychologist and Head, Healthy Brain Ageing Program,
Brain and Mind Research Institute, University of Sydney, Australia

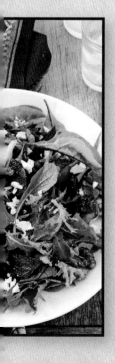

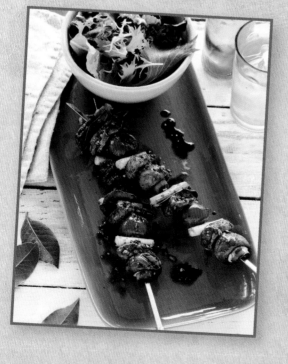

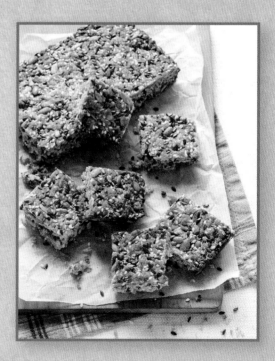

Contents

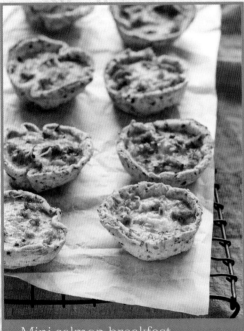

Mini salmon breakfast quiches, 38

Brainy breakfasts 22

Savvy soups and salads 50

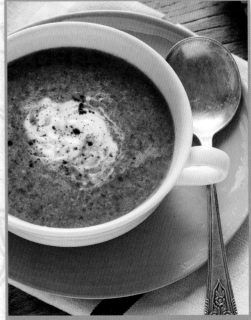

Spinach and lima bean soup with Greek-style yogurt, 61

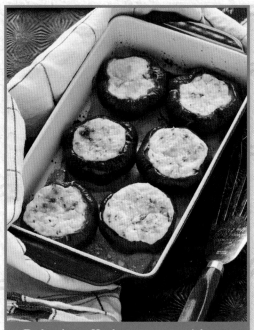

Baked stuffed peppers with herbed ricotta and tomato, 142

Smart snacks, light meals and side dishes 88

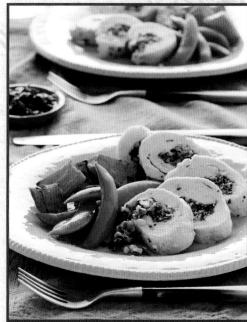

Roasted turkey breast stuffed with quinoa and herbs, 206

Mind-improving main dishes 152

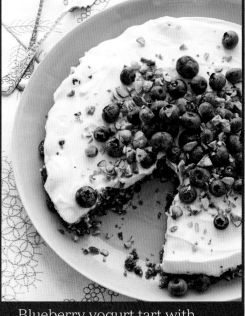

Blueberry yogurt tart with ginger crust, 256

Brain-boosting treats and desserts 228

Food for the brain

We all want to keep our brain in top condition, and it is becoming clear that nutrition makes a big difference. Optimal brain function relies on a good supply of just about every vitamin and mineral you've ever heard of, as well as a healthy cardiovascular system and a reliable fuel source. The best way to guarantee all of these is a healthy, balanced diet, rich in a wide variety of unprocessed foods. Increasingly, research is suggesting that supplements don't give us the same benefits as eating micronutrients in whole foods, so this book has assembled a great collection of recipes based on whole grains, fruits and vegetables, legumes, nuts, seeds, fish and lean meats. Of course they're healthy, but they're also packed with flavor so you can enjoy feeding your brain.

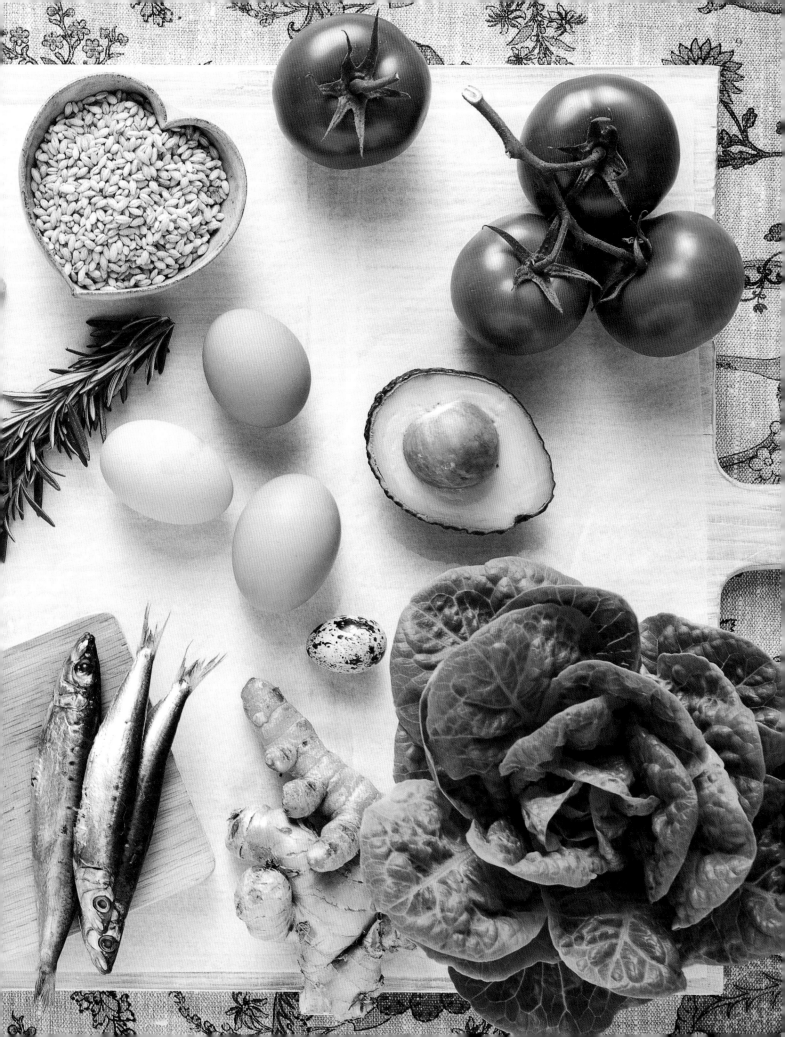

Brain food basics

The brain is at the center of almost everything we do, yet for many years little was known about how the brain actually works. That's changing now, due to technological advances in imaging and scanning that have allowed researchers to watch the brain in action.

Your amazing brain

Inside your skull, your brain is a mass of nerve cells, or *neurons*—twenty billion or more in just the cerebral cortex, the part that thinks. Each neuron has a long tail called an *axon* that acts like a communications cable, covered with a layer of insulation (called *myelin*), and carries electrical signals by branching and linking to perhaps a thousand other neurons. At each junction point, or *synapse*, chemicals called *neurotransmitters* take the message to receptors on the next neuron before being recycled or destroyed. The strength of the message can be increased or decreased by a variety of factors, such as chemical substances, hormones and your own behavior and thinking.

Some foods naturally contain substances that are similar to neurotransmitters in their structure and may have similar effects; other substances may help stimulate neurotransmitter production, block a receptor, or promote or inhibit the destruction of particular neurotransmitters, altering the duration of their action. This can be a very complex process (for an example, see *The effects of caffeine* on page 11).

Many of the substances that travel in our blood are prevented from entering the brain by the blood–brain barrier. This barrier exists thanks to the cells lining the brain's blood vessels, which are wedged tightly together so that their membranes form a wall to exclude intruders. Only substances of a particular size, shape or composition can cross this wall. There are particular doors (transport carriers) that let in hormones, proteins and substances that we need for normal functioning.

Make time for a tea break.
The many flavonoids and antioxidants in tea have been linked to the prevention of dementia.

Mood effects of food

It may seem odd to think that at any given time, your mood is the result of a combination of brain chemicals. Different substances are stimulated by events both in and out of your body. They can be affected by things that happen to you, such as winning a prize, losing your wallet, hearing a favorite song or being shouted at by a passing motorist. They can also be affected by what you eat.

These mood-affecting substances include the monoamines—neurotransmitters such as serotonin, melatonin, dopamine, noradrenaline and adrenaline (sometimes known as epinephrine), as well as related amine chemicals that can also affect neurotransmission. Each of the monoamines is transported into your cells by a specific transporter. Each has a particular role in the body, and each contributes to your overall mood and even perhaps some aspects of your personality.

Eat well to feel happy

The calm, feel-good message of the brain is serotonin. One of the building blocks of protein, an amino acid called tryptophan, is used to produce serotonin, so foods that are high in tryptophan, such as dairy foods, soy foods, eggs, meats and poultry, tend to promote a pleasant, relaxed state ready for sleep. Omega-3 fats also promote the production of serotonin.

Insulin helps tryptophan enter the brain, so foods that contain carbohydrate, which stimulates insulin secretion, may also help boost brain levels of serotonin. Carbohydrate also has the benefit of helping to prevent blood glucose levels from dropping overnight, which can cause a cranky mood and poor sleep. When it gets dark outside, the brain converts serotonin to melatonin, to promote sleep. Vitamin B$_6$ and niacin are involved in serotonin production, too. Some antidepressant medications lift the mood by stopping serotonin from being broken down or removed too quickly.

Dopamine activates the pleasure/reward centers in particular parts of the brain, but it also appears to be involved in regulating the daily sleep–wake cycle, helping to "switch off" melatonin when it is morning and time to be awake.

Adrenaline and noradrenaline are involved in the body's emergency response to danger and promote a "fight or flight" reaction, enabling the heart to beat faster and giving a surge of energy to the muscles. Ideally, this is a short-term process that switches off when the danger has passed. During prolonged stress, this response causes problems as it inhibits the normal digestion of food, interferes with sleep and brain function (such as memory), and prevents a happy, contented mood, increasing the risk of depression.

Altering your neurotransmitters

Individual variations in the production, absorption and destruction of monoamines may contribute to the mood differences between people. Some medications, smoking and foods may also alter these processes.

Substances related to the monoamines occur in foods such as aged cheeses, aged or processed meats, chocolate, alcoholic beverages and older foods that are nearing their use-by date. They can also be produced by gut flora, but normally we do not absorb them in a form that can affect us very much. However, some people do seem to absorb them, and if they cross the blood–brain barrier they can contribute to the mood effects of food in ways that are sometimes undesirable. For example, some people find they become euphoric after eating a lot of chocolate but then feel quite depressed a day or so later. This can be due to loss of serotonin that takes up to 48 hours to be replaced, while noradrenaline is present in higher amounts, resulting in a state similar to chronic stress.

Some vitamin deficiencies are very common among people with depression, highlighting the importance of particular nutrients in maintaining optimal mood. These include vitamin B$_{12}$, thiamine, folate, iron, zinc, selenium and magnesium.

The effects of caffeine

COFFEE, TEA AND COCOA contain caffeine (which is also found as an additive in some soft drinks). The level of caffeine peaks in your bloodstream about an hour after consumption, and lasts about four hours, after which it is metabolized in your liver.

This process produces a variety of other substances with their own power to alter blood pressure and blood composition, and also affect the brain and nervous system. Some of these effects may oppose one another. A major one is adenosine, which is a central nervous system neuromodulator, responsible for putting the brakes on the nervous system's activity. One of the main roles of adenosine is to slow down the brain, ready for sleep. It gives rise to a sleepy feeling and dilates the blood vessels to give the brain a good supply of oxygen while you sleep.

Caffeine blocks adenosine receptors, preventing adenosine from doing its job and therefore delaying sleep. Caffeine also helps to promote the pathway that produces adrenaline, again increasing alertness, and it increases dopamine production. Different people may metabolize caffeine differently, resulting in a different balance of these substances and therefore a different overall effect or one that lasts for a shorter or longer time.

In addition to caffeine, chocolate, tea and coffee contain a range of other substances such as antioxidants that have their own effects, some that also alter brain function.

Quiz

Is your diet brain friendly?

You might already be eating a great diet for brain health. Here's how to tell:
Just answer the following questions by checking **true** or **false**.

		True	*False*
1	I often skip breakfast	☐	☐
2	I tend to have fruit, nuts or yogurt as snacks rather than cookies or candy	☐	☐
3	I get very hungry between meals, especially mid-afternoon when I really "slump"	☐	☐
4	I try to limit fast foods to once every two weeks or less	☐	☐
5	I love crispy fried foods and eat them all the time	☐	☐
6	I usually plan my meals ahead of time and use a shopping list	☐	☐
7	I know vegetables are healthy but I don't always eat them because I don't like them	☐	☐
8	I try to have a variety of different colors and textures at each meal	☐	☐
9	I enjoy salt; it's just how my tastebuds are made	☐	☐
10	I try to eat unprocessed foods and avoid sugary, refined foods	☐	☐

For odd-numbered questions, score 1 for every **false**, and for even-numbered questions, score 1 for every **true**. Add up your score.

Score of 7 or higher: You are doing a good job of eating well to get the best performance from your brain. You can still improve, though, and this book may give you some useful ideas.

Score of 4 to 6: Your brain benefits from some of the things you are already doing, but you have lots of room for improvement. You might enjoy trying some of the suggestions in this book, to improve your diet for better brain health.

Score of 3 or lower: The good news is, you can achieve a significant improvement in brain health by making just a few simple changes to how you eat. You will be able to reduce the level of inflammation in your body and lower your risk of being overweight, having high blood pressure, diabetes and dementia. This book will inspire you to make a start.

The brain needs lots of fuel—it burns up 20 percent
of your energy intake every day—but make sure it is the right fuel.
Slow-release carbohydrates, such as legumes and whole grains,
will give your brain a steady and even supply of glucose,
helping you maintain your concentration.

How your brain gets its energy

Your brain uses up a lot of energy, perhaps 20 percent of your total energy expenditure. Its preferred fuel is glucose, and the brain needs a constant supply in order to maintain optimal activity. We obtain this glucose from the breakdown of carbohydrate foods—sugars and starches. Starch consists of long, branched chains of glucose molecules, which are split up into individual glucose units during digestion. Sugars are single or paired molecules—for example, table sugar or sucrose is a pair consisting of one molecule of glucose and one molecule of fructose (the natural sugar found in fruit). Digesting a slice of bread might produce 15 to 20 grams of glucose, which is then absorbed from the gut into the bloodstream where it can be transported to cells for energy.

Glycemic index

Some foods release this glucose very rapidly, because it is in a form that is quickly digested and absorbed. Pure glucose syrup, which does not need to be digested, is an extreme example; other fast-acting foods include most sugary and refined carbohydrate foods (such as puffed rice cereal or fluffy white bread). The glycemic index (GI) is a measure of each food's effect on blood glucose levels, and these refined foods have a high GI value, meaning the level of glucose in the bloodstream rises very rapidly after these foods are eaten. This triggers a rush of insulin that rapidly lowers glucose over the next hour or two, so that you may feel quite sluggish or hungry after the meal. Because the brain relies on a steady supply of glucose for fuel, it may not perform optimally when you mainly eat high-GI foods and snacks, as this can cause the level of glucose in your blood to fluctuate wildly. A high-GI diet can also have longer-term implications for your health, as repeatedly stressing the body's insulin system is thought to increase the risk of type 2 diabetes and promote inflammation in the body. This could affect the brain, too. A large Dutch study of nearly twenty thousand people found that stroke risk was higher in men consuming a high-GI diet.

Foods that empty more slowly from the stomach, and foods that are digested more slowly, tend to have a low GI value, thanks to a higher content of fiber or starches that are slow to break down, fat or protein that slows stomach emptying or other factors that lower the GI value, such as the presence of acid in the food. Low-GI foods create a steady and slow increase in blood glucose levels, not reaching such high peaks, and lasting longer to keep you going between meals and placing less stress on your body. You may find that this steady supply of blood glucose keeps your brain more alert and performing better.

Essential brain nutrients

Blood glucose levels are not the only factor in fueling brain activity, however. As your cells use oxygen to burn up the glucose for energy, vitamins and minerals are consumed as part of the process. A shortage of any vitamin or mineral can potentially prevent the brain from getting the energy it needs. The brain also relies on a good blood supply to deliver the glucose, as well as the required oxygen, vitamins and minerals. Some of the degenerative conditions that affect the brain are a result of changes in the cardiovascular system rather than in the brain itself, so looking after the heart and blood vessels is an essential part of brain health.

Running out of fuel

If you do not eat sufficient carbohydrate to meet the glucose needs of the brain, it shifts its fuel consumption to use more ketones instead, which are a product of fat breakdown. This might sound like a good idea, but the brain does not work as well when it runs on ketones. Very low carbohydrate diets may cause a slight feeling of euphoria but also a decrease in cognitive ability as the brain tries to make do with a different fuel. These diets can cause other health problems, too, such as loss of bone density, increased cardiovascular disease risk, kidney damage, bad breath and, in recent animal studies, significantly shorter lifespan. Cutting down on refined carbohydrates has many benefits, but it is not recommended to go so low that the brain has to do without its normal fuel source.

Low GI foods

The following foods have a low glycemic index:

LEGUMES—such as lentils, kidney beans, chickpeas

DAIRY FOODS—such as milk and yogurt (including low-fat varieties)

SOY—such as soy milk, soy yogurt

FRUIT—such as apples, pears, peaches, citrus

GRAINS—such as barley, oats, rye

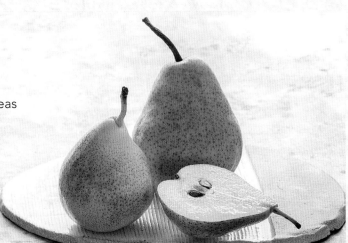

Keeping your brain healthy

Aging brings an overall decrease in body function, but your brain is particularly vulnerable to this process. Of all the body's cells, neurons are the most likely to be attacked by free radicals, which are rogue circulating molecules that damage the cells they encounter as they circulate in the body. Antioxidants help neutralize free radicals, preventing this damage not just in the brain but throughout the cardiovascular system. Many of the colorful pigments in fruits and vegetables are powerful antioxidants, so eating a wide variety of foods means eating a whole rainbow each day.

Micronutrients and your brain

As well as antioxidants, almost all of the known vitamins and minerals are essential for maintaining normal brain function, playing key roles in processes such as conducting nerve messages, supplying blood to the brain, energy metabolism in the brain, or making substances needed in the brain. For example, vitamin B_{12} is important in the production of neurotransmitters, and is also needed to maintain the layer of insulation, called myelin, that protects the neurons. Riboflavin is essential for obtaining energy for your cells, including your brain cells. Folate, pyridoxine (vitamin B_6) and vitamin B_{12} protect against inflammatory homocysteine. Vitamin B_6 promotes the production of mood-boosting serotonin, and some studies have found a connection between memory and vitamin B_6 status.

The consequences of an inadequate intake of many of these micronutrients include brain symptoms such as confusion or irritability, which then improve when the missing vitamin or mineral is provided. What we don't know is whether consuming more than the normal dietary amounts can cause further improvements in brain function or help prevent brain changes that are due to age or to conditions such as dementia. Recent research indicates that micronutrients in supplement form don't help. A 12-year study of nearly six thousand men found no difference in cognitive function with the use of multivitamins compared to no multivitamins.

However, obtaining your nutrients from whole foods is different, a bit like what happens in sports when you have a whole team instead of just a few individual players. Researchers are still investigating whether having more of these precious micronutrients in your diet has potential benefits for the brain.

Your brain's blood supply

Apart from the micronutrients, a key determinant of brain function is the blood supply. Your brain is richly supplied with blood vessels, but the health of your cardiovascular system determines how much glucose, oxygen and nutrients your brain can receive. If your blood vessels are scarred from high pressure, or are constricted and blocked with cholesterol, your brain won't be getting the oxygen and fuel it needs to function, and you will also be at increased risk of dementia and stroke. This means that healthy eating for your heart and blood vessels means better brain health, too—strategies such as choosing healthy types of fat, avoiding salt, and eating plenty of unprocessed foods like fruit and vegetables that are high in fiber and antioxidants. Protein is important, too. Amino acids are the building blocks from which all proteins are made, and some individual amino acids help to form neurotransmitters, the brain's communication chemicals. Protein is also essential for repairing body tissue, which is important to keep your cardiovascular system healthy.

When planning a meal, think in color. Colorful ingredients, such as berries, peppers and carrots, are rich sources of antioxidants that help to protect brain cells from damage.

Good fats

Another key factor in brain function is the type of fat you eat. Your brain is made of very soft tissue, high in fat, and the composition of this fat is altered by the types of fat in your diet as these are incorporated into cell membranes. With a high intake of omega-3 fatty acids, your brain cell membranes become much more flexible and responsive, which seems to improve brain performance. Perhaps because of their anti-inflammatory effect, omega-3 fatty acids also appear to help preserve brain function in the long term. One study of older Americans that measured cognitive decline over six years found significantly better results in those who ate fish twice a week, compared to those who ate no fish. The monounsaturated fats found in olive oil, nuts and seeds (as in the Mediterranean diet) appear to be beneficial in a similar way. However, it's not just the amount of good fats that counts—more significant is the ratio between the beneficial fats and the other kinds, so it is important that these good fats are used instead of other fats, not in addition to them. This is also essential to avoid excessive weight gain from the additional calories.

Junk food

Obesity is another factor that can increase inflammation in the body, but an unhealthy diet might also influence this more rapidly. A recent Australian study found that rats fed junk food for just six days showed a deterioration in some aspects of their memory function although their weight did not increase in this time. The researchers concluded that the high levels of saturated fat, salt and sugar in the diet had caused inflammation in the hippocampus part of the brain, which controls memory and learning, and that this effect was in addition to the effect that is seen with obesity.

Alcohol and your brain

You may think that following a healthy diet means avoiding alcohol, but in fact the relationship between alcohol and the brain is complicated. An occasional drink with a meal actually seems to reduce the risk of dementia and stroke, perhaps by increasing HDL cholesterol—the good kind—and making blood less likely to clot. However, exceeding the current recommendations appears to cause an abrupt increase in risk. The U.S. Department of Health and Human Services recommends no more than one drink per day for women and two drinks per day for men and recommends abstaining from alcohol for pregnant women and adolescents. Heavy drinking alters blood flow to the brain, increases blood pressure and clotting, decreases serotonin, and depletes the body of important vitamins, increasing the risk of stroke, depression, dementia and memory impairment. The Mediterranean diet, with its occasional, moderate use of wine, and particularly red wine—which is high in the antioxidant resveratrol—is associated with a reduced risk of dementia and cardiovascular disease. Drinking small amounts of alcohol with meals seems to be the key to protecting brain function.

What to eat at various life stages

The needs of your brain change as you get older. Here are some tips to optimize brain function throughout your life.

AGE 20–30 Recent research indicates that your brain is still completing the maturing process into your early 20s. Essential fatty acids, found in fish, nuts and seeds, and iodine, found in seaweed, are important in this process. You also need to make sure you have enough zinc and iron, found in shellfish and lean red meat.

AGE 30–60 As your life gets busier, it can be easy to skip meals or grab a quick meal on the run, finding your weight starts to increase. For best performance your brain needs regular, balanced nutrition without any excess calories. Find the time to set aside a couple of hours to make a big batch of soup or pasta sauce with plenty of legumes and vegetables, then freeze it in ready-to-go meal-sized portions.

AGE 60+ It is normal for brain function to change with age, but no one wants unnecessary loss of memory or alertness. The best strategy appears to be controlling weight and blood glucose levels with small, frequent, nutritious meals that have a low glycemic index and low salt content. For interest as well as enjoyment, eat a wide variety of foods, too.

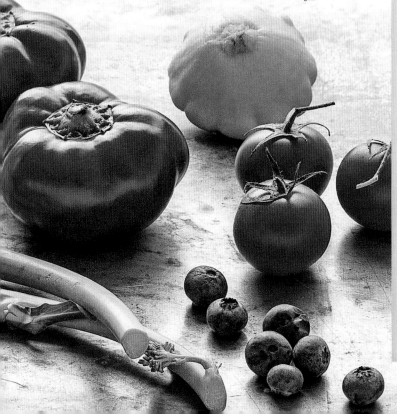

Brain food makeovers

Sometimes it takes only a simple change or two to turn a meal from brain-drain food to brain food that will give your brain the nutrition it needs.

Find and fix your dietary downfalls

✘ **Brain-drain breakfast:** puffed rice cereal with whole milk and sugar, white toast with butter and jam, whole milk latte. This breakfast won't give your brain the long-lasting fuel and the satisfying protein it needs to keep you going until lunchtime.

✔ Brain-food breakfast: whole-grain cereal with fruit and low-fat milk, whole-grain toast with unprocessed peanut butter or an egg, small skim milk coffee.

✔ The fixes: Substitute whole grains for processed carbohydrates to produce a slower and more sustained release of glucose to fuel the brain. Have a serving of high-protein food to help block the production of sleep-inducing serotonin and keep you alert. Improve blood vessel health by increasing fiber and cutting down on saturated fats so that your brain receives a good supply of oxygen and nutrition.

✘ **Brain-drain lunch:** ham and cheese sandwich on white bread, can of cola, piece of cake. After eating all these fast-acting carbohydrates, you will be sleepy and ineffective by mid-afternoon.

✔ Brain-food lunch: lean chicken and salad with a whole-grain roll, fruit salad with low-fat yogurt, water.

✔ The fixes: Stay hydrated with plenty of water for optimal brain function. Improve blood vessel health by increasing fiber and cutting down on salt and saturated fats so that your brain has a good supply of the fuel and nutrition it needs throughout the day. Choose quality

protein foods and avoid large amounts of fast-acting carbohydrates when you need to stay alert. Foods that have a high glycemic index (GI) are the ones that are quickly digested and converted to glucose, sending blood glucose levels up (and then down again) rapidly. What the brain really needs is a steady supply of energy, which will come from low-GI foods that release glucose more gently into the bloodstream. This means choosing foods that contain fiber, complex carbohydrates, healthy fats and protein, which leave the stomach slowly and are digested more gradually. Glucose is then produced over the next few hours instead of a sudden rush, giving the brain a prolonged supply of the fuel it needs for good functioning, improving concentration and memory, as well as keeping mood more stable.

✘ **Brain-drain dinner:** Take-out beef chili with fried noodles, beer, cup of coffee. This dinner might interfere with your well-deserved good night's sleep. Fatty foods take longer to empty from the stomach and they also require more time to digest, which can keep you awake. The large serving of protein and the stimulating effect of chili and coffee will also prevent you from sleeping. Alcohol also alters normal sleep patterns so that you don't wake feeling refreshed.

✔ Brain-food dinner: vegetable stir-fry with a small amount of shredded lean beef, brown rice, chamomile tea or warm milk and honey before bed.

✔ The fixes: Keep your brain's blood supply healthy by increasing fiber and cutting down on saturated fats so that your cardiovascular system remains in good condition. Add small amounts of protein foods rich in tryptophan, which is a key ingredient of a good night's sleep. This amino acid is found in meats and dairy foods, and its absorption is improved when you combine these foods with some carbohydrates such as rice or honey. Dairy foods also help produce dopamine to regulate the sleep–wake cycle. Chamomile is used in alternative medicine to reduce stress and promote sleep.

See **pages 268–279** for recipes that provide food ideas to optimize brain function in the following situations:

🌿 **Kick-start your day:** breakfast ideas for sustained energy throughout the day

🌿 **Boost your performance:** brainpower for exams and tests

🌿 **Avoid the afternoon slump:** lunchbox ideas

🌿 **Keep calm under stress:** brain soothers for stressful situations

🌿 **Think fast:** quiz-night food for fast brain work

🌿 **Sleep well:** nighttime eating before bed

Avoid these foods:
They might harm your brain.

Restricting calorie intake appears to reduce the rate of aging, including the rate at which brain function declines. Maintaining a healthy weight and avoiding overeating could significantly prolong your life. Overweight and obesity are associated with a decline in cognitive function at all ages including childhood, but particularly with increasing age.

It is normal to experience some decline in brain function after about age 65–70, but the rate of decline is steeper and starts earlier in those who are obese. High levels of fats in the blood, high levels of sugars in the blood, and high blood pressure all seem to make this worse. The large Framingham Heart Study, running since 1948 in the US, found that obese men with high blood pressure had the poorest cognitive function, compared to obese people with normal blood pressure, or people of a normal weight who had high blood pressure. This means that overeating of any type of food can be bad for your brain.

Excess salt
Maintaining a healthy blood pressure also means watching your sodium intake, as excess sodium causes blood pressure to increase as you get older. The United States Health and Human Services Department recommendation for American adults is to limit sodium intake to no more than 2,300 mg each day, which is the equivalent of one teaspoon of salt from all sources, but many people eat double this or more.

Refined carbs
Sugar and refined carbohydrates have been associated with poor cognitive function. In a recent study of nearly one thousand adults and another study of over seven hundred Americans who did not have diabetes, there was a notable decline in people with a high intake of refined carbohydrates compared to people who had lower intakes of refined carbohydrates. Carbohydrate foods with a high GI may make it difficult for the brain to receive a steady supply of glucose, as these foods cause a peak then drop in blood glucose level, and this rollercoaster effect can interfere with functioning.

Fatty foods
Not every low-GI food is healthy. Fat causes food to have a lower GI value, so a buttery cake or a deep-fried doughnut may have a lower GI than brown rice, despite being a poor overall choice for health. Also, GI studies measure only the glucose part of the food, so they don't register the effects of other sugar, such as fructose. This means that pure white sugar, also known as sucrose (which is half fructose) has a lower GI than bread. Despite its low GI value, fructose may cause problems if consumed in large quantities. It doesn't have the same effect on appetite, so it's not as satisfying as glucose, making it easier to eat too much of it, and it doesn't trigger an insulin response.

Sugary foods
Fructose has been closely studied due to concerns in the US about high intakes from high-fructose corn syrup (HFCS), which is added in large amounts to a wide variety of foods. Animal studies indicated that very high intakes of fructose or sucrose may have a detrimental effect on brain function, impairing cognitive function and, in particular, memory.

Smaller numbers of human studies have similar findings, again using amounts of fructose that are much larger than is possible in a normal diet unless consuming large amounts of fruit juice or HFCS-sweetened drinks. Study authors make a distinction between "natural" and "non-natural" sources of sugar, as it is very difficult to reach such intakes by eating whole oranges but quite easy with large amounts of orange juice or HFCS-filled orangeade.

The inflammatory effects of a very high sugar intake are thought to be responsible for changes in the brain, but there could also just be some simple effects resulting from the fluctuating energy supply that the brain receives when lots of sugar is consumed. Increased blood fats, formed when a very high sugar intake is converted to fat, could also be responsible for causing insulin resistance, which directly affects the brain by preventing a steady glucose supply.

Junk food
As well as your brain function, your mood can be adversely affected by what you eat. Recent research suggests that the risk of depression increases with the intake of highly processed junk food. One large study conducted by researchers in Melbourne, Australia, followed the diets of over two thousand teenagers for two years and found that the amount of junk food intake was associated with poorer mental health status. Similar results have been obtained in studies involving younger children, adults and pregnant women.

Saturated fat
Unhealthy sources of saturated fat, trans fats and refined carbohydrates may promote inflammation in the body, contributing to decline in brain function, with an increased risk of depression, anxiety and impaired cognition. In addition to this, trans fats and saturated fats have a known effect on the cardiovascular system, which means that the brain does not receive a good supply of glucose, oxygen and micronutrients to work properly. This could explain why high intakes of saturated fat are also associated with poorer performance in cognitive tests and memory tests, and with a higher risk of developing dementia.

Use it or lose it

It was long believed that the brain couldn't change—that brain damage was permanent and unrepairable, that everything in the brain was "hard-wired" like a computer, and that deterioration was the only way the brain could ever alter over time. Unlike, say, a cut on your arm, the human brain does not have a healing process where it gets rid of damaged tissue and regrows new tissue in its place: Damaged areas of the brain become permanently unusable, like a burnt-out electrical circuit. It was thought that this meant there was no way to heal from a brain injury. Not so.

Your changing brain

Thanks to developments in brain imaging technology, it has been possible to see what is really happening in the brain. This new area of research has revealed a concept called *neuroplasticity*, the idea that the brain is constantly changing, altering the way its circuits connect to one another and altering which parts of the brain are used for which functions. It turns out that the brain is flexible, constantly being shaped by our experiences, by practice and training, and by our sensory inputs. Increased firing rates in one part of the brain influence other parts nearby or connected to it, forming new neural pathways or altering existing ones, leading to new ways of processing information and even increasing the size of some parts of the brain. It is now known that new neurons form all the time, even in the elderly.

Grow your brain

You can stimulate the growth of your brain by exposing yourself to new environments and experiences, and by doing physical activity. Physical activity improves brain function by increasing oxygen flow to the brain, but it also increases sensory input to stimulate many areas of the brain directly. Learning new things also reduces the loss of neurons so that the net effect is an increase in mass of that part of the brain.

Visualization has long been promoted as a way to help you achieve your goals, and now this new research on the brain shows us why this works. It is simpler than you might think: Visualizing an object in your mind uses the same part of the brain as actually seeing the object, and mentally practicing an action results in the same physical changes in your brain as actually doing the action. Research studies have demonstrated that those who spend a lot of time mentally practicing, and just a small period physically practicing, can often achieve similar competence when compared to those who only do physical practice. You might think your muscles need physical practice in order to become competent, but a lot of the improvement in competence is actually not occurring at the "muscles" end of the process but instead at the "brain" end: With increased competence, the neural connections involved have become more activated, extra areas of the brain have been recruited to help, and the neural pathways have become more

established as neurons that are repeatedly fired at the same time become more strongly connected. This means neural communication becomes more efficient and the nerve signals become clearer, more precise and faster. This can be useful if you are trying to develop a skill, but it can be inconvenient if the increased efficiency has helped a bad habit to become even more ingrained because it follows the same process.

Keep your brain fit

Neuroplasticity research has found that particular types of exercises or activities may have a stronger effect than others in improving brain function. In particular, brain stimulation occurs the most, and its effects last the longest, when you are challenged by activities where you have to concentrate and focus closely, particularly on sounds, and activities that offer new experiences. Unfortunately, we tend to do fewer of these activities as we get older, at the time of life when they offer most benefit. This creates a vicious cycle, as people with brain deterioration become less confident about going out, traveling or learning new things, so they avoid precisely the activities that could help them maintain brain function. It literally is a case of "use it or lose it."

Sensory stimulation helps to maintain the systems in the brain that regulate brain plasticity. Best of all are activities that require highly focused attention, such as learning a new language, learning a musical instrument, juggling or learning a new dance, but even taking a bus to an unfamiliar place or walking barefoot in grass or sand can encourage the formation of new neurons.

Simple exercises that help to promote brain fitness include retelling stories, using your mental arithmetic skills instead of reaching for the calculator, doing a crossword or sudoku puzzle, and keeping up with and discussing current events. Complete the brain-training exercises and puzzles on pages 280–289. Enlisting for some volunteer work, starting a tricky hobby or making a career change are also effective ways to exercise and stretch your brain. Don't go overboard in challenging yourself, however: Stress is a key factor that reduces brain plasticity. Avoiding stress or reacting to things in a stressful way is very important for good brain health in the long term.

Lifestyle: Put a spring in your step.

Although food has a profound influence on your brain function, the benefits from your healthy diet could be outweighed by other lifestyle factors that can damage your brain. The good news is that when you improve your lifestyle, your whole body will benefit.

Cut down on stress

Stress is the body's short-term response to a challenge, keeping the brain alert with a good supply of adrenaline and fuel for quick thinking and fast reaction. However, constant low-level stress is damaging to the brain over time, as it raises blood glucose levels, increases blood pressure, promotes inflammation and affects your digestion and sleep. It stops the body from carrying out the normal maintenance tasks that keep it repaired and healthy, and increases the risk of depression.

Chronic stress can prevent the brain from saving new memories or being able to retrieve stored ones. For optimal brain health and function, it is important to address and manage stress. You may not be able to do anything about the cause of your stress, but there are strategies that can help to reduce its impact on the health of your body and your brain. Prioritize getting enough sleep and regular exercise. Take your time with the things you need to do, just tackling one task at a time. Smile—it activates some of the brain chemicals that are associated with happy emotions—and take the time to do little kindnesses for others. Remind yourself of all the things you are grateful for, and take some time to enjoy reminiscing. Indulging in happy memories has been shown in several studies to promote positive brain states like optimism and resilience, which help with managing stress. Slow, gentle breathing, relaxation exercises, meditation or yoga are proven to have the ability to counteract the physical and mental effects of stress.

Exercise

Apart from its benefits for cardiovascular health, bone density and joint function, aerobic exercise produces hormones that directly stimulate the production of new neurons, resulting in better memory function and increased size of the hippocampus (the memory part of the brain). Activities that combine social, mental and physical activity are the best—dancing, walking clubs and travel are good examples. Exercise enhances other aspects of mental function, too, such as alertness and concentration, as well as improving mood. This is partly because it promotes blood circulation, but also because it often allows the mind the freedom to roam and relax. Overweight and obese people often think they can't exercise, but this is false—just check with your doctor before starting anything new or vigorous. Obese people who participate in regular exercise tend to have better health outcomes than normal weight people who never do any, and these health outcomes include brain health.

Sleep well

Sleep happens in cycles, alternating between the rapid eye movement (REM) sleep that refreshes your brain, and the deep sleep that rests your body. During REM sleep you dream and consolidate memories, like a clerk sifting through the day's paperwork and filing everything into long-term storage. This is the sleep that leaves you feeling alert and ready for the day. Early in the morning the amount of REM sleep is increasing, so this is the main kind of sleep that you will miss if your sleep is cut short, or if alcohol has disturbed your sleep. The neurotransmitter dopamine is involved in regulating sleep–wake cycles and is responsible for your refreshed feeling of alertness in the morning after REM sleep. In animal studies where dopamine is completely blocked, REM sleep doesn't happen at all. Repeatedly missing your REM sleep makes this worse by decreasing the number of dopamine receptors, so that even after a rare sleep-in you can get up feeling tired, slow, grumpy and unfocused. Some researchers also suspect that dopamine deficiency is responsible for restless legs syndrome, which can lead to a poor night's sleep for some people.

Tips for a good night's sleep

- Get up at the same time every morning.
- Open the curtains or go outside to get light exposure when you wake in the morning.
- If taking a nap during the day, nap just after lunchtime and for no more than 30 minutes.
- Avoid caffeine in the afternoon.
- Avoid heavy meals at night.
- Don't take a bath that is too hot before bedtime.
- Have a light carbohydrate snack or some milk before bed.

7 ways to improve your brain in 7 days

Monday
Plan to get enough sleep.
Organize your evening so that you are ready for bed an hour earlier than usual. Keep your evening meal light and alcohol-free, and have a small carbohydrate snack before bed. Choose a quiet activity for the last thing at night, without any bright screens or lights, or loud noise.

Tuesday
Schedule some exercise.
Adequate aerobic exercise is important for whole-body health, but it also has significant short- and long-term benefits for the brain. Today, schedule your exercise for the week ahead and make it easy for yourself to stick to it, by planning it carefully. For example, pack your gym bag or get out your running gear the night before, or make a date with a friend to go walking or dancing.

Wednesday
Train your brain.
Keep your brain fit with a crossword or sudoku puzzle today, when you have some free time. Try online brain-training exercises. Teach yourself to juggle (start with lightweight handkerchiefs or small beanbags at first). Sign up for a language course. All of these activities stimulate the brain to improve long-term functioning.

Thursday
Make a health plan.
When was the last time you had a complete physical? High blood pressure, smoking, type 2 diabetes and heart disease are all associated with a decline in brain function, so it is important to identify and treat these problems early.

Friday
Plan to be social.
Invite friends for a meal, start a book club, phone a family member or just take your dog to the local dog park and chat to other owners. Oxytocin, the hormone generated by feelings of affection for others, helps to reduce stress and inflammation. Cuddling your cat for 10 minutes can significantly increase your oxytocin levels, if the humans in your life are unavailable.

Saturday
Try something new.
Try a new recipe today, or shop in a different town and buy an ingredient you have never used before. Like any other new experience, unfamiliar flavors stimulate the formation of new neurons. You can also take this opportunity to choose a few foods that are high in brain-boosting antioxidants, healthy fats and unprocessed carbohydrates for optimal brain health.

Sunday
Relax and rejuvenate.
If you have been experiencing stress, take the time to think about what is causing it. Decide whether there are any actions you can take to reduce the stress, or whether you need instead to choose how you will react to the stress. Say no to people who are asking too much, and take some time for yourself. It is important to do this because chronic low-level stress inhibits brain growth and plasticity, and promotes inflammation in the body. Spend time relaxing each day, focusing on a book or quiet hobby or something else that allows you to be reflective and calm. Meditation, yoga or a relaxation exercise can all be helpful here.

Diet and dementia

Are you optimizing your brain health as you get older? Complete this checklist:

- ☐ I'm keeping my weight stable in the healthy range for my age.
- ☐ I stick to small amounts of alcohol, mainly with meals.
- ☐ I choose low-sodium foods when shopping.
- ☐ I don't eat processed foods very often.
- ☐ Most of what I eat is unprocessed vegetables, fruits, legumes, grains, nuts and seeds.
- ☐ I keep my meat lean, and have it in small amounts.
- ☐ I have three servings of low-fat dairy foods each day.
- ☐ I avoid foods high in refined sugar and starch.
- ☐ I avoid adding salt or sugar to my food.
- ☐ I eat small meals frequently rather than a few very large meals.

Staying sharp

It is normal for brain function to start declining after about age 65 to 70, but around one in five older people experiences a dramatic loss of skills in memory, focus, judgement and social ability associated with damage to the brain. Dementia is a progressive and devastating loss of function, caused by blood vessel damage, stroke or Alzheimer's disease. It has been claimed that the incidence of dementia could be halved purely by altering lifestyle factors. This would mean that, apart from getting enough sleep, keeping fit, avoiding smoking and staying mentally active with puzzles and social activities, you could reduce your risk of dementia by the food choices that you make.

The right diet

A diet that is rich in plant foods, with small amounts of alcohol and caffeine (like the Mediterranean diet), may be protective against dementia. This means eating plenty of legumes, vegetables and whole grains, nuts and seeds; eating more fish and olive oil; and eating less vegetable oil, fatty grain-fed meats and salt. The same foods that are important for heart health are also influential in brain health, and this might help to explain why eating excessive saturated and trans fats appears to double the risk of developing dementia. As people get older, vitamin B_{12} becomes more important for health, and unfortunately at the same time, harder to obtain from food as absorption decreases with age. Vitamin B_{12} is found only in animal foods, so it is important to have enough low-fat dairy products, lean meats, fish and eggs; vegans need to take a B_{12} supplement.

Diabetes and the brain

Obesity and type 2 diabetes both appear to significantly increase the risk of dementia, doubling or tripling the risk. And even if you don't have diabetes, high blood glucose could be increasing your dementia risk. The Sydney (Australia) Memory and Aging Study is following over one thousand older people and reviewing their brain function every two years. So far there are worrying indications that people with diabetes are more likely to have signs of brain shrinkage and cognitive decline. More worrying is the fact that people without diabetes but whose fasting blood glucose is raised show similar (but less dramatic) brain changes. Blood glucose levels appear to correlate with the rate of brain atrophy and cognitive decline, particularly in the area of memory. High blood glucose levels cause proteins nearby in the blood to get stuck to a sugar molecule, a process called glycosylation. Glycosylated proteins floating around in the blood increase inflammation and oxidative stress, both of which damage brain cells. Avoiding overeating, controlling weight and getting enough exercise are important ways to reduce this effect.

Controlling blood glucose

Eating less carbohydrate has been suggested as a way of reducing blood glucose levels in order to combat the risk of dementia. The most extreme proponents of this idea have advocated avoiding nearly all carbohydrate, particularly grains, to keep blood glucose levels low. However, completely avoiding carbohydrates is not the best way to lower your blood glucose level while still keeping your brain happy (see *How your brain gets its energy*, page 13). It makes much more sense to avoid sugary and refined carbohydrates and eat plenty of vegetables and fiber so that your blood glucose levels are kept steady at a relatively low level. Controlling your weight and blood pressure is also very important for brain health.

Avoid that afternoon slump. Eat whole-grain breads—the grains are rich in B vitamins, which are vital for nerve function, and the energy is released slowly.

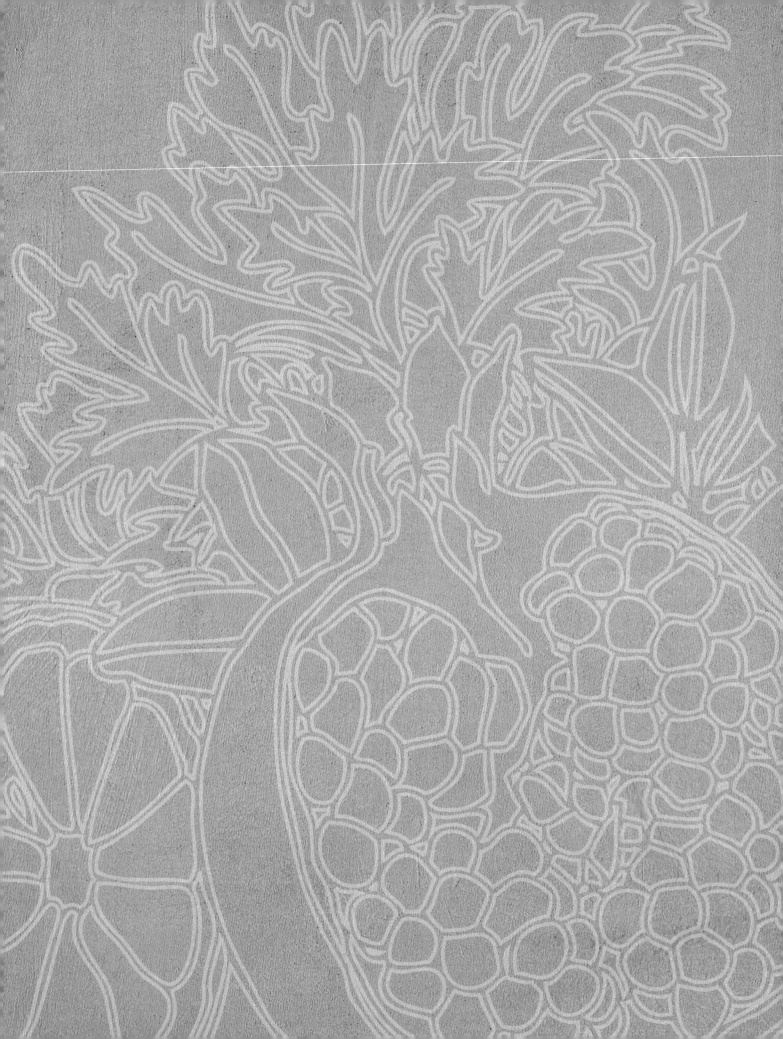

Brainy breakfasts

A balanced start in the morning gives your brain fuel to power you until lunch.

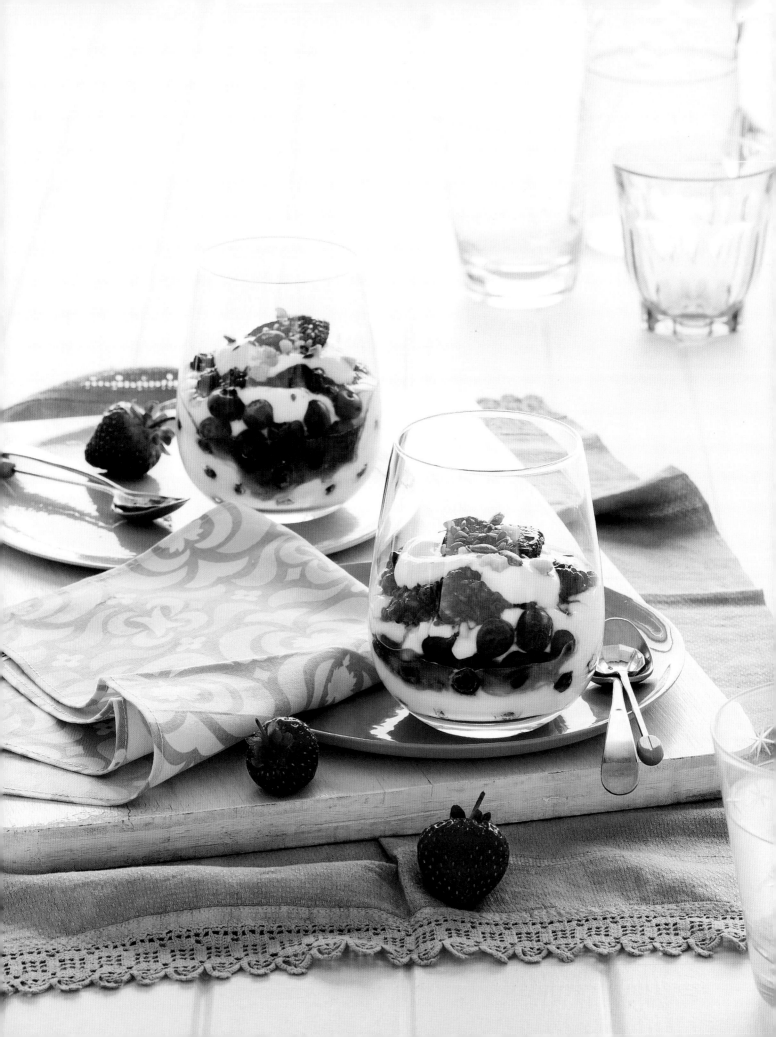

Berry yogurt swirl with walnuts and pepitas

Celebrate berry season with this healthy swirl of goodness. It will give you the energy and nutrients you need in the morning. Use thawed frozen berries if fresh ones aren't available—they're just as nutritious.

PREPARATION **10 MINUTES**
COOKING **5 MINUTES**
SERVES **4**

¼ cup (25 g) walnuts
2 tablespoons (30 ml) pepitas
  (pumpkin seeds)
2 teaspoons (10 ml) honey
½ teaspoon (2 ml) ground cinnamon
3¼ cups (800 ml) low-fat Greek-style yogurt
1 cup (125 g) blueberries
1 cup (125 g) raspberries
1 cup (125 g) strawberries, hulled and sliced
2 teaspoons (10 ml) flaxseeds

1 Preheat the oven to 350°F (180°C). Put the walnuts and pepitas on a large baking pan, keeping them separate. Bake for 5 minutes, until fragrant and lightly toasted. Cool, then chop the walnuts.

2 Gently stir the honey and cinnamon into the yogurt. Divide the blueberries among four serving glasses and top with half the yogurt. Lightly crush the raspberries with a fork and add to the glasses. Spoon in the remaining yogurt and gently swirl together.

3 Add the strawberries to the glasses, and sprinkle with the walnuts, pepitas and flaxseeds. Serve immediately.

Use any combination of berries in this recipe, but include blueberries if possible.

The walnuts and pepitas can be toasted ahead of time. Cool them completely, and store in an airtight container.

EACH SERVING PROVIDES
352 calories, 19 g protein, 14 g fat (5 g saturated fat),
36 g carbohydrate (25 g sugars), 5 g fiber, 305 mg sodium

Walnuts and *flaxseeds* are the main plant sources of omega-3 fats. They also contain antioxidants that are important for brain health.

Sourdough toast with ricotta and fresh fruit

Use any fresh fruit in season for this recipe—sliced bananas, apples, pears, mangoes or strawberries, blueberries, grapes, cherries or mandarin segments would all be good.

PREPARATION **10 MINUTES**   COOKING **2 MINUTES**   SERVES **4**

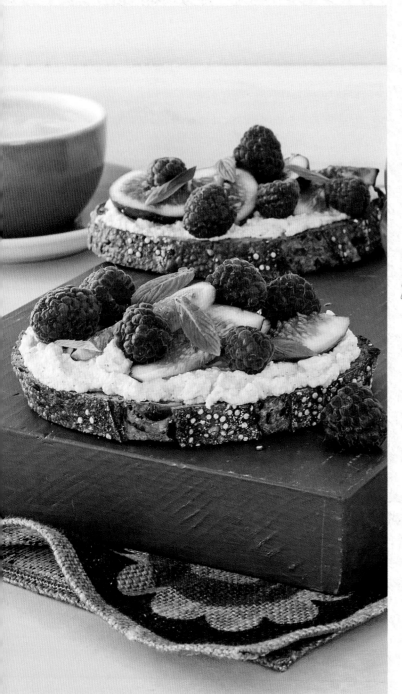

8 slices whole-grain sourdough bread
^{2}/$_3$ cup (150 g) low-fat ricotta
3 teaspoons (15 ml) honey
1 teaspoon (5 ml) ground cinnamon
4 figs, sliced
1 cup (125 g) raspberries
2 tablespoons (30 ml) shredded fresh mint

1   Toast the sourdough bread until golden brown on both sides.

2   Combine the ricotta, honey and cinnamon in a small bowl. Thickly spread the ricotta mixture over the toast.

3   Top the toast slices with the figs and raspberries, and scatter with mint leaves to serve.

Let the bread cool slightly before spreading it with the ricotta. You can use either smooth ricotta from a container or the firm ricotta sold at the deli counter.

When berries are not in season, you could use thawed frozen berries. Thaw the berries on paper towels to help absorb the excess liquid.

EACH SERVING PROVIDES
338 calories, 13 g protein, 7 g fat (3 g saturated fat), 52 g carbohydrate (13 g sugars), 12 g fiber, 326 mg sodium

Using low glycemic index *sourdough bread* helps control blood glucose levels by slowing the release of glucose. This gives the brain a steady energy supply that lasts longer.

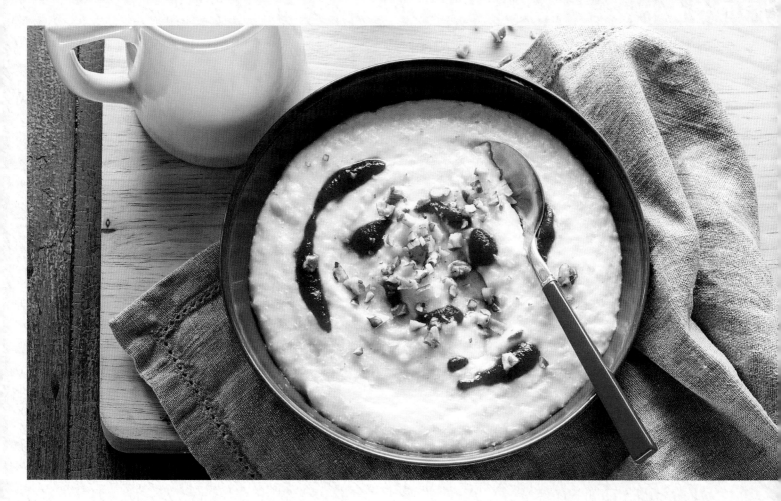

Warm quinoa and cranberry cereal

Cranberries contain many valuable nutrients but they have a limited season so buy a few extra bags when they are available and freeze them.

PREPARATION 10 MINUTES   COOKING 10 MINUTES   SERVES 4

1¼ cups (80 g) quinoa flakes
2 cups (500 ml) low-fat milk
½ cup (60 g) frozen cranberries, thawed
2 teaspoons (10 ml) honey
1 tablespoon (15 ml) chopped pecans

1   Combine the quinoa flakes, milk and 1 cup (250 ml) water in a saucepan. Bring to a boil, reduce the heat to low and gently simmer, stirring occasionally, for 5 minutes, until thick and creamy.

2   Meanwhile, combine the cranberries, honey and 2 tablespoons (30 ml) water in a blender, and blend until almost smooth. Gently warm in a saucepan.

3   Divide the cereal among four serving bowls. Serve topped with the cranberry mixture, sprinkled with the pecans.

Look for quinoa flakes in the health-food section of the supermarket or in a health food store.

Cranberries are naturally very tart in flavor. They have tough skins, so puréeing makes them easier to eat.

EACH SERVING PROVIDES
187 calories, 9 g protein, 5 g fat (2 g saturated fat), 26 g carbohydrate (12 g sugars), 2 g fiber, 78 mg sodium

Cranberries are high in antioxidants, which protect the brain's cells from damage and may reduce the risk of dementia. Animal studies suggest cranberries contain substances that may improve memory and coordination.

Oatmeal with dried fruit compote

Warm your winter mornings with this hearty hot cereal. Its combination of slow-acting carbohydrates and protein will keep your brain fueled for optimal performance despite the cold weather.

PREPARATION **15 MINUTES**
COOKING **10 MINUTES**
SERVES **4**

1¼ cups (125 g) old-fashioned rolled oats
2 tablespoons (30 ml) chopped pistachios, lightly toasted
1 cup (250 ml) skim milk

Dried fruit compote
⅓ cup (40 g) raisins
¼ cup (35 g) diced dried apricots
¼ cup (30 g) dried cranberries
1 tablespoon (15 ml) brown sugar (optional)
½ teaspoon (2 ml) ground cinnamon

1 To make the dried fruit compote, combine the raisins, apricots, cranberries and sugar, if using, in a saucepan. Pour in 1 cup (250 ml) water, and stir to dissolve the sugar. Cover and cook over low heat until simmering, and simmer for 5 minutes. Uncover the pan, slightly increase the heat and cook, stirring occasionally, for another 5 minutes, until the fruit is soft and the liquid has reduced. Stir in the cinnamon and remove from the heat.

2 While the compote is cooking, combine the oats and 3 cups (750 ml) cold water in a saucepan. Slowly bring to a boil over medium–low heat, stirring often. Reduce the heat to low and simmer, stirring often, for 5 minutes, until the oats are soft and creamy.

3 Serve the oatmeal immediately, topped with the dried fruit compote, sprinkled with the pistachios and drizzled with the milk.

You can use any type of dried fruit to make the compote.

EACH SERVING PROVIDES
270 calories, 9 g protein, 8 g fat (2 g saturated fat), 41 g carbohydrate (17 g sugars), 7 g fiber, 50 mg sodium

Oats are high in soluble fiber and are slow to digest, releasing their energy gradually. Milk and fruit have a low glycemic index for a gradual effect on blood glucose levels. This is a great breakfast that provides sustained energy until lunchtime.

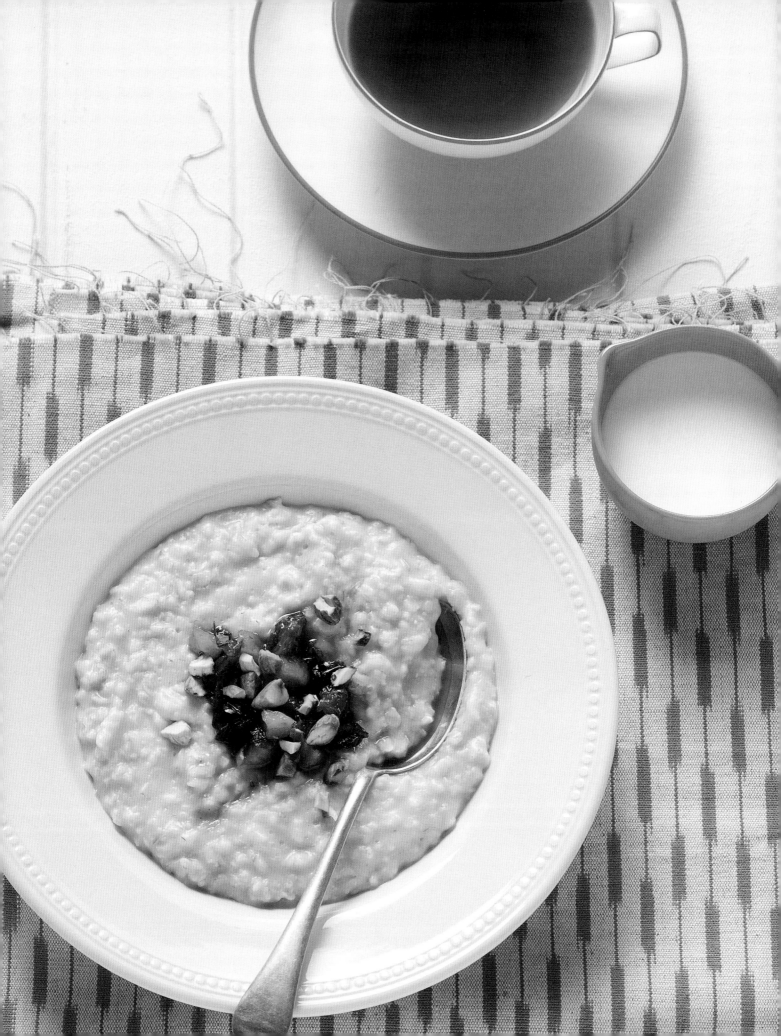

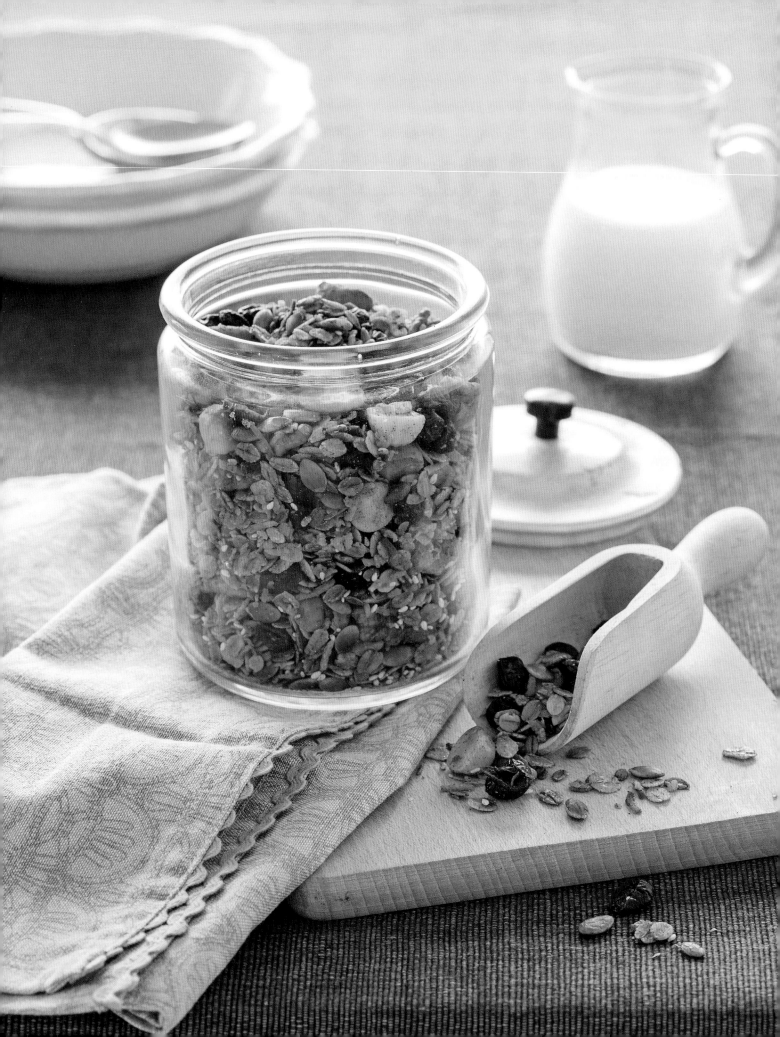

Blueberry and cranberry meusli

Start your day with this healthy mix of fruit, nuts and seeds served with low-fat milk or yogurt. In summer, skip the dried fruit and serve it with fresh berries instead.

PREPARATION **5 MINUTES**
COOKING **25 MINUTES**
SERVES **10 (MAKES ABOUT 5 CUPS)**

2 cups (200 g) five-grain cereal mix
$^{1}/_{2}$ cup (30 g) shredded coconut
$^{1}/_{2}$ cup (70 g) pumpkin seeds
2 tablespoons (30 ml) sesame seeds
$^{1}/_{2}$ cup (50 g) walnuts
$^{1}/_{3}$ cup (50 g) macadamia nuts
1 teaspoon (5 ml) ground cinnamon
1 teaspoon (5 ml) ground cardamom
$^{1}/_{4}$ cup (50 ml) olive oil
$^{1}/_{4}$ cup (50 ml) pure maple syrup
$^{1}/_{4}$ cup (50 g) dried blueberries
$^{1}/_{4}$ cup (50 g) dried cranberries
2 tablespoons (30 ml) chia seeds

1 Preheat the oven to 350°F (180°C). Line two large baking pans with parchment paper.

2 Combine the cereal mix, coconut, seeds, nuts and spices in a large bowl.

3 Heat the oil and maple syrup in a small saucepan over medium heat for 5 minutes, until warmed through. Pour into the cereal mixture and stir until well combined. Spread the mixture out on the prepared pans.

4 Bake the mixture for 20 minutes, stirring several times to be sure it browns evenly. Set aside to cool on the pans.

5 Pour the cooled mixture into a bowl and stir in the dried fruit and chia seeds. Store in an airtight container.

A five-grain cereal mix provides great variety of textures, but you can also use old-fashioned (not instant) rolled oats.

EACH SERVING PROVIDES
318 calories, 6 g protein, 21 g fat (4 g saturated fat),
28 g carbohydrate (9 g sugars), 7 g fiber, 6 mg sodium

Pumpkin seeds, also known as pepitas, are a great source of zinc, one of the most critical nutrients for immune function as well as helping to control the body's response to stress. Zinc is required for normal brain development and may help to protect against depression.

Blueberry and oat breakfast muffins

These muffins are best eaten within a couple of hours of baking, but they can be frozen for up to 1 month. Wrap each muffin individually in foil, place in a large ziplock bag, expel all the air and tightly seal. Thaw the muffins at room temperature and reheat in a low oven.

PREPARATION **15 MINUTES**
COOKING **20 MINUTES**
MAKES **12**

$1^{1}/_{2}$ cups (240 g) whole-wheat
   self-rising flour
$1/_{3}$ cup (60 g) brown sugar
1 teaspoon (5 ml) ground cinnamon
1 cup (100 g) old-fashioned rolled oats
$3/_{4}$ cup (180 ml) skim milk
$1/_{4}$ cup (50 ml) canola oil
2 eggs
1 teaspoon (5 ml) vanilla extract
2 ripe bananas, mashed
$1/_{2}$ cup (50 g) pecans, roughly chopped
1 cup (125 g) blueberries

1   Preheat the oven to 350°F (180°C). Line a 12-hole standard muffin pan with paper liners.

2   Sift the flour, sugar and cinnamon into a large mixing bowl. Add the husks from the sieve into the bowl. Stir in the oats and make a well in the center.

3   Use a fork to whisk the milk, oil, eggs and vanilla in a bowl. Add to the dry ingredients along with the mashed bananas, and fold together until just combined. Gently fold in the pecans and blueberries.

4   Divide the batter among the muffin cups. Bake the muffins for 20 minutes, until risen, golden and springy to a gentle touch. Serve warm or at room temperature.

You'll need 2 large bananas for this recipe. Make sure they are well-ripened—slightly overripe is even better.

EACH SERVING (1 MUFFIN) PROVIDES
222 calories, 6 g protein, 10 g fat (1 g saturated fat),
28 g carbohydrate (10 g sugars), 4 g fiber, 154 mg sodium

Blueberries contain colorful anthocyanins, which protect the heart and nervous system. Anthocyanin pigments are responsible for the red, purple and blue colors of many fruits, vegetables and cereal grains. They are one class of flavonoid compounds that may help improve general cognitive function.

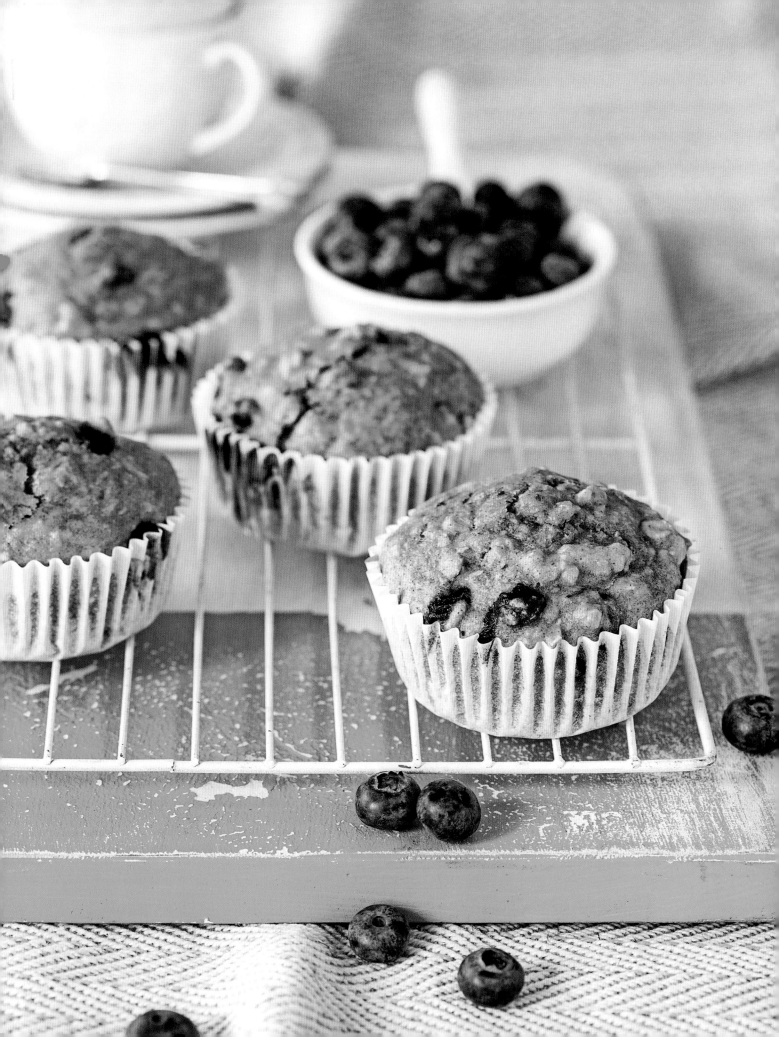

These vitamin-packed drinks make a filling and nutritious breakfast if you are in a hurry. Have some toast or nuts, too, and you'll be satisfied until lunchtime.

Left: Beet and raspberry smoothie
Right: Mixed berry smoothie

Beet and raspberry smoothie

PREPARATION **10 MINUTES**
SERVES **4**

2 cooked beets, cooled and roughly chopped,
    about $^1\!/_2$ cup (125 g) total
$^1\!/_2$ cup (60 g) raspberries, plus extra to garnish
    (optional)
1 cup (250 ml) cranberry juice, chilled
1 cup (250 ml) low-fat plain yogurt or
    low-fat Greek-style yogurt

1 Purée the beets, raspberries and cranberry juice
in a food processor or blender.

2 Strain the purée into a large bowl to remove the
raspberry seeds, then whisk in most of the yogurt.

3 Pour the smoothie into four glasses and spoon
in the remaining yogurt. Gently swirl in the yogurt,
and garnish with the extra raspberries, if desired.
Serve immediately.

To cook fresh beets, trim and wash them, leaving the
skin, roots and leaf stems intact. Place in a saucepan,
cover with water and bring to a boil. Reduce the heat,
cover and simmer for 30 minutes, until tender. Drain and
cool under cold running water. Rub off the skins and
drain the beets on paper towels. You can also use the
preboiled, vacuum-packed beets available in most
supermarkets. Just don't use the pickled beets preserved
in vinegar for this recipe.

If you prefer your smoothie with a thinner consistency,
add a little bit of water.

EACH SERVING PROVIDES
83 calories, 5 g protein, <1 g fat (<1 g saturated fat),
15 g carbohydrate (15 g sugars), 2 g fiber, 69 mg sodium

Beets may help improve blood flow to the brain
in older people, especially to the frontal lobe—
a part of the brain that often experiences
reduced blood flow in age-related dementia
and cognitive decline.

Mixed berry smoothie

PREPARATION **5 MINUTES**
SERVES **2**

1 cup (125 g) mixed berries
1 ripe banana, chopped
1 cup (250 ml) low-fat milk
1 cup (250 ml) low-fat plain yogurt
pinch of ground cinnamon

1 Combine all the ingredients in a blender. Blend
until smooth and well mixed.

2 Divide the smoothie between two glasses and
serve immediately.

Use fresh or frozen berries—any type or combination
you like. For an icy cold smoothie, use frozen berries
straight from the freezer.

Use the type of milk that suits you: Cow's milk, soy milk,
rice milk and almond milk will all work well.

EACH SERVING PROVIDES
208 calories, 15 g protein, <1 g fat (<1 g saturated fat),
33 g carbohydrate (28 g sugars), 4 g fiber, 170 mg sodium

Staying hydrated is important to brain function,
as a dehydrated brain has less effective circulation
of energy and precious nutrients. This energy
drink combines protein, calcium and antioxidants
for a great start to the day.

Berries

Berries (including raspberries, blueberries, blackberries, cranberries, black currants and even cherries) are one of nature's superfoods. They contain extremely high levels of antioxidants within a great-tasting, low-calorie, high-fiber fruit.

From left: strawberries, blueberries, cherries, raspberries, blackberries

Berries are especially high in vitamin C, which is required in large quantities in the brain and the nervous system as part of the antioxidant system, and is also needed for the synthesis of noradrenaline and for vitamin E to work. During stress, vitamin C requirements are increased. A deficiency of vitamin C can lead to fatigue and depression, and oxidative damage in the brain. Vitamin C aids in the absorption of iron from plant sources, making it useful for vegetarians.

Blueberries contain anthocyanins, which have been used in laboratory studies of memory loss. Aging rats that were fed blueberry extract for two months performed better on maze tests. According to the researchers, this is the result of enhanced neuron signaling due to the antioxidant power found in berries.

Berries can be expensive when they are not in season, but frozen berries can be enjoyed all year round. Nutritionally, frozen berries are actually better for you than out-of-season fruit, as they contain more vitamins and antioxidants when they are picked at their peak of ripeness and flash-frozen instead of being stored. Frozen berries can be blended into smoothies or added to cake and pancake batters right from the freezer, which keeps them whole, or you can cook them to make a sauce or coulis to stir into a recipe or drizzle on a finished dish. Berries aren't just for desserts, either. A vinegary raspberry dressing is perfect on a warm salad with grilled chicken or pork, and a handful of blueberries is always a wonderful addition to a pilaf or green salad.

Mini salmon breakfast quiches

To make breakfast a little faster and easier in the morning, you can bake the bread shells for these quiches a day in advance. Allow them to cool completely, and store in an airtight container until required. Fill and bake the quiches as close as possible to serving time.

PREPARATION **20 MINUTES**
COOKING **25 MINUTES**
SERVES **4 (MAKES 12)**

olive oil spray
12 slices whole-grain bread
7$\frac{1}{2}$ ounces (210 g) canned salmon, drained and flaked
1 tablespoon (15 ml) snipped fresh chives
1 tablespoon (15 ml) chopped fresh dill
4 eggs, lightly beaten
1 tablespoon (15 ml) finely grated parmesan

1   Preheat the oven to 350°F (180°C). Spray a 12-hole standard muffin pan with olive oil.

2   Use a rolling pin to flatten out the bread slices, and use a 4-inch (10-cm) biscuit cutter to cut a round from each slice. Press the bread rounds into the muffin pan and lightly spray with olive oil. Bake for 10 minutes, until the bread shells are very lightly browned and slightly dried out. Transfer to a wire rack to cool.

3   Return the bread shells to the muffin pan. Combine the salmon and herbs, and divide the mixture among the bread shells. Carefully pour the eggs into the shells over the salmon and sprinkle with the parmesan.

4   Bake the quiches for 12–15 minutes, until set and golden brown. Serve warm or at room temperature.

It is best to use day-old bread rather than very fresh bread for the shells.

EACH SERVING (3 QUICHES) PROVIDES
333 calories, 26 g protein, 15 g fat (4 g saturated fat), 19 g carbohydrate (1 g sugars), 10 g fiber, 450 mg sodium

Salmon is one of the best sources of brain-boosting omega-3 fats. Increase the omega-3 content of this dish even more by choosing omega-3-enriched eggs.

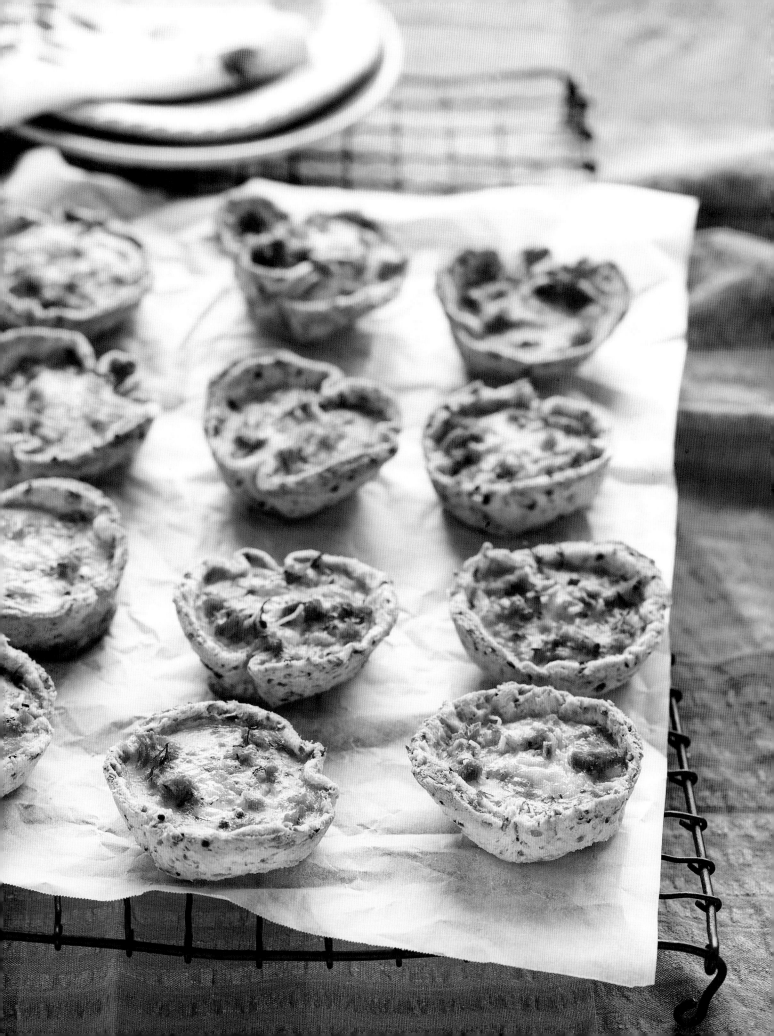

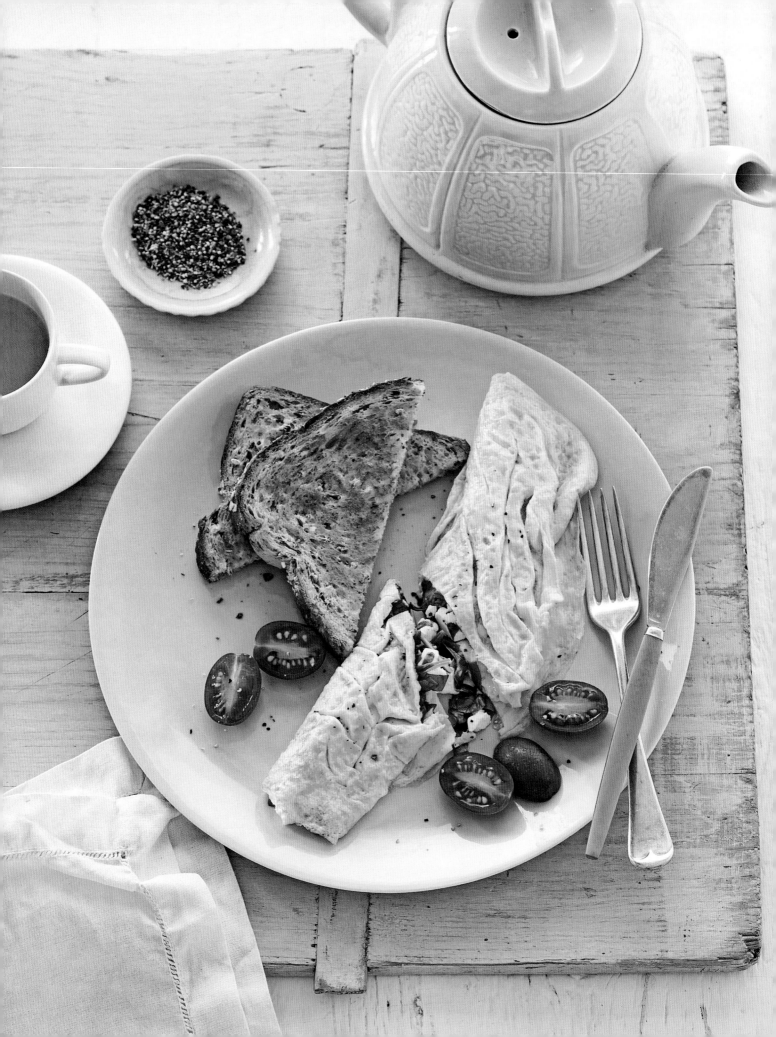

Spinach and feta omelets

This high-protein breakfast will help sustain your energy levels for hours. For extra fiber, serve the omelet with whole-grain toast. Add a green salad for a nutritious brunch or lunch.

PREPARATION **10 MINUTES**
COOKING **10 MINUTES**
SERVES **4**

1 tablespoon (15 ml) olive oil
8 eggs, lightly whisked
1/2 cup (100 g) baby spinach leaves, shredded
1/2 cup (125 g) low-fat feta, crumbled
1 cup (250 g) red baby plum or cherry
   tomatoes, halved
freshly ground black pepper

1 Heat 1 teaspoon (5 ml) of the oil in a 10-inch (25-cm) nonstick frying pan over medium heat. Pour in one-quarter of the eggs and swirl to make an even layer.

2 Use a spatula to draw the egg into the center of the pan from the side as it begins to set. After about 1 minute, the egg will be set around the side and bottom but moist on top. Sprinkle with the spinach and feta. Fold one-third of the omelet towards the center, and fold over again to enclose the filling.

3 Slide the omelet onto a plate and serve immediately with the tomatoes, seasoned with freshly ground black pepper. Repeat to make three more omelets.

If you prefer, cook the tomatoes in a little oil in a frying pan over medium heat for about 5 minutes, until the skins just start to split. Keep them warm while you cook the omelets.

EACH SERVING PROVIDES
266 calories, 22 g protein, 19 g fat (7 g saturated fat), 2 g carbohydrate (2 g sugars), 1 g fiber, 493 mg sodium

Vitamin K is thought to help limit neuron damage in the brain, and good sources such as spinach are currently being researched for their potential in lessening the effects of dementia.

Quinoa pancakes with raspberry compote

Quinoa flour has a distinctive flavor, stronger than the flavor of quinoa when it is used as a whole grain. It is a useful flour for baking in place of wheat flour as it's gluten-free and also very high in protein.

PREPARATION 25 MINUTES
COOKING 20 MINUTES
SERVES 4 (MAKES 12)

$1^1/_2$ cups (200 g) quinoa flour
1 teaspoon (5 ml) baking powder
1 tablespoon (15 ml) superfine sugar
$^1/_2$ teaspoon (2 ml) ground cinnamon
$1^1/_2$ cups (375 ml) buttermilk
2 eggs
1 teaspoon (5 ml) vanilla extract
$^2/_3$ cup (150 ml) low-fat plain yogurt

Raspberry compote
2 cups (250 g) fresh or frozen raspberries
1 tablespoon (15 ml) superfine sugar

1 To make the compote, put the raspberries and sugar in a small saucepan. Gently stir over low heat until the sugar has dissolved and the mixture is heated through.

2 Sift the flour, baking powder, sugar and cinnamon into a bowl and make a well in the center. Whisk the buttermilk, eggs and vanilla together. Pour the mixture into the well in the dry ingredients and stir to combine.

3 Lightly grease a large heavy-bottom frying pan and heat over medium–low heat. For each pancake, drop 2 slightly heaping tablespoons (35 ml) of batter into the pan and spread into a neat 4-inch (10-cm) round. Repeat with more batter, depending on the size of your pan.

4 Cook the pancakes for about 2 minutes, until golden brown underneath, turn over and cook the other side for 1–2 minutes, until golden. Remove from the pan and keep warm while you cook the remaining pancakes.

5 Serve three pancakes for each person, with the yogurt and raspberry compote.

To keep the pancakes warm, place them on a baking pan in a very low oven, loosely covered with foil.

EACH SERVING (3 PANCAKES) PROVIDES
370 calories, 18 g protein, 8 g fat (2 g saturated fat), 52 g carbohydrate (19 g sugars), 7 g fiber, 192 mg sodium

Quinoa contains more protein than any other grain, important for maintaining brain health. Unlike many other plant foods, the protein in quinoa is a good-quality complete protein that can be readily used by the body.

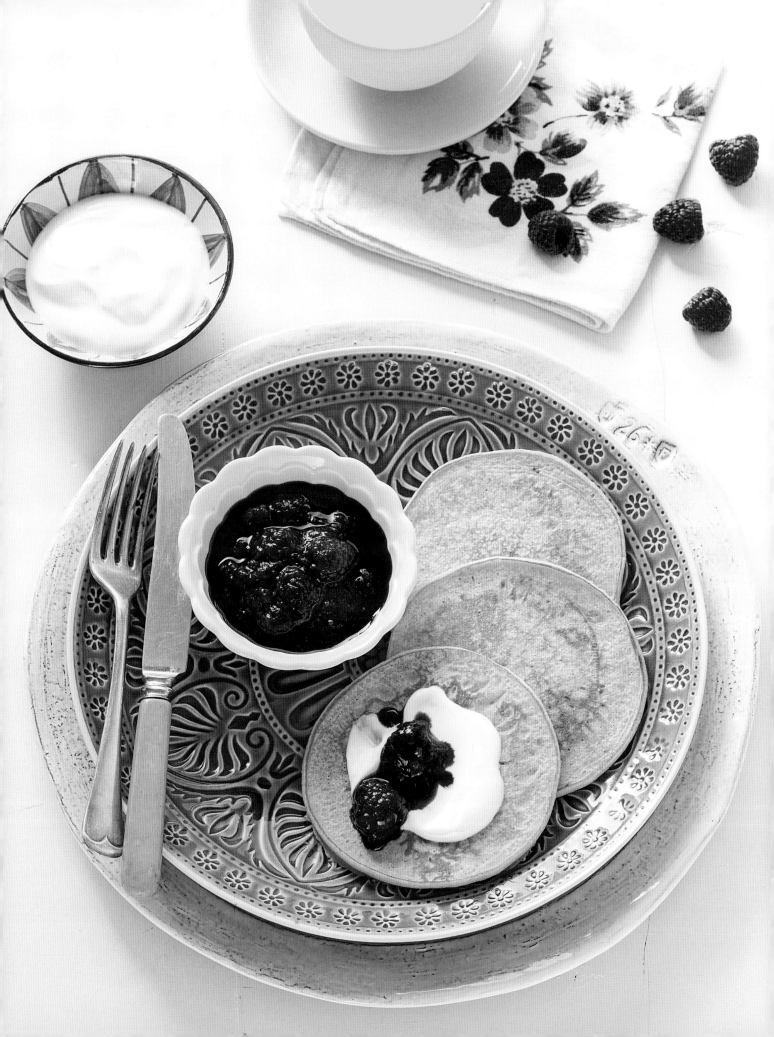

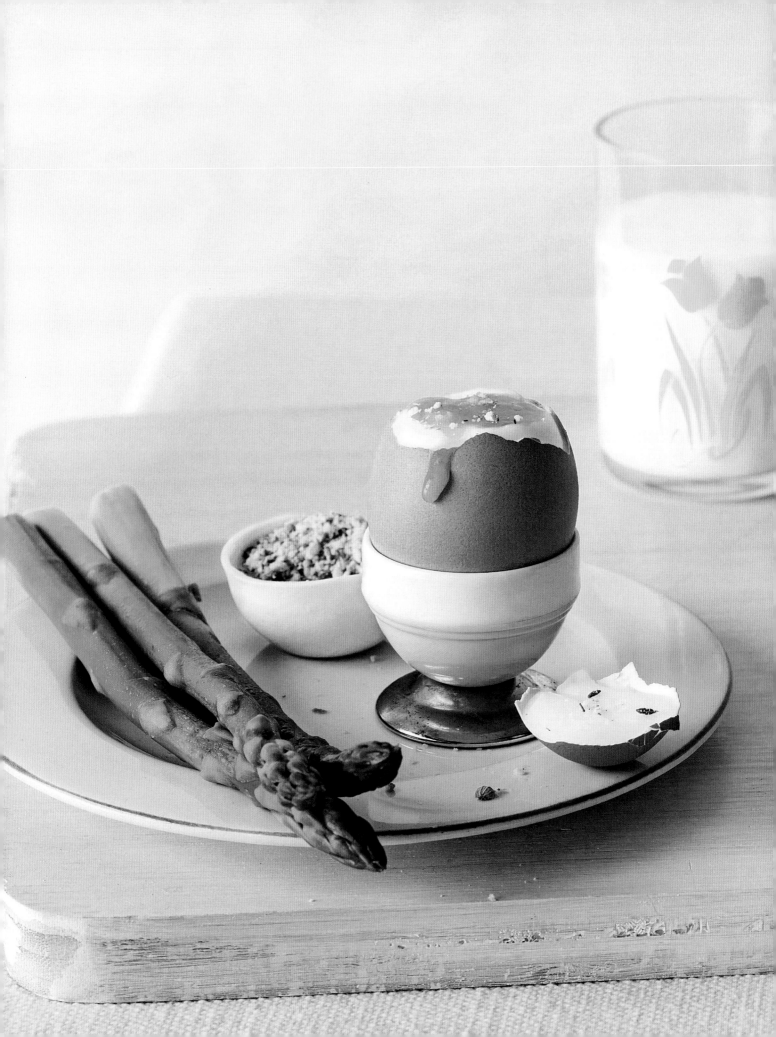

Boiled eggs with dukkah and asparagus spears

Dukkah is an Egyptian nut and spice mix that can be sprinkled over vegetables or used as a dip. The nuts and spices vary, so feel free to experiment to make your own version. You can buy ready-made dukkah in jars, but it usually contains quite a lot of salt.

PREPARATION **15 MINUTES**
COOKING **10 MINUTES**
SERVES **4**

12 asparagus spears, trimmed
4 eggs

Dukkah
2 tablespoons (30 ml) pistachios,
  roughly chopped
1 tablespoon (15 ml) sesame seeds
2 teaspoons (10 ml) coriander seeds
2 teaspoons (10 ml) cumin seeds

1   To make the dukkah, toast the pistachios in a dry frying pan over medium heat, stirring occasionally, for 2 minutes. Transfer to a plate to cool. Repeat with the sesame seeds, cooking them for 1 minute, then the coriander and cumin seeds, cooking them for 1 minute, until fragrant. When the nuts and seeds are completely cool, coarsely grind them in a spice grinder, clean coffee grinder or mortar and pestle.

2   Place the asparagus in a heatproof bowl. Cover with boiling water and let stand for 2 minutes, drain and pat dry with paper towels.

3   Put the eggs in a saucepan, cover with cold water and bring to a boil over high heat. As soon as the water boils, time the eggs to cook for 3 minutes. Drain the water from the pan and let the eggs cool slightly.

4   Place the eggs in egg cups and slice off the tops. Serve with the asparagus spears for dipping, and 1 teaspoon (5 ml) of the dukkah each for sprinkling.

Store the remaining dukkah in an airtight container for up to 3 weeks.

To check if your eggs are fresh, gently lower whole uncooked eggs into a saucepan of cold water. Fresh eggs will sink to the bottom; eggs that float to the top should be discarded.

EACH SERVING PROVIDES
92 calories, 8 g protein, 6 g fat (2 g saturated fat),
1 g carbohydrate (<1 g sugars), <1 g fiber, 68 mg sodium

In recent animal studies, *pistachios* helped assure the supply of oxygen to the brain by maintaining the levels of healthy fats and inhibiting inflammatory substances in brain cells.

Roasted tomato, cannellini and avocado salad with pan-fried eggs

Tomatoes and white beans are a classic Italian combination that makes a perfect base for fried eggs. This dish is rich in antioxidants from the tomatoes and greens. Roasting the tomatoes adds a layer of sweetness to the dish, and the egg provides a protein boost any time of day.

PREPARATION **20 MINUTES**
COOKING **20 MINUTES**
SERVES **4**

1 cup (250 g) red cherry tomatoes
14$\frac{1}{2}$ ounce (400 ml) can cannellini beans,
    rinsed and drained
1 avocado, diced
1$\frac{1}{3}$ cups (60 g) baby arugula
1 tablespoon (15 ml) snipped fresh chives
1 tablespoon (15 ml) lemon juice
2 teaspoons (10 ml) olive oil
4 eggs
freshly ground black pepper

1   Preheat the oven to 375°F (190°C). Line a baking pan with parchment paper. Arrange the tomatoes on the pan. Roast the tomatoes for 15 minutes, until softened and lightly browned. Cool slightly.

2   Combine the roasted tomatoes with the cannellini beans, avocado, arugula, chives and lemon juice. Arrange on four serving plates.

3   Heat the olive oil in a large nonstick frying pan over medium–high heat. Crack the eggs into the pan and cook for 3 minutes, until the whites have set, or until done to your liking.

4   Serve the eggs on top of the bean mixture, sprinkled with freshly ground black pepper.

If you prefer your eggs poached, bring a saucepan of water to a simmer. Crack an egg into a cup. Stir the water to create a whirlpool, then gently slide the egg into the water. Repeat with another egg. Simmer for 2 minutes for a soft yolk, or until done to your liking. Use a slotted spoon to lift the egg out. For best results, cook no more than 2 eggs at a time. Use the freshest eggs you can find. Adding 1 tablespoon (15 ml) white vinegar to the water will help set the egg.

EACH SERVING PROVIDES
276 calories, 12 g protein, 21 g fat (5 g saturated fat),
9 g carbohydrate (3 g sugars), 6 g fiber, 240 mg sodium

Tomatoes are a source of uridine, which according to some animal studies, appears to act as an antidepressant. Uridine is essential for making and maintaining healthy brain tissue.

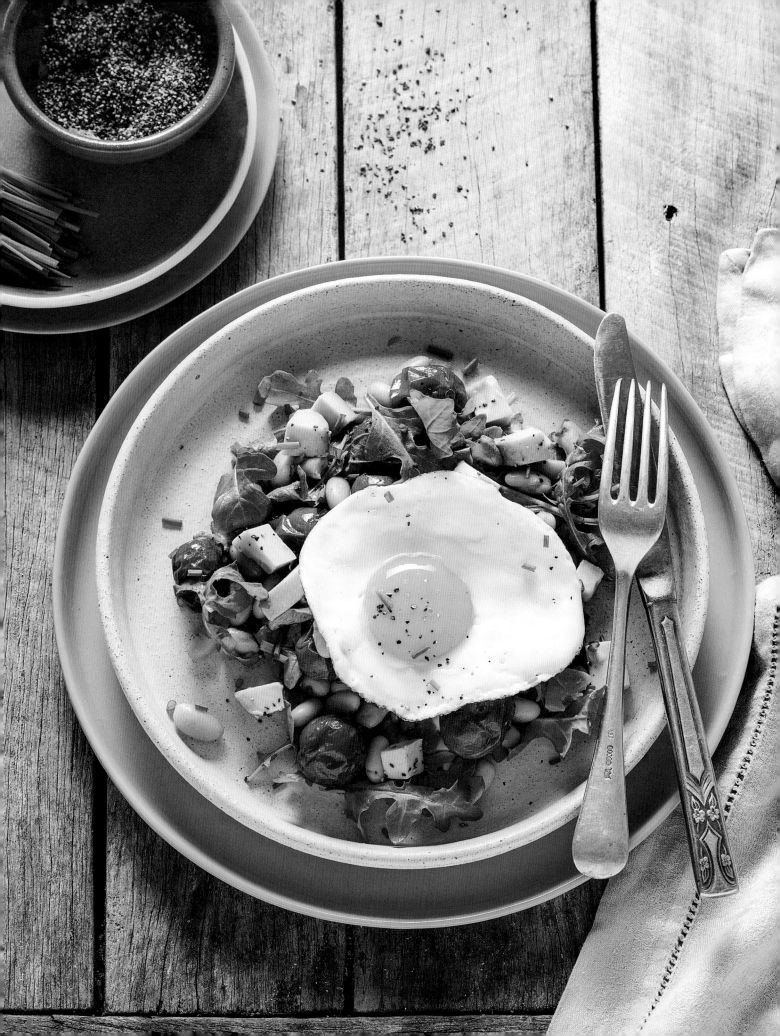

Eggs

As the first complete nutrition source for a developing chicken, eggs contain all the protein and micronutrients needed for growth. This makes them a nutritious ingredient, as well as being extremely versatile in cooking.

From left: hen eggs, bantam egg, quail eggs

Eggs possess many unique culinary qualities, including coagulation properties (for sticking food together or setting it solid); holding large amounts of air (to aerate or raise foods); and emulsification. On its own, an egg can form the basis of many quick and easy meals that provide balanced, complete protein as well as most vitamins and minerals. Both the yolk and egg white are nutritious, but most of the vitamins and minerals are concentrated in the yolk. There is no reason to worry about limiting your intake of egg yolks unless you already have a cholesterol problem.

One lesser-known nutrient found in eggs is choline. Although not a vitamin, choline is very closely related to the B-group vitamins and is essential for the synthesis of neurotransmitters and maintaining the myelin sheath that protects the nerves, as well as being a component of cell membranes. Choline is the precursor for the neurotransmitter acetylcholine, important for memory and muscle control. Choline deficiency means you have less acetylcholine available when you need to think clearly or to remember

something. During growth, choline deficiency results in cognitive problems and impaired memory function. Researchers are investigating the possibility that choline may help prevent memory loss associated with aging. Choline is found in a wide variety of foods, but eggs are the richest source. Eggs also provide tryptophan, a precursor for serotonin.

Vitamin B_{12} is found only in animal foods, including eggs. It is needed for maintaining myelin, for producing normal blood cells and for converting inflammatory homocysteine into another amino acid. Deficiency is more common with aging, as absorption declines, and many of the symptoms are brain-related, including memory loss, difficulty concentrating, disorientation and sensory numbness.

Eggs are also one of the best known sources of pantothenic acid (vitamin B_5). Cooked eggs are a good source of biotin, formerly known as vitamin B_7. Biotin is involved in the metabolism of fats and proteins, important in brain function as shown by the fact that biotin deficiency results in numbness, lethargy and depression.

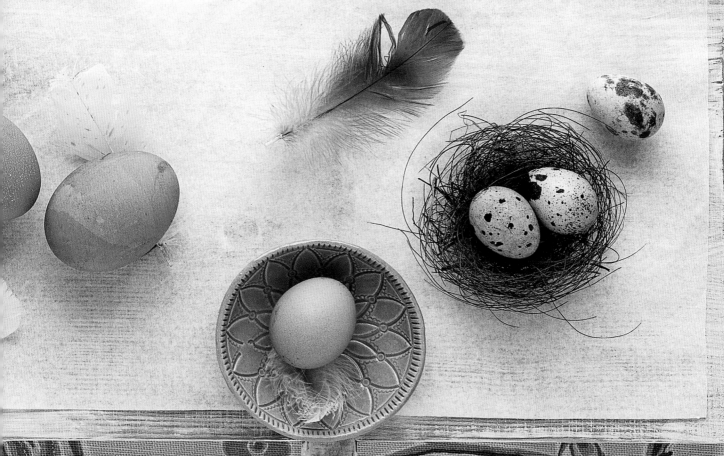

Savvy soups and salads

Choose from these tempting new ways to give your brain the nutrients it needs.

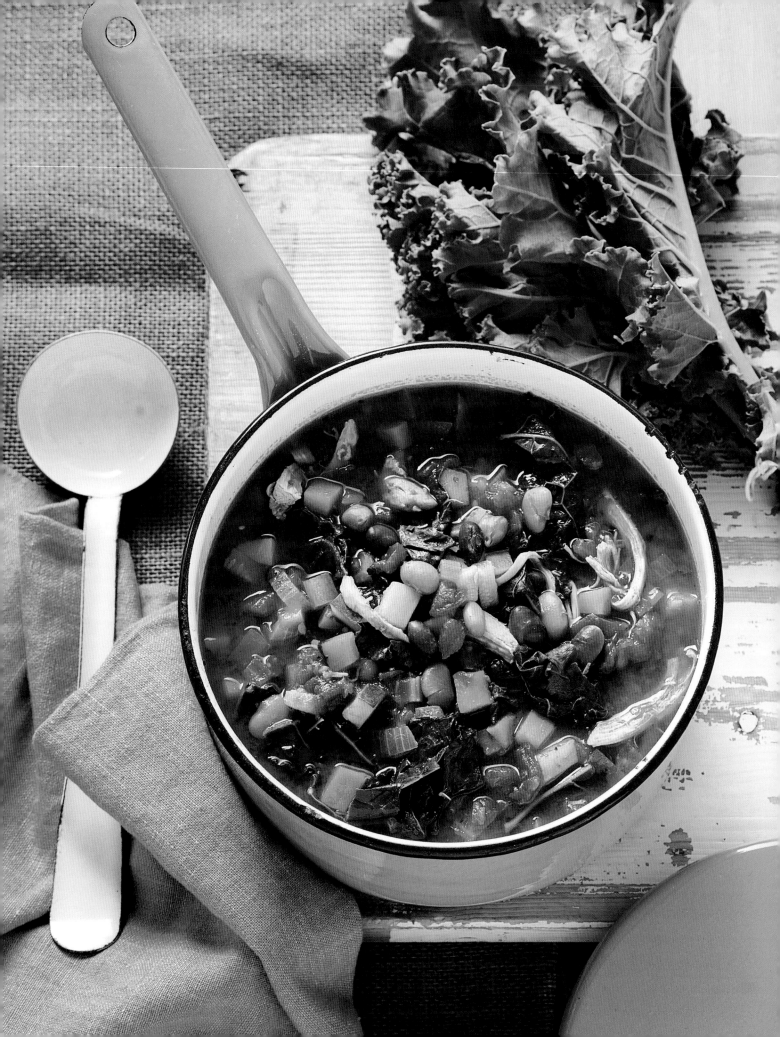

Tuscan-style chicken, bean and tomato soup

This is a great winter soup that freezes well, too. Simply divide it into individual portions before freezing. You can use any kind of beans in this recipe, or try a mix—chickpeas, lentils, red kidney beans, cannellini beans and baby lima beans are all good options.

PREPARATION **15 MINUTES**
COOKING **40 MINUTES**
SERVES **4**

1 tablespoon (15 ml) olive oil
1 onion, chopped
1 carrot, chopped
2 stalks celery, chopped
1 zucchini, chopped
14$^{1}/_{2}$ ounce (400 ml) can low-sodium
  diced tomatoes
15 ounce (425 ml) can beans,
  rinsed and drained
$^{2}/_{3}$ pound (300 g) boneless, skinless chicken
  thighs, trimmed and thinly sliced
4 cups (1 L) low-sodium chicken stock
1 bay leaf
1 teaspoon (5 ml) dried oregano
grated zest of 1 lemon (optional)
$^{2}/_{3}$ cup (150 g) chopped kale or
  baby spinach leaves

1   Heat the oil in a large saucepan over medium heat and cook the onion for 10 minutes, until soft and golden. Add the carrot and celery, and cook for 5 minutes, until just soft.

2   Stir in the zucchini, tomatoes, four-bean mix, chicken, stock and 1 cup (250 ml) water. Add the bay leaf, oregano and lemon zest, if using. Simmer for 20 minutes, until the vegetables are tender and the chicken is cooked through.

3   Stir in the chopped kale or baby spinach leaves and cook for 2 minutes, until wilted.

4   Spoon the soup into four bowls and serve immediately.

Replace the canned beans with 2 cups (500 g) cooked beans made from $^{2}/_{3}$ cup (150 g) dried beans.

EACH SERVING PROVIDES
252 calories, 23 g protein, 9 g fat (2 g saturated fat),
20 g carbohydrate (10 g sugars), 6 g fiber, 1030 mg sodium

The *beans* bulk up this dish with extra protein and fiber without adding fat, making it satisfying and beneficial for your cardiovascular system. Your brain relies on a healthy heart and blood vessels for its supply of oxygen and precious nutrients.

Leek soup with oysters and whole-grain flatbreads

You can include any seeds or nuts in these easy flatbreads. Try using sesame seeds, chia seeds, flaxseeds or finely chopped Brazil nuts. You can also include garlic, herbs or spices to vary the flavors.

PREPARATION **20 MINUTES**
COOKING **25 MINUTES**
SERVES **4**

2–3 whole leeks, about 1^2/$_3$ pounds (800 g)
2 tablespoons (30 ml) olive oil
^{2}/$_3$ pound (300 g) potatoes, unpeeled, roughly diced
2 cups (500 ml) low-sodium chicken or vegetable stock
12 fresh oysters
2 tablespoons (30 ml) snipped fresh chives
cracked black pepper

Whole-grain flatbreads
2 teaspoons (7 g) dry yeast
^{3}/$_4$ cup (120 g) whole-wheat all-purpose flour, plus extra for dusting
^{1}/$_3$ cup (50 g) poppyseeds
2 tablespoons (30 ml) olive oil

1   To make the flatbreads, pour ^{1}/$_3$ cup (75 ml) lukewarm water into a large bowl and sprinkle with the yeast. Let stand for a few minutes to rehydrate, then add the flour. Mix well to form a soft dough, and knead the poppyseeds into the dough until the seeds are incorporated and the dough has formed a smooth, sticky ball. Let the dough rest while you prepare the soup.

2   Preheat the oven to 480°F (250°C). Line a baking pan with parchment paper.

3   Cut the leeks in half lengthwise, wash well and then thinly slice the white and tender green parts, discarding the rest. Heat the olive oil in a large saucepan and cook the leeks over low heat for 5 minutes, until soft.

4   Add the potatoes and stock to the pan, and simmer for 15 minutes, until the potatoes are very soft.

5   Meanwhile, divide the flatbread dough into four pieces and roll each portion into a ball. Dust a work surface and rolling pin with flour and roll each ball into a long oval, as thin as possible, about ^{1}/$_8$ inch (0.25 cm). Place the ovals on the prepared pan, spaced apart, and brush with the oil. Bake for 10–15 minutes, until crisp and golden.

6   Allow the soup to cool slightly, transfer to a blender or food processor and purée until smooth. Thin the soup with stock, water or milk to your desired consistency, and reheat if necessary.

7   Spoon the soup into four bowls and top each with three oysters. Sprinkle with the chives and cracked black pepper. Serve with the flatbreads.

You can use a pasta machine instead of a rolling pin to roll out the flatbreads for a crisp, thin result. This will make two flatbreads per person.

Seeds and *nuts* contain beneficial fats that are good for the brain and cardiovascular system.

EACH SERVING PROVIDES
474 calories, 20 g protein, 27 g fat (4 g saturated fat), 39 g carbohydrate, (10 g sugars), 14 g fiber, 505 mg sodium

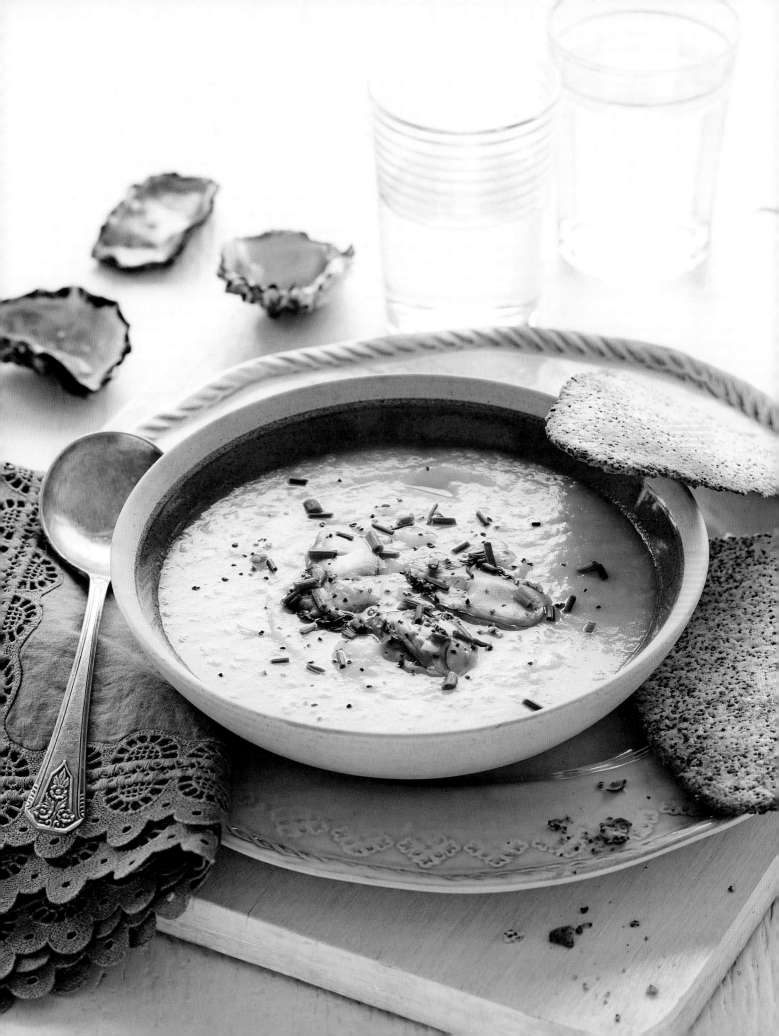

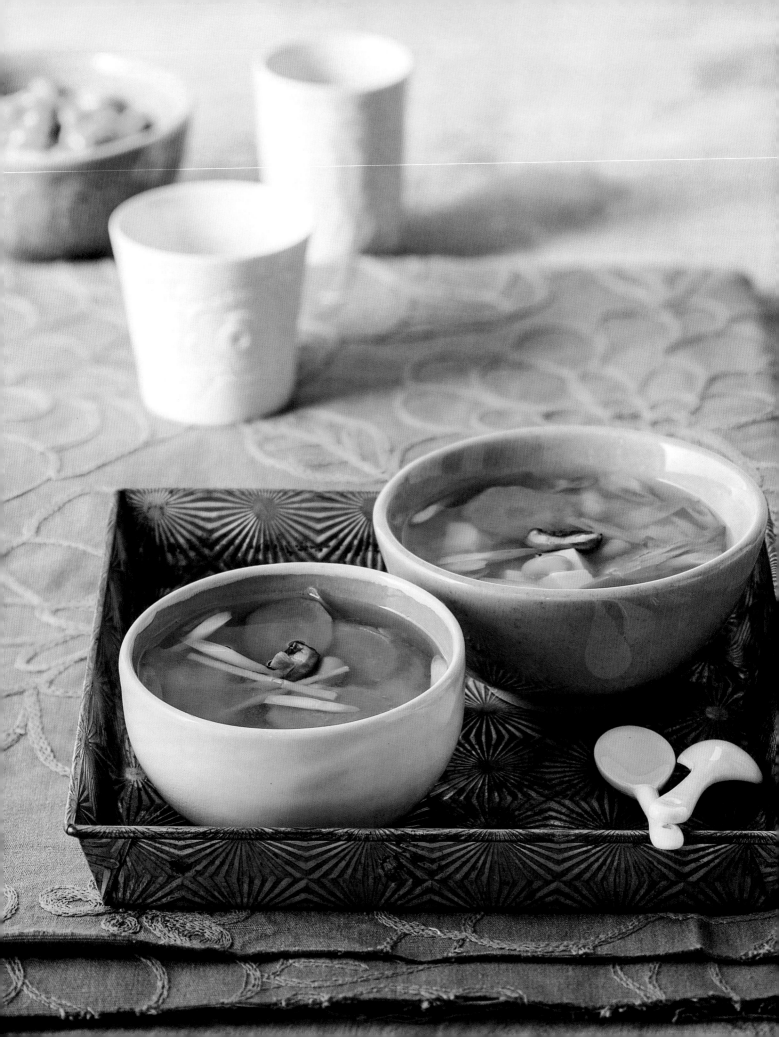

Japanese tofu miso soup with edamame and ginger

It is very important that you don't boil the miso after you add it to the soup, or it will destroy the health-giving enzymes in the miso. Shiro miso is a light-colored miso that is less salty than darker miso.

PREPARATION **10 MINUTES**
COOKING **25 MINUTES**
SERVES **4**

4 scallions, thinly sliced on the diagonal
1 carrot, thinly sliced
1 daikon radish, thinly sliced
6 dried shiitake mushrooms, broken into small pieces
2-inch (5-cm) piece fresh ginger, peeled and cut into thin matchsticks
2 tablespoons (30 ml) shiro miso
³/₄ cup (175 g) shelled edamame
5 ounces (150 g) silken firm tofu, cut into small cubes

1   Pour 5 cups (1.25 L) water into a large saucepan. Add the scallions, carrot, daikon, dried mushrooms and ginger. Bring to a boil, reduce the heat and simmer for 15 minutes.

2   Spoon out 2 tablespoons (30 ml) of the hot liquid and blend it with the miso. Stir the miso back into the pan. Do not allow the soup to boil.

3   Add the edamame and tofu to the soup, cook for 5 minutes, until the edamame are bright green and tender.

4   Divide the tofu and vegetables among four bowls, and ladle on the hot stock.

Edamame are available in the freezer sections of most supermarkets and Asian food stores.

EACH SERVING PROVIDES
148 calories, 10 g protein, 4 g fat (<1 g saturated fat), 20 g carbohydrate (6 g sugars), 6 g fiber, 377 mg sodium

Miso is made by fermenting soy and sometimes grains such as rice or buckwheat. The fermentation process releases beneficial nutrients. Unpasteurized miso contains live probiotic bacteria that can promote healthy digestive and immune systems. Because miso is a high-sodium food, use it in small quantities.

Beef and vegetable soup

One of the secrets to a great-tasting soup is the aromatic vegetables such as onion, carrot and celery. This is a thick and hearty soup, but you can add more stock or water if you like it thinner.

PREPARATION **20 MINUTES**
COOKING **1 HOUR 15 MINUTES**
SERVES **4**

1 tablespoon (15 ml) oil
$^{2}/_{3}$ pound (350 g) boneless chuck steak,
   fat trimmed, chopped
1 leek, white part only, sliced, or
   1 yellow onion, finely chopped
2 cloves garlic, crushed
1 carrot, halved and sliced
2 stalks celery, thinly sliced
14$^{1}/_{2}$ ounce (400 ml) can diced tomatoes
   or 3 finely diced tomatoes
2 cups (500 ml) low-sodium vegetable
   or beef stock
1 bay leaf
1 zucchini, halved and sliced
$^{1}/_{4}$ cabbage (1 cup/200 g), shredded
2 tablespoons (30 ml) chopped fresh parsley

1   Heat half the oil in a stock pot or large saucepan over high heat. Cook the beef in batches, stirring often, for 2–3 minutes, until browned. Transfer the beef to a plate.

2   Heat the remaining oil in the pot and cook the leek and garlic over low heat for 3–5 minutes, until soft.

3   Add the carrot and celery to the pot, then add the beef, tomatoes, stock, bay leaf and 2 cups (500 ml) water. Bring to a boil, reduce the heat and simmer for 1 hour, until the beef and vegetables are tender. Add more water if the soup is too thick. Skim any scum from the surface of the soup.

4   Stir in the zucchini and cabbage and cook for 5 minutes, until the vegetables are tender. Discard the bay leaf.

5   Sprinkle the soup with the chopped parsley. Ladle into four bowls to serve.

EACH SERVING PROVIDES
206 calories, 22 g protein, 9 g fat (2 g saturated fat),
10 g carbohydrate (9 g sugars), 5 g fiber, 665 mg sodium

Iron and *zinc* are important nutrients for brain function and maintaining energy levels and immunity. Lean red meat is one of the best sources of these two valuable minerals.

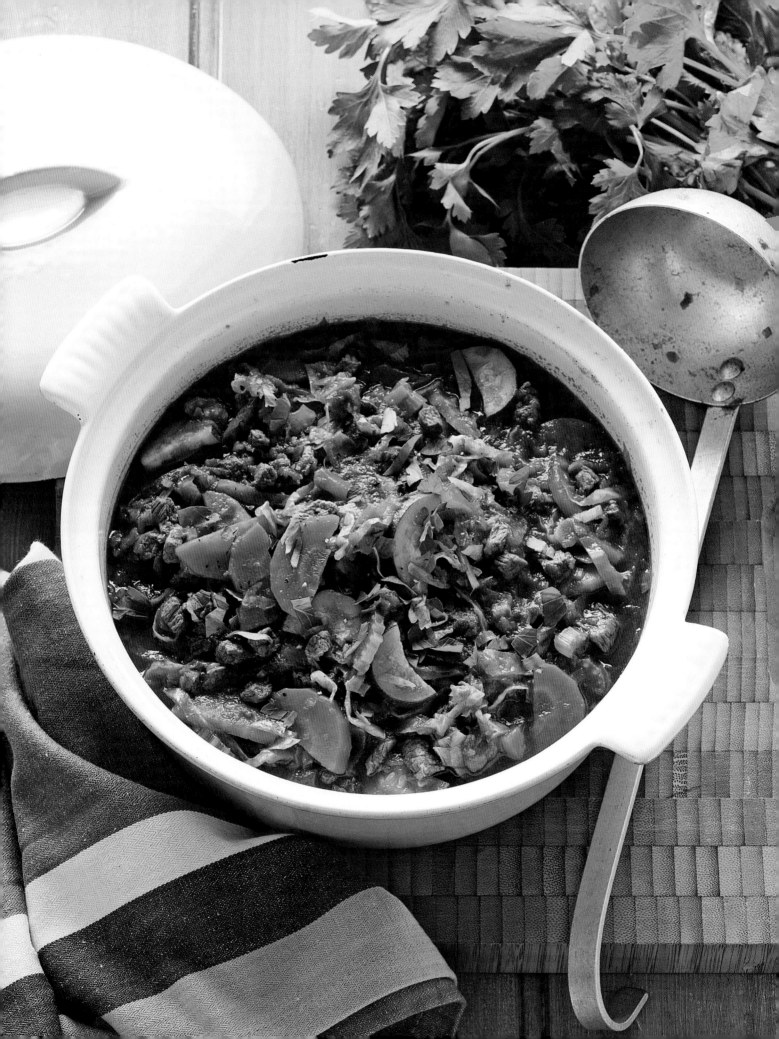

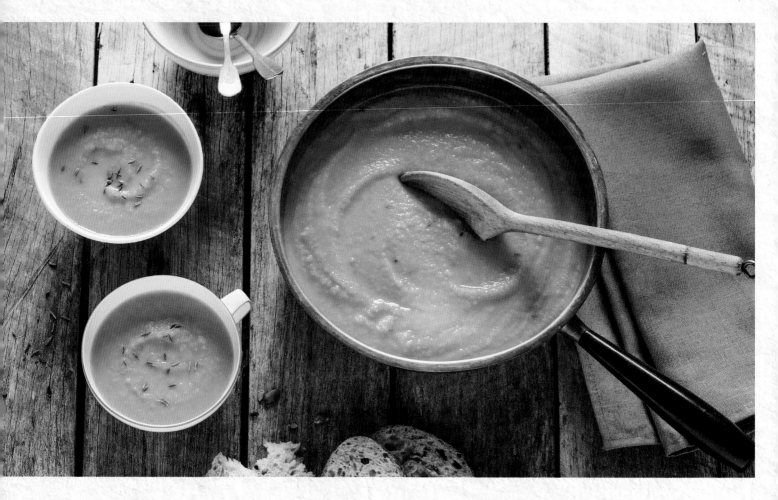

Roasted carrot and caraway soup

Roasting the carrots enhances their natural sweetness in this aromatic soup. The caraway seeds complement the carrots beautifully.

PREPARATION **20 MINUTES**   COOKING **55 MINUTES**   SERVES **4**

2 pounds (1 kg) carrots
1 tablespoon (15 ml) olive oil
1 onion, finely chopped
2 cloves garlic, crushed
1½ tablespoons (22 ml) low-sodium
  vegetable stock
freshly ground black pepper
4 slices whole-grain bread, to serve

1 Preheat the oven to 350°F (180°C). Line a large baking pan with parchment paper. Peel the carrots, cut into quarters lengthwise, and place in the pan. Roast for 45 minutes, until tender and browned.

2 Heat the oil in a large saucepan. Cook the onion over medium heat for 4 minutes, until soft. Stir in the garlic and caraway seeds, and cook for 1 minute. Add the roasted carrots, stock and 1 cup (250 ml) water.

3 Use a stick blender to purée the soup. Bring to a boil, reduce the heat and simmer for 5 minutes. Season with freshly ground black pepper.

4 Spoon the soup into bowls and garnish with the extra caraway seeds. Serve with whole-grain bread.

EACH SERVING PROVIDES

153 calories, 4 g protein, 6 g fat (<1 g saturated fat), 21 g carbohydrate (18 g sugars), 9 g fiber, 1141 mg sodium

High-fiber *carrots* actually provide more brain-boosting antioxidants when cooked, as the cooking process makes these special substances more available for absorption into the body.

Spinach and lima bean soup with Greek-style yogurt

This silky soup can be served chilled in hot weather. Vary it by using your choice of legumes (try chickpeas or lentils) and by adding fresh herbs for a different flavor.

PREPARATION **15 MINUTES**   COOKING **10 MINUTES**   SERVES **4**

1 tablespoon (15 ml) olive oil
1 onion, chopped
2 cloves garlic, crushed
3$^{1}/_{2}$ cups (875 ml) low-sodium vegetable
  or chicken stock
2 cans lima beans, 15 ounces (425 ml) each,
  rinsed and drained
1$^{1}/_{4}$ pounds (600 g) spinach, trimmed
$^{1}/_{3}$ cup (90 ml) low-fat Greek-style yogurt
$^{1}/_{4}$ teaspoon (1 ml) paprika

1   Heat the oil in a large saucepan. Add the onion and cook over medium heat for 4 minutes, until soft. Stir in the garlic and cook for 1 minute.

2   Stir in the stock and lima beans, and bring to a simmer. Add the spinach and cook until wilted.

3   Use a stick blender to purée the soup.

4   Ladle the soup into serving bowls. Top each with a spoonful of yogurt and a light dusting of paprika.

If you don't have a stick blender, allow the soup to cool slightly, then purée in batches in a food processor. Return to the pan and gently reheat.
   Replace the canned lima beans with 3 cups (750 g) cooked beans made from 1 cup (250 g) dried beans.

EACH SERVING PROVIDES
274 calories, 19 g protein, 7 g fat (1 g saturated fat),
28 g carbohydrate (10 g sugars), 13 g fiber, 951 mg sodium

> *Green leafy vegetables* such as spinach are an important brain-boosting food, rich in essential vitamins, minerals and antioxidants.

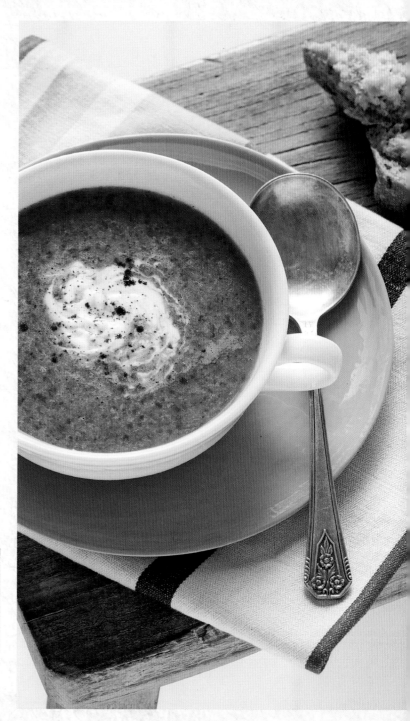

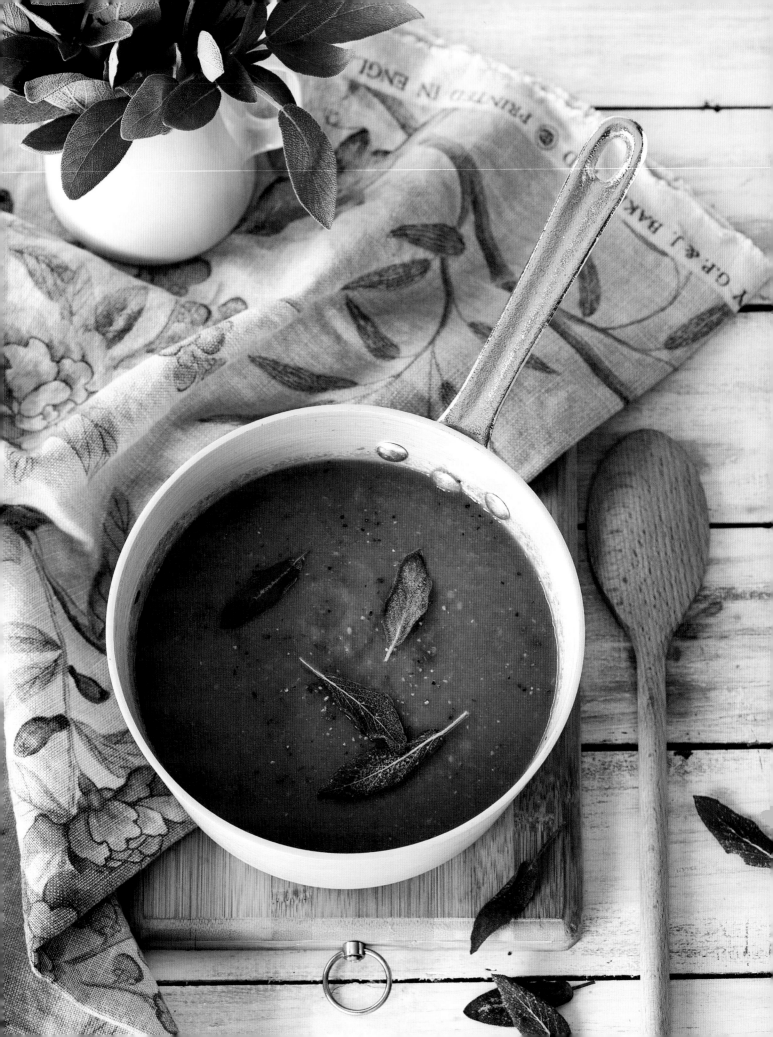

Roasted red pepper and tomato soup

This gorgeous red soup will brighten any autumn meal. Its rich color reflects its high antioxidant content. Roasting enhances the natural sweetness of vegetables such as peppers, tomatoes and onions.

PREPARATION **20 MINUTES**
COOKING **1 HOUR 10 MINUTES**
SERVES **4**

4 large red peppers
8 large plum tomatoes, halved lengthwise
1 red onion, cut into 6 wedges
4 large cloves garlic, unpeeled
1½ tablespoons (22 ml) olive oil
3 cups (750 ml) low-sodium vegetable
  or chicken stock
2 teaspoons (10 ml) finely chopped
  fresh sage
16 fresh sage leaves
freshly ground black pepper

1 Preheat the oven to 375°F (190°C). Line two large baking pans with parchment paper. Put the whole peppers on one of the pans. Arrange the tomatoes, cut side up, on the other pan. Bake for 20 minutes.

2 Add the onion and garlic to the pans. Drizzle the onion with 2 teaspoons (10 ml) of the olive oil. Bake, turning the peppers once, for 40 minutes, until the peppers and tomatoes are very soft and the onion is tender. Set aside to cool.

3 Peel the peppers, and discard the seeds and white membrane. Peel the tomatoes. Put the pepper and tomato flesh in a food processor with the onion. Squeeze the garlic pulp from the skins into the food processor, and purée the vegetables until smooth.

4 Transfer the vegetable purée to a saucepan and stir in the stock and chopped sage. Heat until the soup is simmering.

5 Meanwhile, heat the remaining olive oil in a small frying pan over medium heat. Add the whole sage leaves and cook for a few seconds, until crisp. Drain on paper towels. Set the oil aside to cool slightly.

6 Serve the soup topped with the fried sage leaves, drizzled with the reserved sage oil and sprinkled with freshly ground black pepper.

If you prefer, put the roasted vegetables in a saucepan with the stock and purée them using a stick blender rather than a food processor. Serve the soup with toasted whole-grain bread.

EACH SERVING PROVIDES
157 calories, 6 g protein, 9 g fat (1 g saturated fat), 14 g carbohydrate (9 g sugars), 8 g fiber, 492 mg sodium

Red peppers are high in beta-carotene and vitamin C, with minimal fat and sodium. As the precursor of vitamin A, beta-carotene is essential for healthy vision and also plays a role in the body's immune function.

Spicy lentil soup with butternut squash, tomatoes and green beans

You can use any type of Indian curry paste, from a mild korma to a spicy vindaloo, or leave it out altogether for a simple vegetable and lentil soup. Toss in a handful of leafy greens such as baby spinach or kale at the end of cooking for an extra boost of vegetables.

PREPARATION **15 MINUTES**
COOKING **50 MINUTES**
SERVES **6**

1 tablespoon (15 ml) olive oil
1 onion, chopped
2 stalks celery, chopped
2 carrots, chopped
2 cloves garlic, crushed
2 tablespoons (30 ml) korma curry paste
2 pounds (1 kg) butternut squash, chopped
14$^{1}/_{2}$ ounce (400 ml) can diced tomatoes
3 cups (750 ml) low-sodium vegetable or chicken stock
14$^{1}/_{2}$ ounce (400 ml) can brown lentils, rinsed and drained
$^{1}/_{2}$ cup (125 g) green beans, cut into short lengths
$^{1}/_{2}$ cup (125 ml) low-fat Greek-style yogurt, to serve

1   Heat the oil in a large saucepan over low heat. Cook the onion, celery and carrots for 10 minutes, until golden brown and very soft. Stir regularly to prevent sticking and burning.

2   Stir in the garlic and curry paste, and cook for 1 minute. Add the squash, tomatoes and stock. Cover and bring to a boil, reduce the heat to low and cook for 30 minutes, until the squash is soft.

3   Stir in the lentils and beans, and cook for 5 minutes, until the beans are tender.

4   Spoon the soup into six serving bowls and serve topped with the yogurt.

Replace the canned lentils with 1$^{1}/_{2}$ cups (375 g) cooked lentils made from $^{1}/_{2}$ cup (100 g) dried lentils.

EACH SERVING PROVIDES
197 calories, 7 g protein, 6 g fat (<1 g saturated fat),
31 g carbohydrate (10 g sugars), 7 g fiber, 695 mg sodium

Lentils help to stabilize blood glucose levels as they have a very low glycemic index. Adding lentils to any recipe decreases the glycemic load of the whole meal, ensuring that the brain receives a steady supply of fuel for much longer.

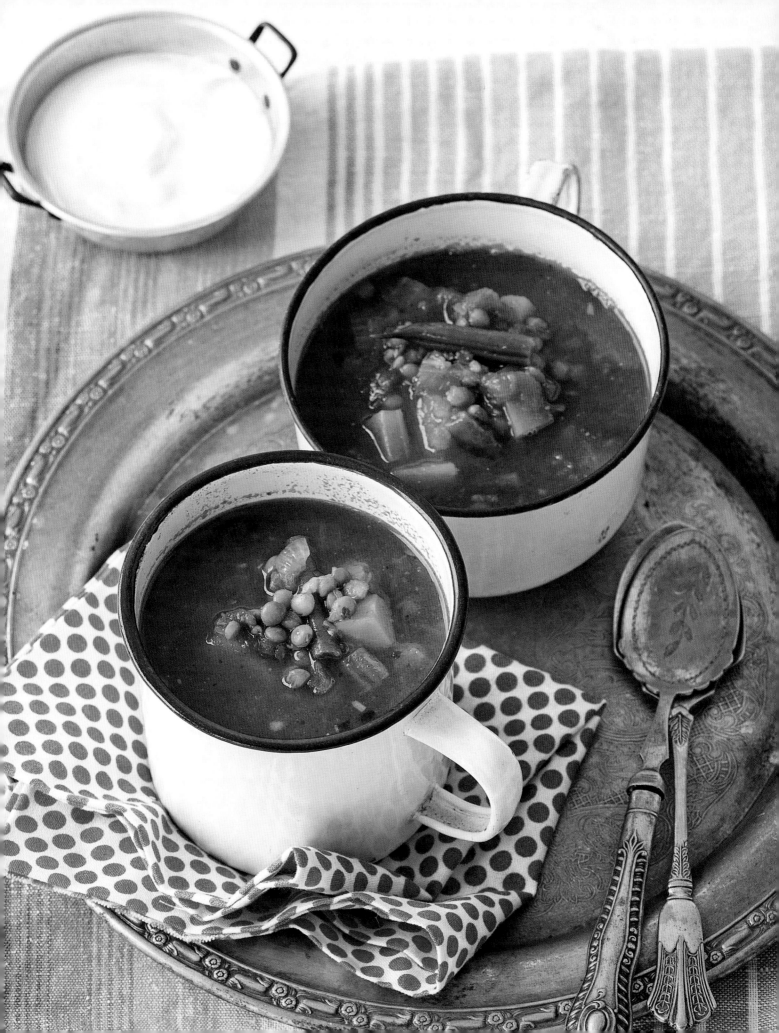

Legumes

Legumes, the seeds of beans, peas and lentils, are a vegetarian protein source that is low in fat and rich in nutrients. Legumes are also high in soluble fiber, which helps to control blood glucose and cholesterol levels.

Unlike animal protein foods, legumes do not contain all the essential amino acids. However, combining them with grains, nuts or seeds produces a complete protein mixture that can be used for all the body's growth and healing needs. Also unlike animal protein foods, legumes are high in fiber and contain low glycemic index (low GI) carbohydrate. This is important because persistently high blood glucose levels are thought to promote inflammation and allow oxidative free radicals to damage cells and lead to some degenerative conditions of the brain, such as dementia.

Adding legumes can reduce the glycemic load of an entire meal, which helps to keep blood glucose levels low and maintain a steady supply of fuel for optimal brain function between meals. There is no need to dig into a big bowl of lentils to achieve this effect—the glycemic load will be reduced and the nutritional value boosted just by adding some kidney beans to a chili, or cannellini beans or chickpeas to a soup. Adding legumes is an economical way to bulk up your meals.

The fiber found in legumes is important for good cardiovascular health: Soluble fiber helps to take cholesterol out of the body, preventing damage and blockage in blood vessel walls as well as promoting a good supply of blood for optimal brain function. Legumes are high in phytonutrients and are also a good source of magnesium, which helps control blood pressure and appears to be needed by the brain to ease stress and to maintain the normal function of neurotransmitters. Optimal magnesium levels seem to promote memory storage and recall.

Clockwise from far left: peas, green beans, lima beans, fava beans, chickpeas, green lentils, red kidney beans, red lentils, four-bean mix (red kidney beans, baby lima beans, chickpeas and cannellini beans).

Legumes provide a good source of calcium and B-group vitamins, especially folate. Niacin, which is also known as vitamin B_3, is found in rich amounts in meat, fish and poultry, but legumes are also a good source. Even a slight deficiency in niacin can lead to changes in mood and brain function. Legumes also provide thiamine—used in the body's energy generation processes and for maintaining normal neurological function—and choline, needed for producing neurotransmitters and for maintaining brain cell membranes.

Iron and zinc, often low in vegetarian diets, are found in legumes in reasonable amounts. However, the zinc from legumes is absorbed by the body reasonably well although the iron is not. Zinc is important in many processes of cell metabolism, and is also required in large amounts for the brain to function optimally. Zinc plays a role in neurotransmission, and a deficiency causes an impairment in brain function. An inadequate zinc supply during pregnancy leads to suboptimal learning, memory and attention in the baby. Iron is essential for normal brain development and function because it is needed for myelin as well as neurotransmitter synthesis, and is also at the center of the body's energy system that fuels every brain cell. To maximize absorption of the plant form of their iron, legumes, should be eaten with a food that is rich in vitamin C, or combined with an animal form of iron, such as meat. For example, add some red peppers or tomatoes to a dish containing legumes, or add some lentils to a meaty pasta sauce or soup.

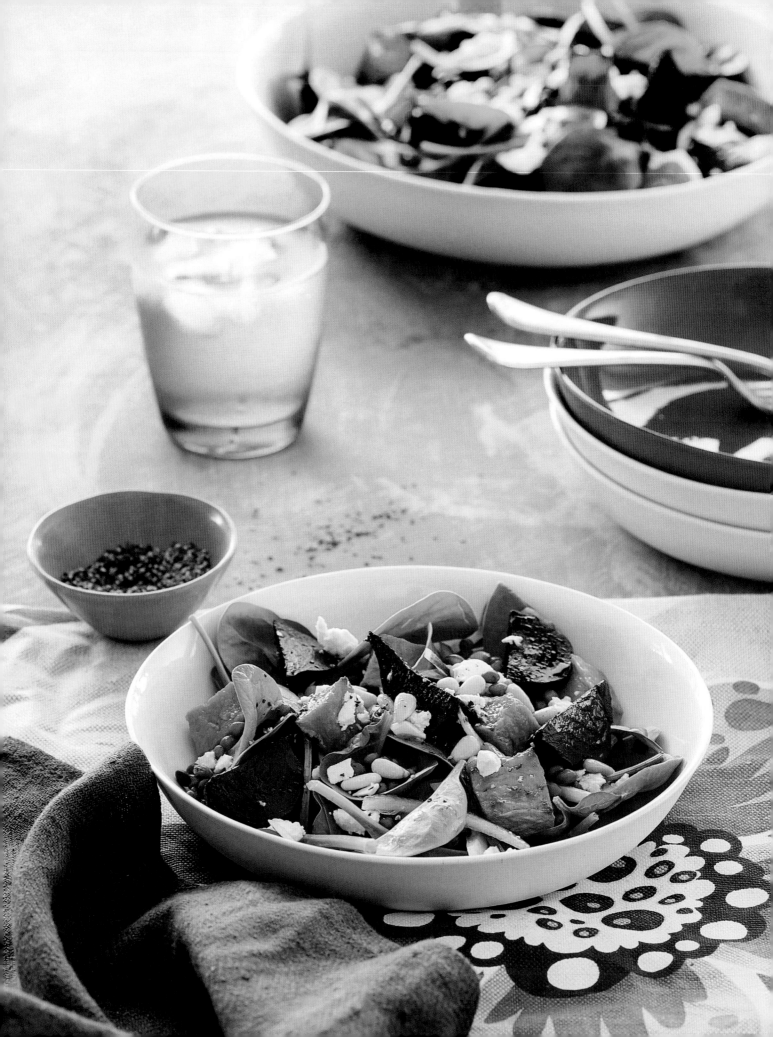

Roasted butternut squash, beet and lentil salad

This elegant salad is easy to prepare and you can roast the squash and beets while you cook other dishes. Serve it with some crusty whole-grain bread for a light but balanced meal.

PREPARATION **20 MINUTES**
COOKING **1 HOUR 5 MINUTES**
SERVES **4**

1½ pounds (750 g) butternut squash, cut into chunks
olive oil spray
4 baby beets, about ½ pound (250 g) total, scrubbed
2 tablespoons (30 ml) pine nuts
14½ ounce (400 ml) can brown lentils, rinsed and drained
1 small red onion, halved and thinly sliced
¼ cup (60 g) baby spinach leaves
1 tablespoon (15 ml) red wine vinegar
1 tablespoon (15 ml) extra virgin olive oil
⅔ cup (100 g) crumbled low-fat feta
freshly ground black pepper

1 Preheat the oven to 400°F (200°C). Line a baking pan with parchment paper.

2 Spread the squash on the prepared pan and spray with olive oil. Wrap the beets in a large sheet of foil. Bake the beets for 15 minutes, then add the squash and bake for 45 minutes, until the squash is tender and lightly browned and the beets are tender when pierced with a small, sharp knife. Unwrap the beets and set aside with the squash to cool to room temperature.

3 Meanwhile, spread the pine nuts on a baking pan. Bake for 3 minutes, until lightly golden. Transfer to a plate to cool.

4 Slip the skins off the cooled beets and cut each into six wedges.

5 Combine the lentils, onion and spinach in a large serving bowl. Drizzle with the vinegar and oil, and toss to combine. Top with the squash and beets, sprinkle with the feta and pine nuts, and season with freshly ground black pepper.

Wear rubber gloves when handling cooked beets to avoid staining your hands.

Replace the canned lentils with 2 cups (500 g) cooked lentils made from ⅔ cup (130 g) dried lentils.

EACH SERVING PROVIDES
307 calories, 13 g protein, 15 g fat (3 g saturated fat), 34 g carbohydrate (10 g sugars), 8 g fiber, 509 mg sodium

This salad provides an excellent combination of *beneficial fats* and different types of *fiber* for optimal cardiovascular health, which provides a good blood supply to the brain.

Tuna, tomato and bean salad

PREPARATION **20 MINUTES**
COOKING **2 MINUTES**
SERVES **4**

$^{1}/_{3}$ pound (150 g) whole green beans, trimmed
1 baby romaine lettuce
15 ounce (425 ml) can tuna, drained and flaked
15 ounce (425 ml) can red kidney beans,
    rinsed and drained
3 scallions, sliced
1 cup (200 g) baby plum tomatoes
    or red cherry tomatoes, halved
freshly ground black pepper

Dressing
1 tablespoon (15 ml) lemon juice
1$^{1}/_{2}$ tablespoons (22 ml) extra virgin olive oil
1 clove garlic, halved

1 To make the dressing, combine the lemon juice,
oil and garlic in a small bowl. Whisk and set aside.

2 Drop the green beans into a saucepan of boiling
water and cook for 2 minutes. Drain and refresh in
ice water. Drain and pat dry with paper towels.

3 Separate the lettuce leaves and arrange them
on a platter. Top with the green beans, tuna, kidney
beans, scallions and tomatoes.

4 Discard the garlic clove and whisk the dressing
again. Drizzle over the salad and season with freshly
ground black pepper.

The kidney beans can be replaced with chickpeas or
cannellini beans. Other vegetables, such as red peppers
or celery, can be added, too.

Replace the canned kidney beans with 1$^{1}/_{2}$ cups (375 g)
cooked beans made from $^{1}/_{2}$ cup (100 g) dried beans.

EACH SERVING PROVIDES
248 calories, 28 g protein, 10 g fat (2 g saturated fat),
12 g carbohydrate (4 g sugars), 7 g fiber, 282 mg sodium

> The color of *kidney beans* comes in part from
> the anthocyanins, a group of antioxidants that are
> thought to improve brain function.

Grilled tuna with avocado

PREPARATION **20 MINUTES, PLUS MARINATING**
COOKING **4 MINUTES**
SERVES **4**

2 cloves garlic, crushed
1 teaspoon (5 ml) dried oregano
2 teaspoons (10 ml) olive oil
freshly ground black pepper
4 tuna steaks, $^{1}/_{3}$ pound (150 g) each
$^{1}/_{4}$ cup (60 g) mixed baby spinach and
    arugula leaves
15 ounce (425 ml) can chickpeas, rinsed
    and drained
1 red pepper, chopped
1 small red onion, halved and thinly sliced
1 avocado, sliced
2 tablespoons (30 ml) lemon juice
2 tablespoons (30 ml) extra virgin olive oil

1 Combine the garlic, oregano and olive oil in a
shallow dish, and season with freshly ground black
pepper. Add the tuna steaks and turn to coat. Cover
and refrigerate for 15 minutes.

2 Preheat a grill pan over medium–high heat. Cook
the tuna steaks for 2 minutes on each side, until just
cooked through. Set aside to cool slightly, then use a
fork to break the tuna into chunks.

3 Combine the spinach and arugula, chickpeas,
red pepper, onion, avocado and tuna in a serving
dish. Serve drizzled with the lemon juice and extra
virgin olive oil.

Replace the canned chickpeas with 1$^{1}/_{2}$ cups
(375 g) cooked chickpeas made from $^{1}/_{2}$ cup (110 g)
dried chickpeas.

EACH SERVING PROVIDES
536 calories, 44 g protein, 30 g fat (8 g saturated fat),
12 g carbohydrate (3 g sugars), 5 g fiber, 226 mg sodium

> *Choline* appears to be involved in nourishing
> the brain as well as helping to form healthy cell
> membranes. Tuna is a good source of choline,
> and spinach provides some choline as well.

The tuna salad makes a filling and healthy meal, thanks to the protein-packed tuna and beans. The grilled tuna can be cooked ahead of time and served cold, too.

Left: Tuna, tomato and bean salad
Right: Grilled tuna with avocado

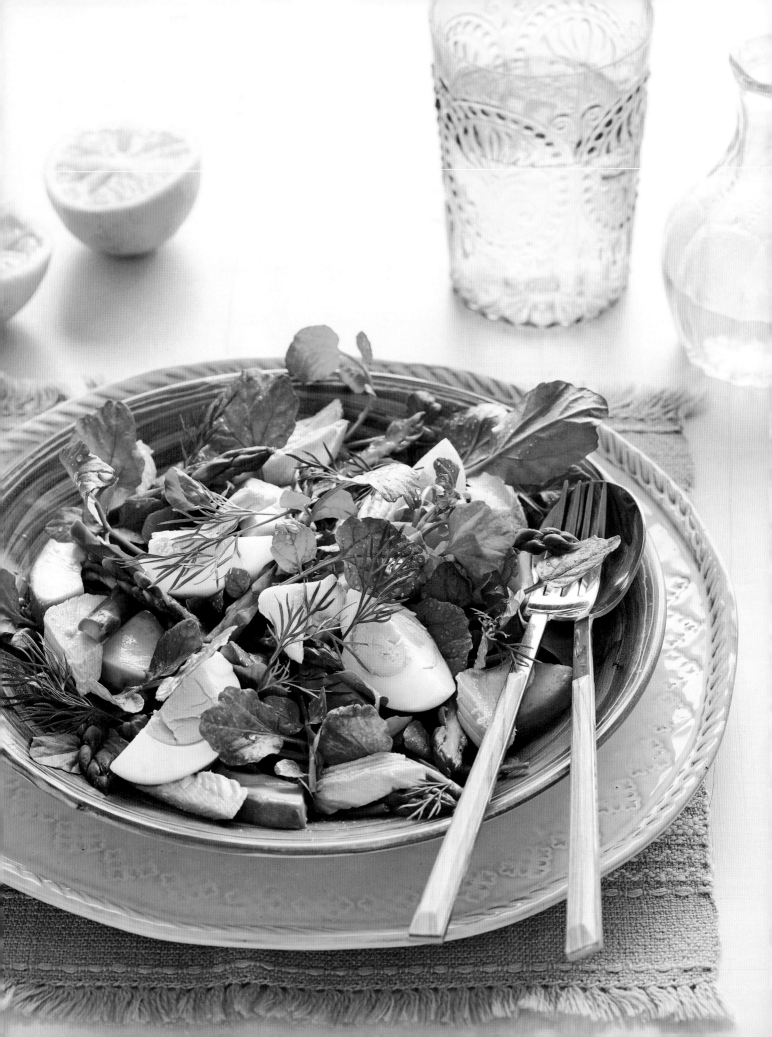

Trout, egg and asparagus salad

Protein and healthy fats make this salad very satisfying as a light meal, served with a side of grains or a whole-grain roll. It can also be used as the filling for a whole-grain wrap.

PREPARATION **15 MINUTES**
COOKING **10 MINUTES**
SERVES **4**

4 eggs
$^2/_3$ pound (350 g) rainbow trout, cleaned and scaled
$^2/_3$ pound (300 g) asparagus, trimmed
2 cups (60 g) watercress sprigs, trimmed
1 avocado, chopped
2 tablespoons (30 ml) lemon juice
1 tablespoon (15 ml) macadamia nut or olive oil
2 tablespoons (30 ml) fresh dill sprigs

1 Place the eggs in a saucepan, cover with cold water and bring to a boil over high heat. As soon as the water boils, time the eggs to cook for 8 minutes. Drain, then cool under cold water.

2 Meanwhile, half-fill a deep frying pan with water. Bring to a simmer, and add the trout. Return to a simmer, cover and gently poach for 8 minutes, until just cooked through. Lift out the trout with a slotted spoon and transfer to a plate. Cool slightly, slip off the skin and pull the meat from the bones in large flakes.

3 Put the asparagus in a heatproof bowl and cover with boiling water. Let stand for 2 minutes, drain and plunge into a bowl of ice water. Drain and pat dry with paper towels. Cut each spear in half lengthwise, and cut each half into three pieces.

4 Peel and quarter the eggs. Arrange the watercress on four serving plates. Top with the avocado, asparagus, trout and egg quarters.

5 Drizzle the lemon juice and oil over the salad, sprinkle with the dill and serve immediately.

If the asparagus spears are thin, don't cut them in half lengthwise; simply cut each spear into three pieces.

EACH SERVING PROVIDES
338 calories, 27 g protein, 25 g fat (6 g saturated fat), 2 g carbohydrate (2 g sugars), 3 g fiber, 139 mg sodium

Omega-3 fats, found in trout and watercress, appear to improve mood as well as enhancing brain and cardiovascular function. Eggs also provide omega-3 fats; the amount depends on how the hens are fed—check the label on your egg carton. In general, free-range eggs and those labelled "omega-3" have a higher content of omega-3 fats than other eggs.

Purple potato and pumpkin salad

If you have trouble finding purple potatoes, you can substitute fingerling potatoes, which are a similar shape but don't contain the same brain-benefiting nutrients.

PREPARATION **20 MINUTES**   COOKING **40 MINUTES**   SERVES **4**

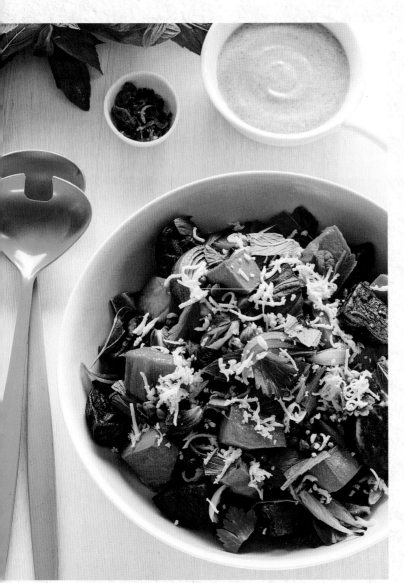

³/₄ pound (400 g) purple potatoes, scrubbed
³/₄ pound (400 g) pumpkin or kabocha squash
1 red onion, cut into thin wedges
1 tablespoon (15 ml) olive oil
2 eggs
¹/₄ cup (5 g) fresh mint leaves, torn
¹/₄ cup (5 g) fresh flat-leaf parsley,
    roughly chopped
2 tablespoons (30 ml) capers, rinsed and dried
2 tablespoons (30 ml) fried Asian shallots

Dressing
¹/₄ cup (50 ml) low-fat Greek-style yogurt
2 teaspoons (10 ml) dijon mustard
¹/₂ teaspoon (2 ml) smoked paprika

1   Preheat the oven to 400°F (200°C). Line a large baking pan with parchment paper. Cut the potatoes and pumpkin into large pieces and arrange in the pan with the onion. Drizzle with the oil and bake for 40 minutes, until soft.

2   Meanwhile, place the eggs in a small saucepan, cover with cold water and bring to a boil over high heat. As soon as the water boils, time the eggs to cook for 5 minutes. Drain, and cool before peeling.

3   Allow the potatoes and pumpkin to cool slightly, transfer to a bowl and add the mint and parsley.

4   To make the dressing, whisk the yogurt, mustard and smoked paprika in a small bowl.

5   Just before serving, spoon the dressing over the salad and gently toss to combine. Alternatively, serve the dressing on the side. Grate the eggs over the salad and sprinkle with the capers and shallots.

Crispy fried Asian shallots are available in Asian food stores and some supermarkets.

EACH SERVING PROVIDES
214 calories, 10 g protein, 8 g fat (2 g saturated fat),
24 g carbohydrate (8 g sugars), 4 g fiber, 181 mg sodium

Many important brain-protecting *antioxidants* are actually the pigments found in brightly colored varieties of fruit and vegetables. Purple and blue potatoes are a great example, containing much higher levels of flavonoids than white potatoes.

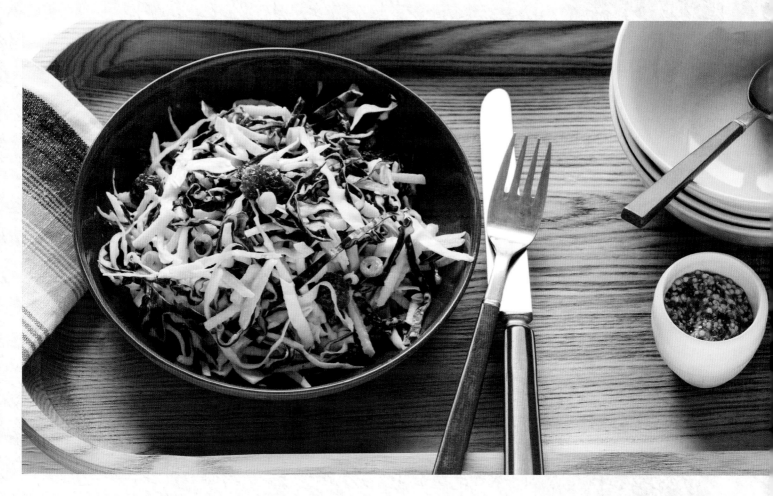

Apple and raisin coleslaw

Yogurt is a healthier alternative to mayonnaise in this coleslaw's dressing. It's not only lower in fat but delivers probiotic benefits, too.

PREPARATION 20 MINUTES   SERVES 6

$^1/_3$ cup (40 g) raisins
1 tablespoon (15 ml) lemon juice
2 green apples
$^3/_4$ cup (175 g) white cabbage, shredded
$^3/_4$ cup (175 g) red cabbage, shredded
2 scallions, thinly sliced

Dressing
$^1/_2$ cup (125 ml) low-fat Greek-style yogurt
2 teaspoons (10 ml) dijon or whole-grain mustard
2 teaspoons (10 ml) olive oil
2 teaspoons (10 ml) lemon juice

1 Place the raisins in a bowl with the lemon juice. Coarsely grate the apples, leaving the skin on, and add to the bowl. Turn to coat in the lemon juice to prevent browning.

2 To make the dressing, stir the yogurt, mustard, oil and lemon juice together.

3 Just before serving, combine the apple mixture, cabbage and scallions in a large bowl, and toss with the dressing.

EACH SERVING PROVIDES
97 calories, 3 g protein, 3 g fat (<1 g saturated fat), 16 g carbohydrate (14 g sugars), 4 g fiber, 84 mg sodium

> Both *white* and *red cabbage* are high in antioxidants, as are all other members of the cruciferous vegetable family. Red cabbage also contains a pigment called flavin, one of the anthocyanin group of antioxidants, giving it additional brain-protective benefits not found in white cabbage.

Salmon and potato salad

Cooled potatoes have a low glycemic index, making them a satisfying source of long-lasting fuel for the brain and body. This salad combines them with brain-boosting salmon and a low-fat dressing.

PREPARATION **20 MINUTES**
COOKING **20 MINUTES**
SERVES **4**

$^3/_4$ pound (400 g) boneless,
   skinless salmon fillets
$1^1/_4$ pounds (600 g) small
   new potatoes
$^2/_3$ cup (150 g) snow peas
2 celery stalks, thinly sliced
1 red pepper, thinly sliced
freshly ground black pepper

Dressing
$^1/_2$ cup (125 ml) buttermilk
1 clove garlic, crushed
1 teaspoon (5 ml) dijon mustard
2 tablespoons (30 ml) lemon juice
1 teaspoon (5 ml) finely grated
   lemon zest

1   Preheat the oven to 325°F (160°C). Place the salmon on a large sheet of parchment paper. Wrap the salmon in the paper and fold the edges to seal. Place the parcel on a baking pan and bake for 20 minutes. Set aside to rest and cool slightly.

2   Meanwhile, cook the potatoes in a large saucepan of boiling water for 10 minutes, until tender when tested with a knife. Drain and cool.

3   Place the snow peas in a large heatproof bowl, cover with boiling water and let stand for 2 minutes. Drain the snow peas and plunge them into a bowl of ice water. Drain well. Trim the tops, and thinly slice lengthwise.

4   To make the dressing, combine the ingredients in a small bowl and whisk until smooth.

5   Flake the salmon into large chunks and cut the potatoes into quarters. Arrange on a serving platter with the snow peas, celery and pepper. Drizzle with half of the dressing and sprinkle with freshly ground black pepper. Serve the remaining dressing on the side.

EACH SERVING PROVIDES
285 calories, 26 g protein, 8 g fat (2 g saturated fat),
25 g carbohydrate (5 g sugars), 5 g fiber, 114 mg sodium

Despite its rich, fatty-sounding name, *buttermilk* is actually a very low-fat product, useful in cooking as an alternative to cream. The brain relies on a healthy cardiovascular system for its blood supply, so for optimal brain function, cut down on saturated fat.

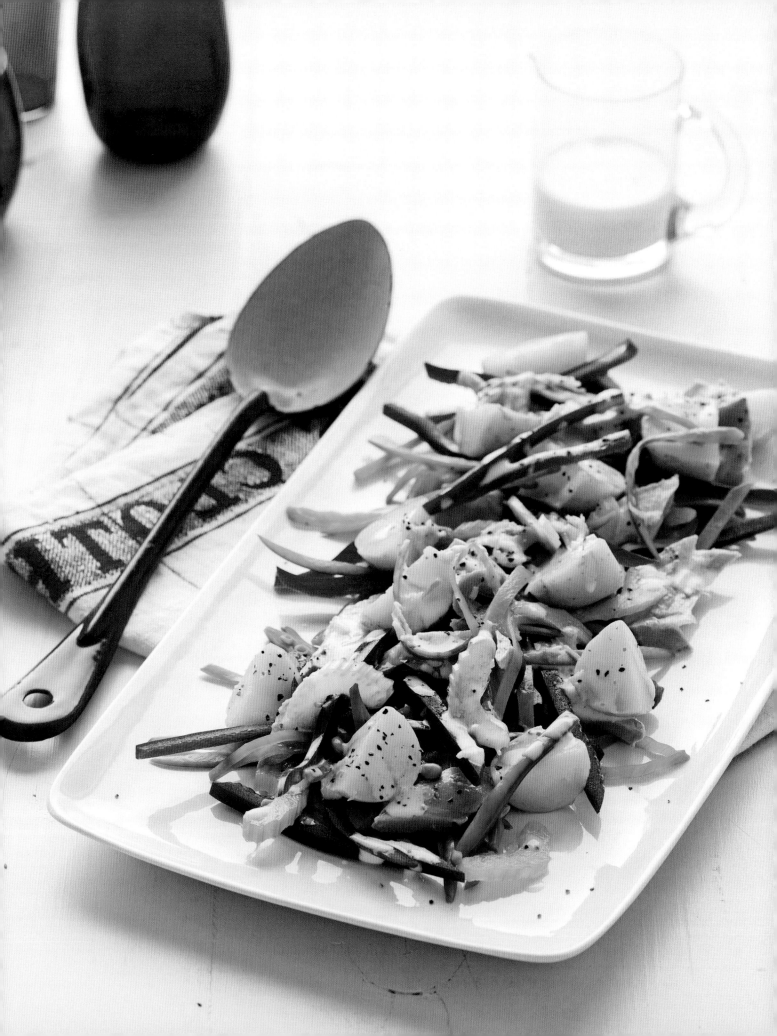

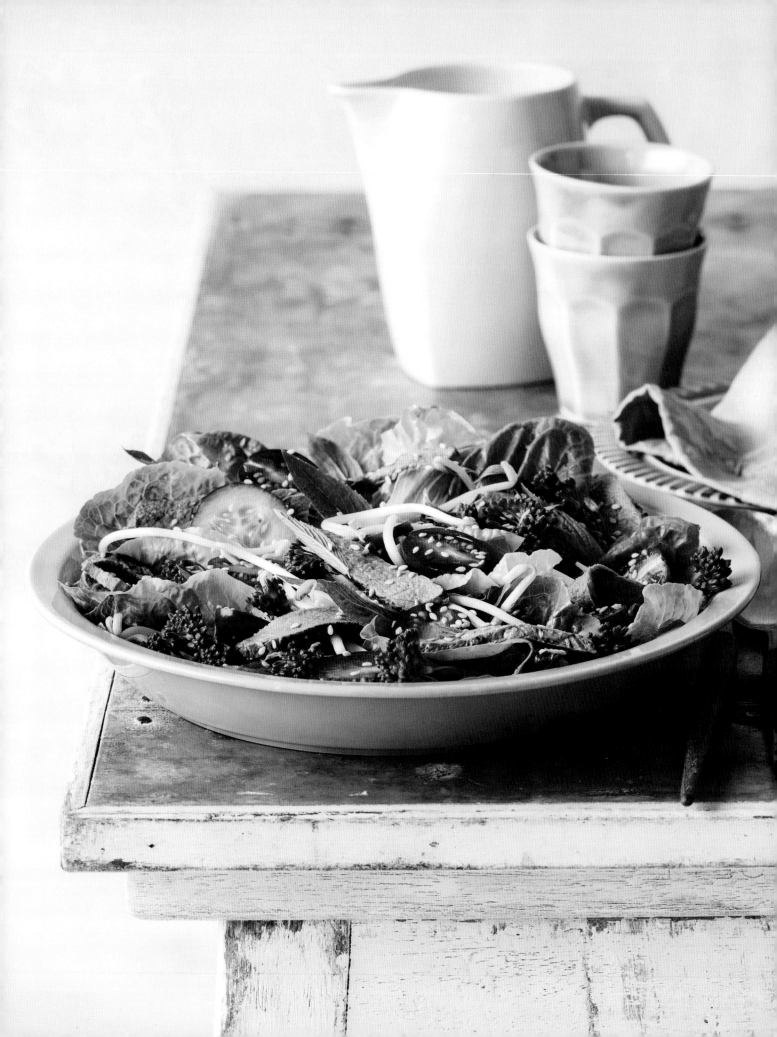

Beef and broccolini salad

Tender lean beef is combined here with antioxidant-rich greens. You can use your choice of vegetables in this salad. Instead of broccolini, try steamed snow peas or asparagus.

PREPARATION **20 MINUTES**
COOKING **15 MINUTES**
SERVES **4**

$^2/_3$ pound (300 g) beef round steak
ground white pepper
1 tablespoon (15 ml) olive or canola oil
1 cup (200 g) broccolini, cut into
   short lengths
$^1/_4$ pound (100 g) baby romaine,
   roughly torn
1 cucumber, thinly sliced
$^1/_2$ cup (100 g) bean sprouts
1 cup (250 g) baby plum tomatoes
   or red cherry tomatoes, halved
$^1/_2$ cup (10 g) fresh mint
2 tablespoons (30 ml) toasted
   sesame seeds

Dressing
few drops of sesame oil
2 tablespoons (30 ml) lime juice
2 tablespoons (30 ml) fresh apple juice
1 tablespoon (15 ml) low-sodium soy sauce

1 Heat a grill pan over medium–high heat. Rub the steak with white pepper and the oil. Cook in the hot pan for 3–5 minutes each side, until medium-rare. Remove from the pan, cover and let rest while you assemble the salad.

2 Steam the broccolini over a saucepan of simmering water for 5 minutes, until bright green and tender.

3 Arrange the lettuce leaves in a serving bowl. Top with the broccolini, cucumber, bean sprouts, tomatoes, mint and half the sesame seeds.

4 Slice the meat and arrange it over the top of the salad.

5 To make the dressing, whisk the sesame oil, lime juice, apple juice and soy sauce in a small bowl.

6 Drizzle the dressing over the salad and serve sprinkled with the remaining sesame seeds.

Make sure you give the meat time to rest—this will allow it to retain all of its juices—and slice the meat across the grain, just before serving.

EACH SERVING PROVIDES
222 calories, 22 g protein, 12 g fat (3 g saturated fat),
8 g carbohydrate (5 g sugars), 4 g fiber, 249 mg sodium

Iron-rich *lean beef* is a source of high-quality protein. Substitute venison for a leaner meat with less calories and more iron than beef.

Soba noodle and salmon salad

Soba noodles are traditionally made from buckwheat or a combination of buckwheat and regular wheat flour. If you want to avoid wheat, be sure to check the label. Pure buckwheat noodles are commonly available in health food stores.

PREPARATION **25 MINUTES**
COOKING **15 MINUTES**
SERVES **4**

$3/4$ pound (400 g) boneless, skinless
   salmon fillets
1 cup (200 g) snow peas, trimmed
9 ounces (270 g) soba noodles
4 scallions, thinly sliced on the diagonal
1 carrot, finely shredded
1 red pepper, cut into thin strips
1 small cucumber, cut into thin strips
$1/4$ cup (10 g) fresh cilantro leaves,
   roughly torn

Dressing
$1^{1}/_{2}$ tablespoons (22 ml) rice wine vinegar
1 tablespoon (15 ml) canola oil
2 teaspoons (10 ml) sesame oil
2 teaspoons (10 ml) low-sodium soy sauce

1 Half-fill a deep frying pan with water and bring to a simmer. Add the salmon and return to a simmer. Cover and gently poach for 10 minutes, until the salmon is just cooked through. Lift out with a slotted spoon and transfer to a plate. Let cool slightly, then use a fork to break the salmon into large flakes.

2 Meanwhile, bring a large saucepan of water to a boil over high heat. Add the snow peas and cook for 1 minute. Using a slotted spoon, transfer the snow peas to a bowl of ice water. Drain and pat dry with paper towels, then thinly slice on the diagonal.

3 Return the water to a boil. Add the noodles and cook for 4 minutes. Drain in a colander, and rinse under cold running water.

4 To make the dressing, whisk the vinegar, canola oil, sesame oil and soy sauce in a small bowl.

5 Combine the noodles and vegetables in a large bowl. Drizzle with the dressing, gently toss to combine, and fold in the salmon and cilantro. Serve immediately, or refrigerate and serve chilled.

EACH SERVING PROVIDES
484 calories, 30 g protein, 15 g fat (2 g saturated fat), 53 g carbohydrate (5 g sugars), 5 g fiber, 773 mg sodium

Despite its name, *buckwheat* is not related to wheat. It is a gluten-free grain, high in copper, zinc, magnesium and manganese, all used by the brain to maintain normal processes.

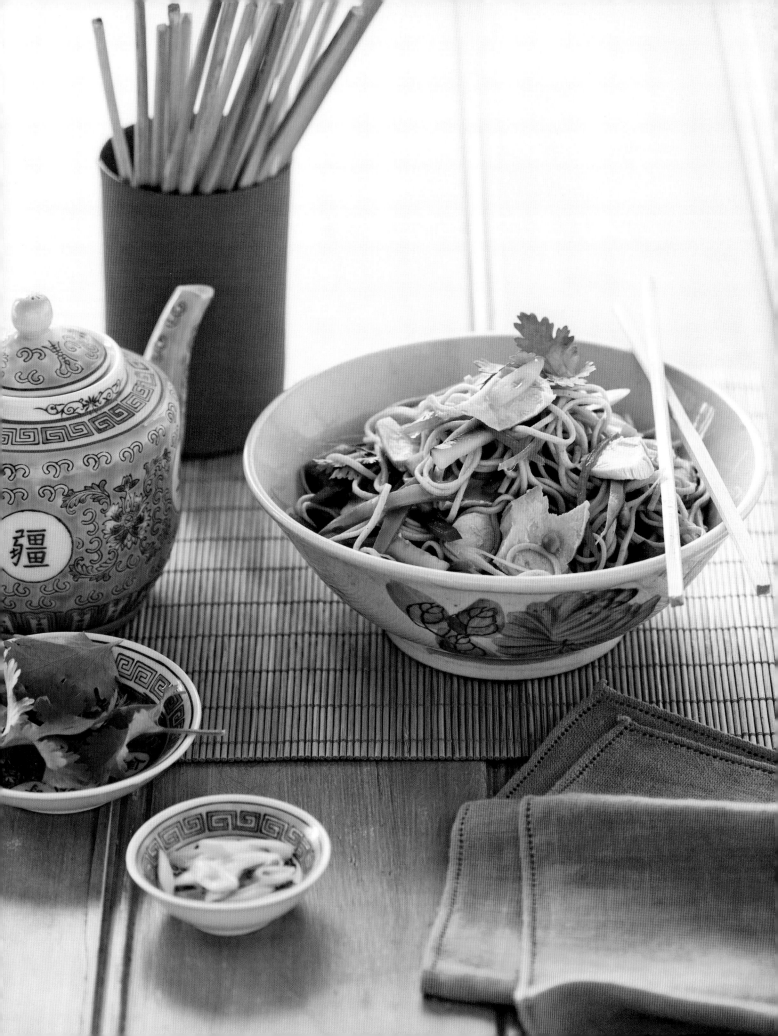

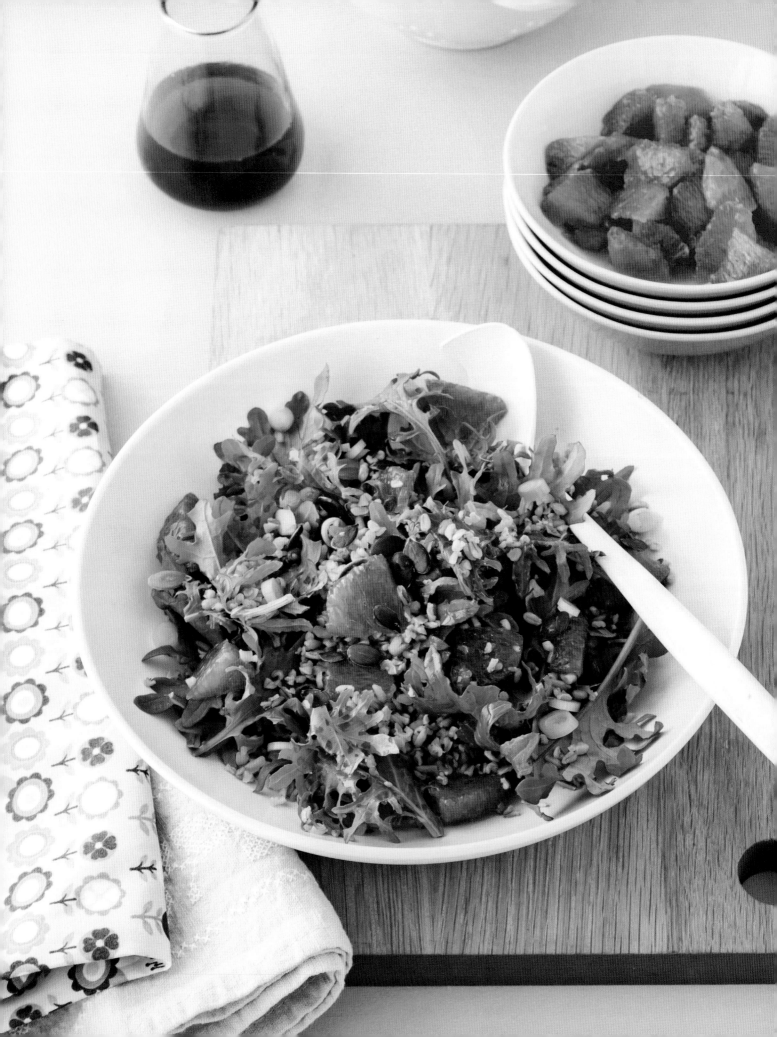

Freekeh and baby kale salad with pepitas and ruby red grapefruit

Freekeh is wheat grain that is harvested while still green, then dried and roasted. Available at health food stores, you can buy it as a whole grain or in the cracked form used here, which gives it a texture similar to bulgur. It makes a lovely side dish with barbecued meats.

PREPARATION **15 MINUTES**
COOKING **20 MINUTES**
SERVES **6**

1 cup (175 g) cracked freekeh
2 ruby red grapefruit
2 ounces (60 g) baby kale, larger leaves torn
3 scallions, thinly sliced
1 tablespoon (15 ml) extra virgin olive oil
1 tablespoon (15 ml) red wine vinegar
1/4 cup (30 g) pepitas (pumpkin seeds), lightly
   toasted

1 Cook the freekeh in a large saucepan of boiling water for 20 minutes, until tender. Drain well and set aside to cool.

2 Slice the top and bottom from each grapefruit so they sit flat. Using a small, sharp knife, cut downwards to remove the skin, taking off the white pith. Hold the grapefruit in the palm of your hand and remove the segments by carefully cutting on either side of the membrane. Cut each segment in half crosswise.

3 Combine the freekeh, grapefruit, kale and scallions in a large bowl. Drizzle with the oil and vinegar, and toss to combine. Sprinkle with the pepitas and gently toss.

To toast the pepitas, preheat the oven to 325°F (160°C). Spread the pepitas on a baking pan and bake for 5 minutes. Transfer to a plate to cool.

EACH SERVING PROVIDES
184 calories, 6 g protein, 6 g fat (<1 g saturated fat),
26 g carbohydrate (4 g sugars), 6 g fiber, 11 mg sodium

Freekeh is high in protein and fiber and has a low glycemic index, which means your brain receives a steady supply of fuel for optimal functioning.

Wilted Swiss chard salad with caramelized onions, walnuts and feta

This colorful salad features Swiss chard, drizzled with a sweet, vinegary dressing and sprinkled with feta. The orange provides vitamin C, which helps your body absorb the iron from the chard.

PREPARATION **20 MINUTES**
COOKING **20 MINUTES**
SERVES **4**

1¼ pounds (600 g) Swiss chard
1 orange
1 tablespoon (15 ml) olive oil
2 red onions, cut into thin wedges
1 cup (100 g) walnut halves
¼ cup (30 g) pepitas (pumpkin seeds)
1 teaspoon (10 ml) ground cumin
1 teaspoon (10 ml) ground cinnamon
1 teaspoon (10 ml) maple syrup
1 red apple, thinly sliced
3½ ounces (100 g) feta

Dressing
2 tablespoons (30 ml) extra virgin olive oil
1 tablespoon (15 ml) red wine vinegar
1 teaspoon (10 ml) maple syrup
1 teaspoon (10 ml) dijon mustard
1 small clove garlic, crushed

1   Remove the tough white stems from the chard and thinly shred the green leaves. Pour a little water into a large saucepan. Put the chard in a metal colander. Place over the pan, cover and steam, tossing occasionally, for 5 minutes, until the chard is just wilted. Rinse under cold water to stop the wilting.

2   Slice the top and bottom from the orange so it sits flat. Using a small, sharp knife, cut downwards to remove the skin, taking off the white pith. Hold the orange in the palm of your hand and remove the segments by carefully cutting on either side of the membrane.

3   Heat the olive oil in a large frying pan. Cook the onions over medium heat for 10 minutes, until caramelized. Stir in the walnuts, pepitas and spices, and cook until the spices are fragrant. Add the maple syrup and cook, stirring, for 1 minute. Remove from the heat.

4   To make the dressing, whisk the oil, red wine vinegar, maple syrup, mustard and garlic in a small bowl.

5   Arrange the wilted Swiss chard on a platter and top with the caramelized onion mixture, apple and orange segments. Drizzle with the dressing and gently toss to coat. Crumble the feta over the top and serve.

Watch the Swiss chard carefully as it can quickly overcook. Cook it in batches if it doesn't fit in your colander.

EACH SERVING PROVIDES
507 calories, 15 g protein, 42 g fat (9 g saturated fat),
17 g carbohydrate (14 g sugars), 8 g fiber, 485 mg sodium

This salad is a feast of *antioxidants* and *healthy fats* for optimal brain function and protection against inflammation.

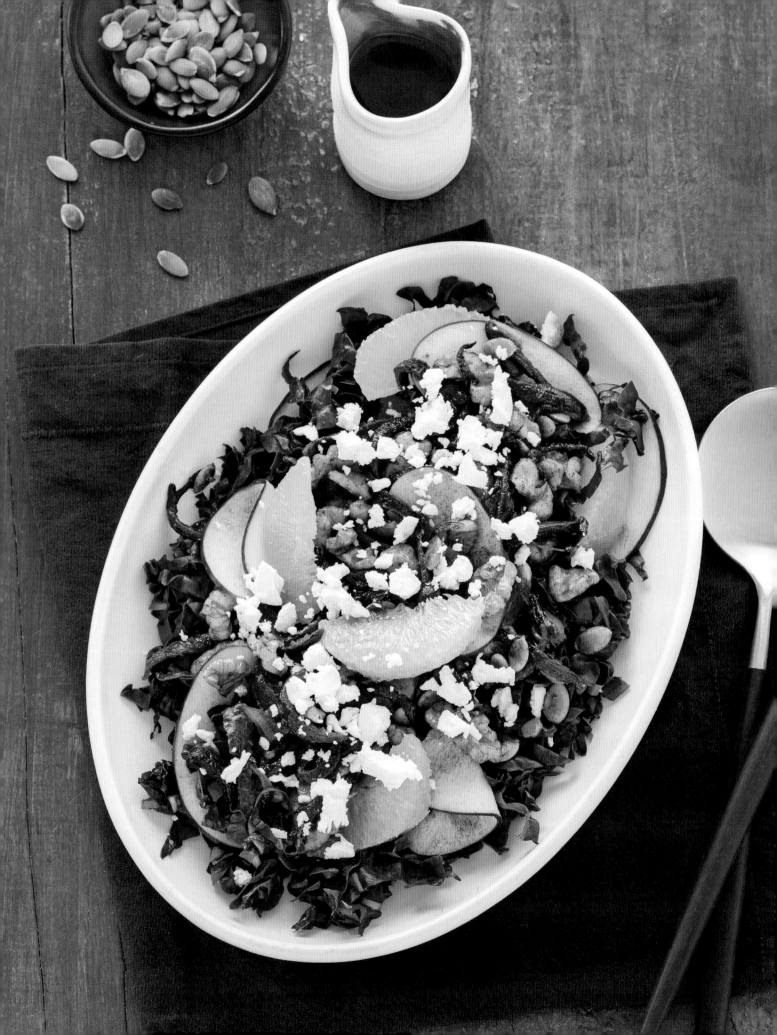

Green leafy vegetables

Your mother most likely told you to eat your greens, and we now know that there are so many good reasons—and endless great-tasting ways—to do so.

Clockwise from above: broccoli, baby romaine lettuce, brussels sprouts, Swiss chard, kale, baby spinach, Tuscan kale

Apart from providing a low-calorie source of fiber, green leafy vegetables are nature's antioxidant powerhouses, rich in many different substances that are known to be beneficial for health. Green leafy herbs are valued for their concentrated flavors and aromas. Herbs such as parsley, basil, oregano and mint have concentrated nutrients, too. The types of vitamins, minerals and antioxidants found in herbs are similar to those in green leafy vegetables, but in higher quantities. This is balanced by the smaller amounts typically used in recipes so that their contribution is quite similar. Some of these substances are destroyed in cooking, and some are fat-soluble, so it's a great idea to have at least some of your greens raw, in the form of a salad, with a healthy fat source such as olive oil dressing, or some nuts, seeds or avocado. You can also add a handful of chopped raw greens to soups just before serving. A quick stir-fry with a small amount of oil and/or nuts is good because it minimizes heating time, leaving many of the heat-sensitive nutrients intact.

Green leafy vegetables are a good source of vitamin C, choline and folate. Folate, which is named after the green foliage that is its best source, works so closely together with vitamin B_{12} that it wasn't discovered as a separate entity until the middle of the 20th century. Folate is unable to do its job when vitamin B_{12} is lacking. Together, they help to process inflammatory homocysteine and they are involved in DNA synthesis, which is an essential part of making normal blood cells. Folate is also required for the synthesis and breakdown process of several neurotransmitters, including noradrenaline, serotonin and dopamine. Folate deficiency in an adult causes problems with mood, memory and sleep.

Calcium, potassium and magnesium are also found in greens, and all are important for your brain. They all help keep blood pressure under control, reducing the risk of stroke. Magnesium takes part in hundreds of the body's essential reactions, and many of these occur in the brain to maintain normal function. It is important for the body to maintain steady magnesium levels because an excess can cause drowsiness and a deficiency can lead to spasms and seizures. Restless legs and migraine are associated with a transient lack of magnesium in some cases, and magnesium supplementation has been used to treat these conditions by relaxing the nerves and muscles, and promoting serotonin production. Magnesium requirements seem to be higher during periods of stress, so it is important to be sure you have enough in your diet at these times. Magnesium is currently being researched for its role in slowing down cognitive aging, and has also been used to improve mood and memory.

Among the antioxidants that are found in green leafy vegetables are carotenoids, which include lutein, important in preventing macular degeneration. This degeneration is a significant cause of visual impairment in older adults, so it is worth keeping up your intake of greens.

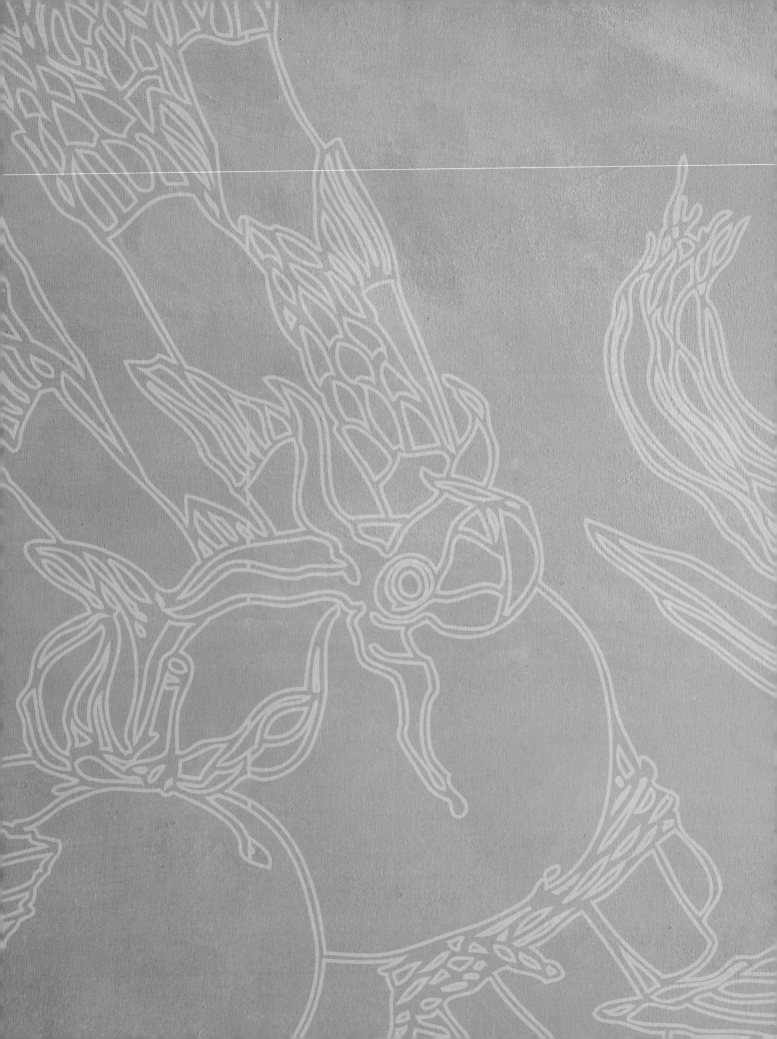

Smart snacks, light meals and side dishes

Give your brain a boost with these easy, light dishes and snacks.

Snack platters

These easy snack ideas provide complete protein along with fiber and a variety of vitamins and minerals to keep your brainpower fully charged until dinnertime. Combine two of them or add a salad and you'll have a balanced light meal that's ready in a flash.

Baked beans with corn chips

2 large corn tortillas, cut into wedges
14½ ounce (400 ml) can low-sodium baked beans
2 tablespoons (30 ml) grated low-fat cheddar
2 tablespoons (30 ml) spicy Mexican salsa

Cook the tortilla wedges in the microwave until crisp, about 3 minutes (watch carefully to avoid scorching). Microwave the baked beans in a heatproof bowl until heated through. Top the beans with the cheese and salsa, and serve with the tortilla wedges.

SERVES 2–4 AS A SNACK

Avocado ricotta toasts

4 slices whole-grain bread
⅓ cup (90 g) low-fat ricotta
grated zest and juice of 1 lemon
1 small ripe avocado, cut into quarters
cracked black pepper
2 tablespoons (30 ml) mixed seeds

Toast the bread until golden brown. Meanwhile, combine the ricotta with the lemon zest and juice. Top each toast slice with an avocado quarter and use a fork to flatten it on the toast; don't mash it too much. Top with the lemon ricotta and cracked black pepper, and finish with a sprinkle of seeds.

SERVES 2–4 AS A SNACK

Spiced roast chickpeas and nuts

1 cup (220 g) dried chickpeas
½ cup (80 g) raw almonds
½ cup (80 g) raw Brazil nuts
½ cup (80 g) raw cashew nuts
olive oil spray
½ teaspoon (2 ml) ground cumin
½ teaspoon (2 ml) ground coriander
¼ teaspoon (1 ml) cayenne pepper

Put the chickpeas in a large bowl and cover with plenty of cold water. Soak for 8 hours, or overnight. Drain the chickpeas, place in a large saucepan and cover with fresh water. Bring to a boil and cook for 1 hour, until tender. Drain and cool. Preheat the oven to 400°F (200°C). Line a large rimmed baking pan with parchment paper. Transfer the cooled chickpeas to the pan and roast for 30 minutes. Remove from the oven and add the nuts. Spray with olive oil, sprinkle with the spices and mix well. Roast for 15 minutes. Let cool completely in the pan. Store in an airtight container for up to 2 weeks.

SERVES 14 (MAKES 3½ CUPS/840 g)

Although nuts contain "good" fat, they are high in calories. Limit your intake of this mix to no more than a small handful a day.

For lasting brainpower and balanced nutrition, snacks should contain a *protein*—such as low-fat yogurt or ricotta, legumes, canned fish, hummus, peanut butter or egg—or be served with a glass of low-fat dairy or soy milk. If pressed for time, simply cut up carrots, celery or apples and dip them into some hummus.

Mexican corn cobs

4 corn cobs in their husks
1 tablespoon (15 ml) vegetable oil
1/2 teaspoon (2 ml) smoked paprika
2 tablespoons (30 ml) toasted sesame seeds
2 tablespoons (30 ml) finely chopped pepitas
  (pumpkin seeds)

Microwave the corn until tender, about 15 minutes. When cool enough to handle, remove the husks and snap each corn cob in half. Brush the corn with the combined oil and paprika, then roll in the pepitas and sesame seeds.

SERVES 4 AS A SNACK

Fruit yogurt wedges

2 red apples, red or white nectarines, or fruit
  of your choice
1 cup (250 ml) low-fat Greek-style yogurt
1 cup (130 g) crunchy cereal or muesli

Cut the fruit into thick wedges. Serve separate bowls of yogurt and muesli. Dip the wedges into the yogurt then into the muesli.

SERVES 2–4 AS A SNACK

Celery nut boats

1/3 cup (90 g) peanut or almond butter
1/4 cup (50 g) low-fat ricotta
4 celery stalks, cut into 4-inch (10-cm) lengths
1 tablespoon (15 ml) raisins
1 tablespoon (15 ml) sunflower seeds

Combine the nut butter and ricotta. Spoon into the hollow of the celery and firmly press the raisins and sunflower seeds into the mixture.

SERVES 2–4 AS A SNACK

Egg and tomato crackers

8 large whole-grain crackers
2 tablespoons (30 ml) pesto
2 ripe plum tomatoes, sliced
4 hard-boiled eggs, thinly sliced or mashed
freshly ground black pepper
torn fresh basil leaves

Thinly spread the crackers with the pesto, top with the sliced tomatoes and eggs, and finish with a good grinding of black pepper and some basil.

SERVES 2–4 AS A SNACK

Clockwise from left: Mexican corn cobs, Fruit yogurt wedges, Celery nut boats

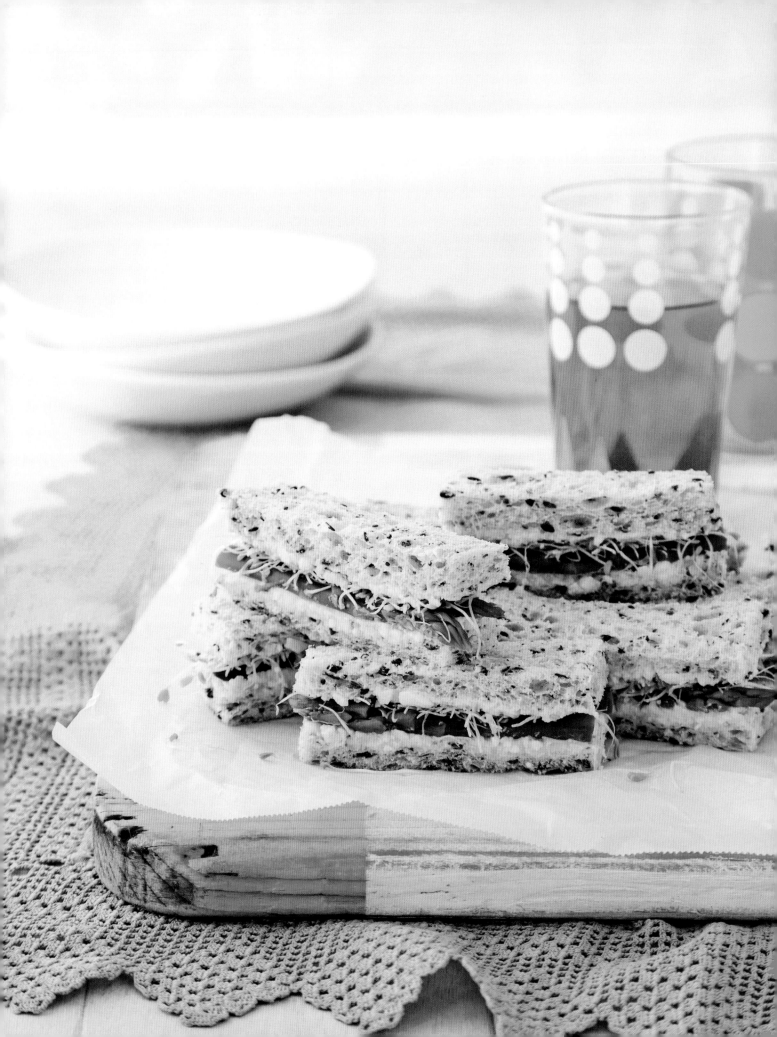

Asparagus finger sandwiches with mustard egg spread

Choose young, thin asparagus for this recipe. Trim the woody ends and cut them through the middle so they will sit flat on top of the egg. Don't overcook asparagus—they should be bright green and tender.

PREPARATION **10 MINUTES**
COOKING **15 MINUTES**
SERVES **4**

3 eggs, at room temperature
12 thin asparagus spears, about ¼ pound (125 g)
1 tablespoon (15 ml) low-fat Greek-style yogurt
1 teaspoon (5 ml) whole-grain mustard
8 thick slices whole-grain bread, crusts removed
¼ cup (60 g) alfalfa sprouts

1   Place the eggs in a saucepan, cover with cold water and bring to a boil over high heat. As soon as the water boils, time the eggs to cook for 8 minutes. Drain and cool under cold water before peeling the eggs.

2   Cut the asparagus spears in half lengthwise, and cut them to fit the bread. Half-fill a frying pan with water, add the asparagus and cook over medium heat for 2 minutes, until the asparagus are bright green and tender. Drain and plunge into ice water to cool, or rinse under cold water, and pat dry on paper towels.

3   In a small bowl, mash the boiled eggs with a fork, then add the yogurt and mustard, and mix to combine.

4   Place the bread slices on a clean chopping board and spread with the egg mixture. Top half the slices with a row of asparagus, then the alfalfa sprouts. Sandwich together with the remaining bread slices. Cut each sandwich into three fingers before serving.

EACH SERVING PROVIDES
256 calories, 17 g protein, 9 g fat (2 g saturated fat), 22 g carbohydrate (2 g sugars), 11 g fiber, 273 mg sodium

Asparagus is packed with antioxidants and brain-boosting vitamins such as folate. It also provides chromium, which helps insulin to move glucose into the brain cells for energy.

Savory beef and vegetables on whole-grain toast

Keep this beef mixture in the fridge for a quick snack on a slice of whole-grain toast. It can also be used as a filling for savory pies and sandwiches, or wrapped in lettuce leaves and eaten as a snack.

PREPARATION **10 MINUTES**   COOKING **35 MINUTES**   SERVES **6 AS A SNACK**

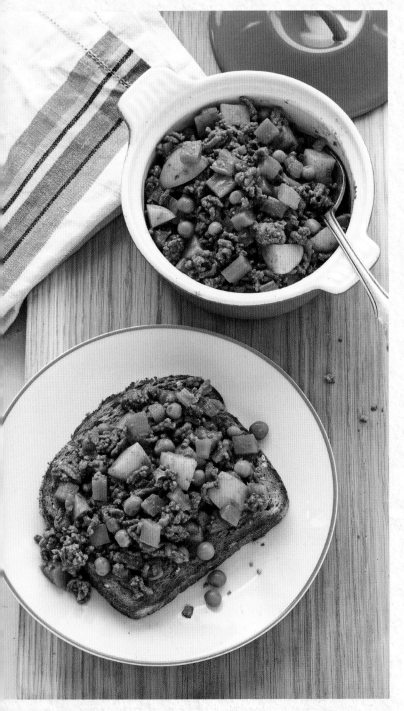

1 tablespoon (15 ml) olive oil
1 small onion, finely chopped
1 pound (500 g) lean ground beef
1 carrot, finely chopped
2 celery stalks, finely chopped
1/4 pound (125 g) new potatoes, chopped
1/2 cup (125 ml) low-sodium beef stock
1 tablespoon (15 ml) worcestershire sauce (optional)
1 tablespoon (15 ml) tomato paste
1/2 cup (80 g) frozen peas
4 thick slices whole-grain bread

1   Heat the oil in a large frying pan and cook the onion over medium heat for 10 minutes, until soft and golden. Add the beef and cook for 5 minutes, until browned.

2   Add the carrot, celery, potatoes and a splash of the beef stock, and cook for 10 minutes, until the vegetables are just soft.

3   Stir in the worcestershire sauce, if using, tomato paste and remaining stock. Cook, stirring constantly, until the mixture boils and thickens slightly. Stir in the peas and cook for 5 minutes, until the peas are bright green and tender.

4   Toast the bread until golden. Serve the beef and vegetables on the toast.

EACH SERVING PROVIDES
239 calories, 23 g protein, 11 g fat (3 g saturated fat), 12 g carbohydrate (2 g sugars), 5 g fiber, 235 mg sodium

Lean beef is an excellent source of iron and zinc, in readily absorbable form. Both are important for getting a good supply of energy to your brain cells.

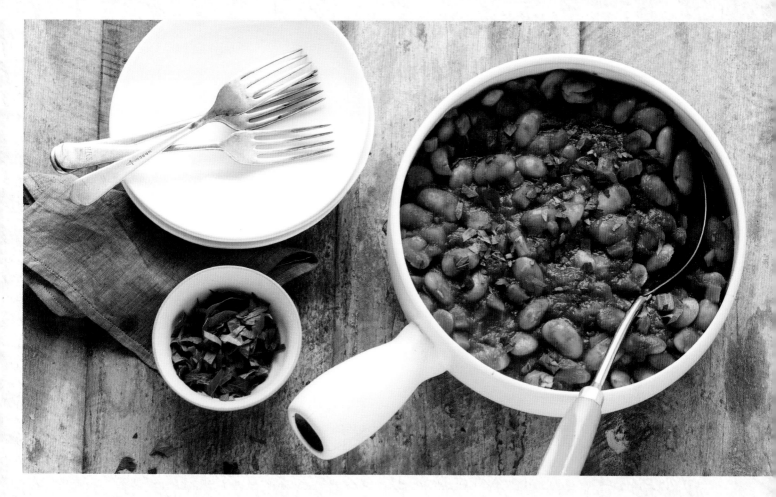

Boston baked beans

These beans are good in a wrap with an omelet and baby spinach,
or on whole-grain toast. They will keep in the fridge for up to a week.

PREPARATION **10 MINUTES**   COOKING **1 HOUR**   SERVES **6 AS A SNACK**

1 tablespoon (15 ml) olive oil
1 onion, finely chopped
1 carrot, finely chopped
2 celery stalks, finely chopped
2 teaspoons (10 ml) smoked paprika
1 tablespoon (15 ml) molasses or brown sugar
3 cans lima beans, 15 ounces (425 ml) each, rinsed
and drained
3 cups (750 ml) tomato purée
2 tablespoons (30 ml) chopped fresh parsley

1   Preheat the oven to 425°F (220°C).

2   Heat the oil in a 10 cup (2.5 L) flameproof dish and
cook the onion over medium heat for 10 minutes,
until soft and golden.

3   Add the carrot and celery, and cook for 5 minutes,
until just soft. Stir in the paprika and molasses or
sugar, and cook for 2 minutes.

4   Stir in the beans and tomato purée. Bring to a
boil, remove from the heat, cover and transfer to the
oven for 40 minutes. Serve sprinkled with parsley.

You can replace the canned beans with 4$\frac{1}{2}$ cups
(1.1 kg) cooked lima beans made from 1$\frac{1}{3}$ cups (250 g)
dried beans.

EACH SERVING PROVIDES

238 calories, 13 g protein, 4 g fat (<1 g saturated fat),
32 g carbohydrate (15 g sugars), 12 g fiber, 813 mg sodium

Legumes are low in fat and high in protein and
fiber, perfect for maintaining cardiovascular
health for optimal blood supply to the brain.

Yogurt cups

Each of these quick snack ideas makes enough for a single serving, ideal for taking to work or school in a small, airtight container for a nutritious breakfast on the go. You can vary the fruits and nuts to your own taste.

Banana, cinnamon and dark chocolate

¾ cup (175 ml) low-fat Greek-style yogurt
½ teaspoon (2 ml) ground cinnamon
1 small banana, chopped
5 walnut halves, roughly chopped
1 ounce (25 g) dark chocolate, at least
  70% cocoa, grated

Combine the yogurt and cinnamon. Gently fold in the banana. Top with the walnuts and finish with the grated chocolate.

SERVES 1

From left: Banana, cinnamon and dark chocolate; Pomegranate, pistachio and mint; Honey, apricot and almonds

Pomegranate, pistachio and mint

3 tablespoons (45 ml) pomegranate seeds
¾ cup (175 ml) low-fat Greek-style yogurt
¼ cup (50 g) raw pistachios, roughly chopped
1 teaspoon (5 ml) fresh small mint leaves

Stir the pomegranate seeds into the yogurt, lightly crushing the seeds to release their juice. Sprinkle with the pistachios and mint leaves.

SERVES 1

Maple muesli with pepitas

1 teaspoon (5 ml) vanilla extract
¾ cup (175 ml) low-fat Greek-style yogurt
¼ cup (50 g) muesli
1 tablespoon (15 ml) pepitas (pumpkin seeds)
1 teaspoon (5 ml) pure maple syrup

Stir the vanilla extract into the yogurt. Combine the muesli, pepitas and maple syrup, and spoon on top of the yogurt.

SERVES 1

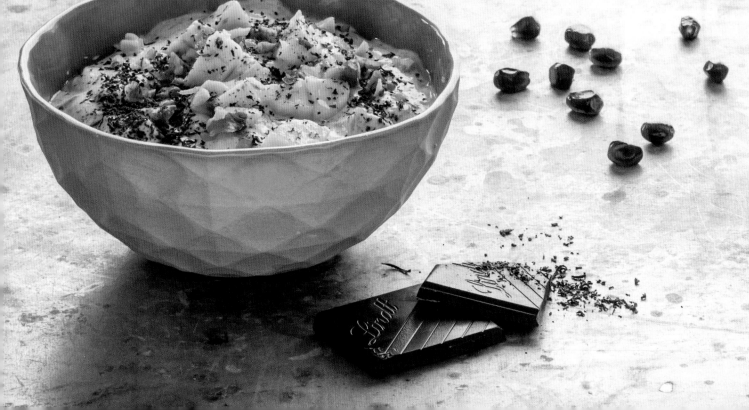

Berries and walnuts

2–3 strawberries, quartered
¾ cup (175 ml) low-fat Greek-style yogurt
1 tablespoon (15 ml) blueberries or blackberries
1 tablespoon (15 ml) walnut halves, roughly
    chopped
honey, to taste (optional)

Stir the strawberries into the yogurt. Scatter the blueberries or blackberries over the yogurt and top with the walnuts. Drizzle with honey, if using.

SERVES 1

Honey, apricot and almonds

1 teaspoon (5 ml) honey
1 teaspoon (5 ml) rosewater or orange
    blossom water
¾ cup (175 ml) low-fat Greek-style yogurt
5 dried apricot halves, diced
2 tablespoons (30 ml) slivered raw almonds

Mix the honey and rosewater or orange blossom water into the yogurt. Scatter the apricots and almonds on top of the yogurt.

SERVES 1

Spicy dates and figs

½ teaspoon (2 ml) ground ginger
½ teaspoon (2 ml) ground cinnamon
¾ cup (175 ml) low-fat Greek-style yogurt
1 tablespoon (15 ml) sesame seeds
5 dried pitted dates, finely diced
5 dried figs, stems removed, finely diced

Stir the ginger and cinnamon into the yogurt until well blended. Combine the sesame seeds, dates and figs, and gently swirl through the yogurt.

SERVES 1

These quick *yogurt* recipes provide protein and a low glycemic-index snack for sustained energy to keep you going until your next meal.

Huevos rancheros with green salsa

An ideal light meal, this is also a great breakfast dish—omit the green chile if you don't like anything spicy in the morning. You can use spinach or Swiss chard instead of kale.

PREPARATION **15 MINUTES**
COOKING **30 MINUTES**
SERVES **4**

1 tablespoon (15 ml) olive oil
1 onion, finely chopped
1 long green chile, finely chopped
1 green pepper, finely chopped
2 tablespoons (30 ml) pickled jalapeños, chopped (optional)
1 teaspoon (5 ml) ground cumin (optional)
1 pound (500 g) green tomatoes, chopped
$1/2$ cup (125 g) kale, finely shredded
2 tablespoons (30 ml) chopped fresh cilantro, plus extra to garnish
4 eggs
4 warm corn tortillas, to serve
Tabasco sauce, to serve

1 Heat the olive oil in a large frying pan over medium heat. Add the onion, chile and pepper, and the jalapeños and cumin, if using. Cook for 10 minutes, until the onion is soft and golden.

2 Add the green tomatoes and cook for 10 minutes, until the tomatoes are soft and pulpy. Stir in the kale, cilantro and $1/4$ cup (50 ml) water, and cook for 3 minutes, until the kale has wilted.

3 Make four small indentations in the top of the tomato mixture with the back of a spoon, leaving space between them. Crack the eggs into the holes, cover and cook for 3 minutes, until the egg whites are cooked but the yolks are still soft.

4 Serve topped with the extra cilantro, the warm corn tortillas and the Tabasco sauce.

Alternatively, fry the eggs in a nonstick frying pan. Put the warm tortillas on four serving plates, top each with the green tomato mixture and a fried egg, scatter with some cilantro and serve with Tabasco.

You can also use red tomatoes if you don't have green ones.

EACH SERVING PROVIDES
150 calories, 9 g protein, 10 g fat (2 g saturated fat), 7 g carbohydrate (4 g sugars), 3 g fiber, 89 mg sodium

Manganese, found in *kale*, is important for making the fats that form the structure of a healthy brain. Kale also contains tyrosine, used for making the neurotransmitters dopamine and noradrenaline.

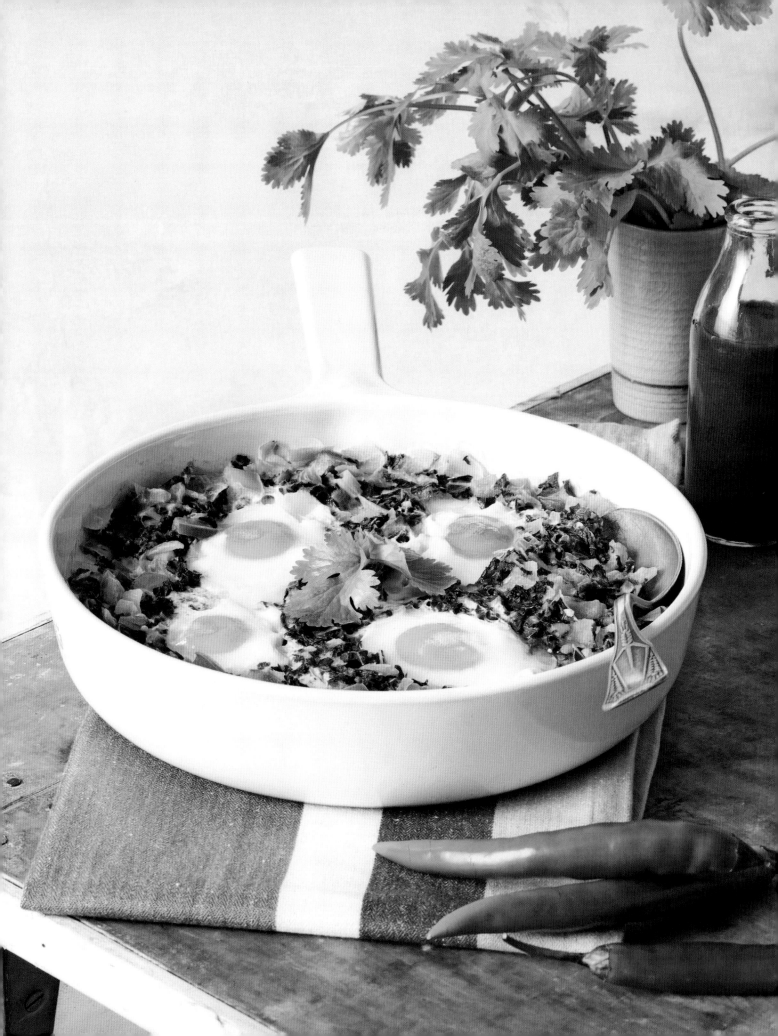

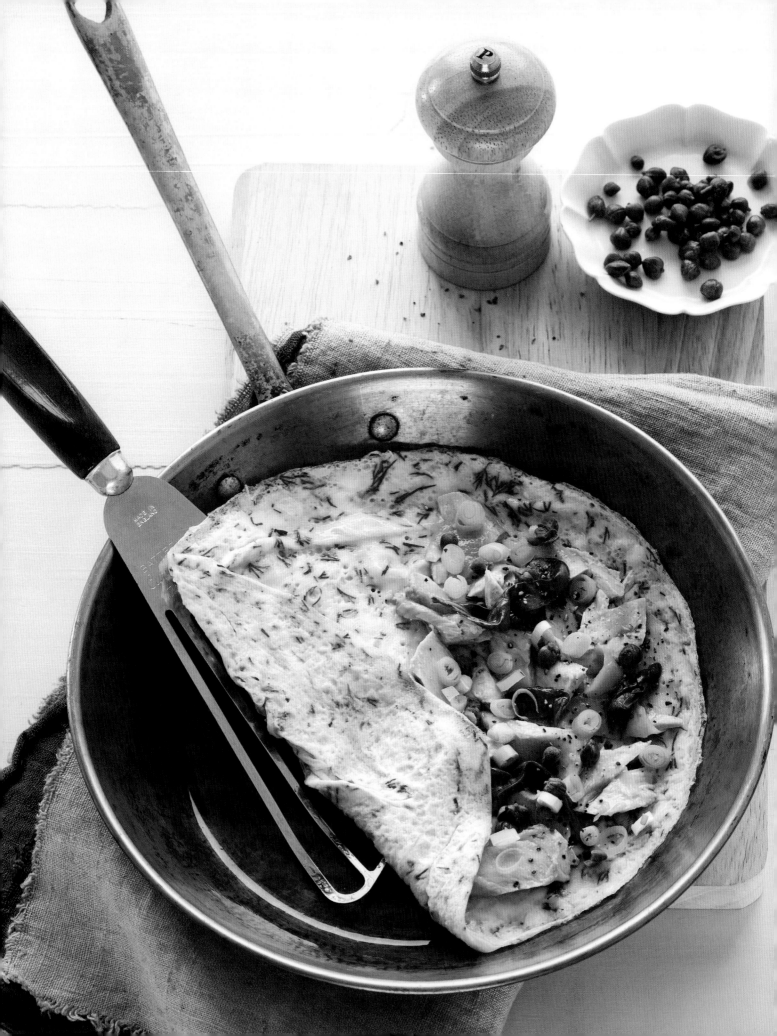

Rainbow trout, spinach and caper omelet

Remove any bones from the fish before you cook it. Cook the trout with the skin on, and gently peel it off when it's done cooking.

PREPARATION **15 MINUTES**
COOKING **35 MINUTES**
SERVES **4**

^{3}/$_4$ pound (400 g) rainbow trout fillet
1 lemon, sliced
1^1/$_3$ cups (60 g) baby spinach leaves
8 eggs
2 tablespoons (30 ml) chopped fresh dill
olive oil, for brushing or spraying
3 scallions, sliced
2 tablespoons (30 ml) baby capers, rinsed
   and squeezed dry
cracked black pepper

1 Put the trout and lemon slices in a large frying pan, cover with water and gently simmer over medium–low heat for 15 minutes, until the trout is tender. Do not let the water boil.

2 Drain the fish on paper towels. Let it cool, discard the skin and flake the flesh into large pieces.

3 Put the baby spinach in a heatproof bowl and cover with boiling water to wilt it. Drain and let cool, then squeeze out the excess water. Roughly chop the spinach.

4 Whisk 2 eggs and 2 teaspoons (10 ml) of the dill in a small bowl until well combined.

5 Lightly brush or spray a 10-inch (25-cm) nonstick frying pan with olive oil, place over medium heat and pour the egg mixture into the pan. Lift the edges of the egg once it starts to set and allow any uncooked egg to run underneath.

6 Sprinkle half of the omelet with a quarter of the scallions, trout, spinach and capers. Generously season with cracked black pepper.

7 Gently fold the omelet over to enclose the filling, and cook for 3 minutes, until the omelet is set. Remove and keep warm while you cook the remaining eggs and filling.

You can use a small brown trout or lake trout if rainbow trout aren't available.

EACH SERVING PROVIDES
277 calories, 33 g protein, 15 g fat (4 g saturated fat),
2 g carbohydrate (2 g sugars), 1 g fiber, 242 mg sodium

Docosahexaenoic acid—DHA for short—is the most abundant omega-3 fat in the brain. Food sources with good amounts of DHA, such as trout, help to maintain healthy brain structure.

Swiss chard, almond and ricotta frittata

Swiss chard and almonds are a winning combination of flavors and textures in this frittata. Serve it hot or cold with some crusty whole-grain bread and a simple salad.

PREPARATION **25 MINUTES**
COOKING **20 MINUTES**
SERVES **4**

¼ cup (30 g) slivered almonds
1¾ pounds (900 g) Swiss chard
1 tablespoon (15 ml) olive oil
1 small onion, finely chopped
2 cloves garlic, crushed
½ cup (125 g) low-fat dry ricotta, crumbled
1 tablespoon (15 ml) chopped fresh dill
1 teaspoon (5 ml) finely grated lemon zest
6 eggs, lightly beaten

1 Stir the almonds in a dry frying pan over medium heat for 2 minutes, until lightly toasted. Transfer to a plate to cool.

2 Trim the white stems from the chard. Wash and dry, and roughly shred the leaves. Place in a heatproof bowl and cover with boiling water to wilt. Drain and cool, then squeeze out as much liquid as you can. Place in a large bowl.

3 Heat 2 teaspoons (10 ml) oil in a 7-inch (18-cm) nonstick ovenproof frying pan. Cook the onion over medium heat for 5 minutes, until soft. Add the garlic and cook for 1 minute. Add the garlic and onions to the bowl with the chard and cool slightly. Add the ricotta, dill, lemon zest and toasted almonds; use your hands to combine the ingredients.

4 Wash and dry the frying pan. Brush with the remaining oil, add the chard mixture and pour in the eggs. Use a fork to distribute the eggs and spread the mixture over the pan. Cook over medium heat for 3–4 minutes, until the frittata is set underneath and around the edges.

5 Preheat the broiler to medium. Cook the frittata under the broiler for 4 minutes, until set (test with a fork to be sure the egg underneath is not still raw).

6 Let the frittata stand for 5 minutes, slide it onto a cutting board and cut into wedges to serve.

To wash the Swiss chard thoroughly, submerge the leaves in a large bowl or sink of cold water and swirl with your hands. Let it soak for 5 minutes, and lift out (any grit will have fallen to the bottom). Use a salad spinner to dry thoroughly.

You can substitute kale or any leafy green for the Swiss chard.

Swiss chard, also known as silverbeet, is related to beets and contains excellent amounts of folate, essential for healthy brain function.

EACH SERVING PROVIDES
273 calories, 18 g protein, 20 g fat (5 g saturated fat),
4 g carbohydrate (4 g sugars), 5 g fiber, 637 mg sodium

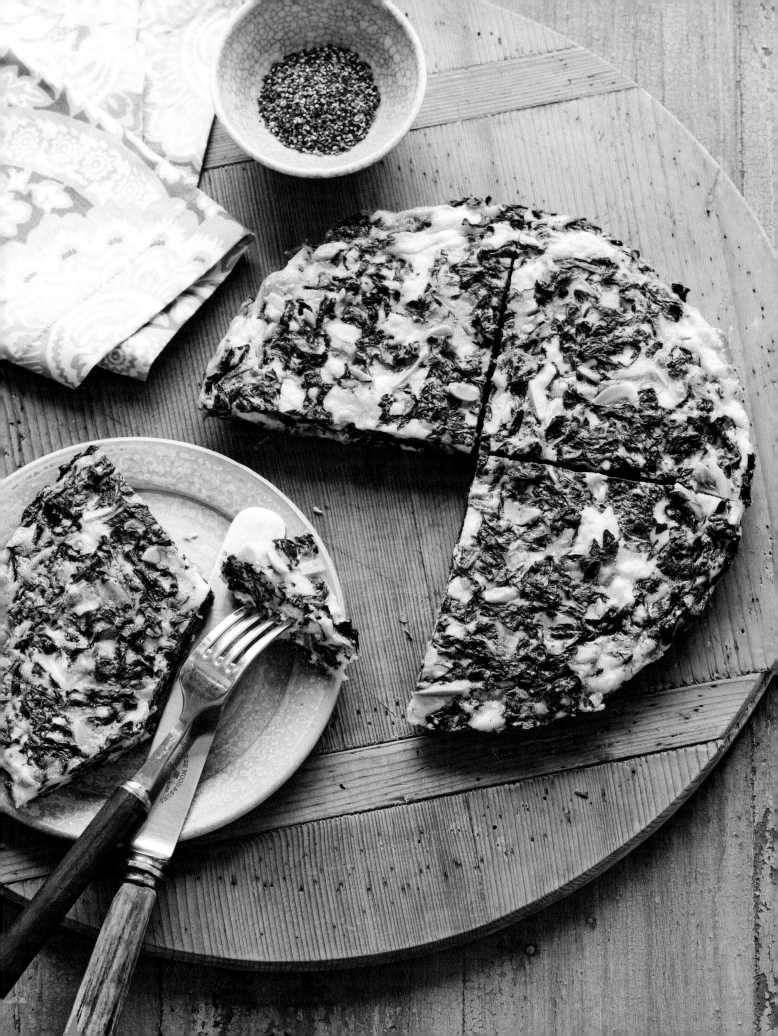

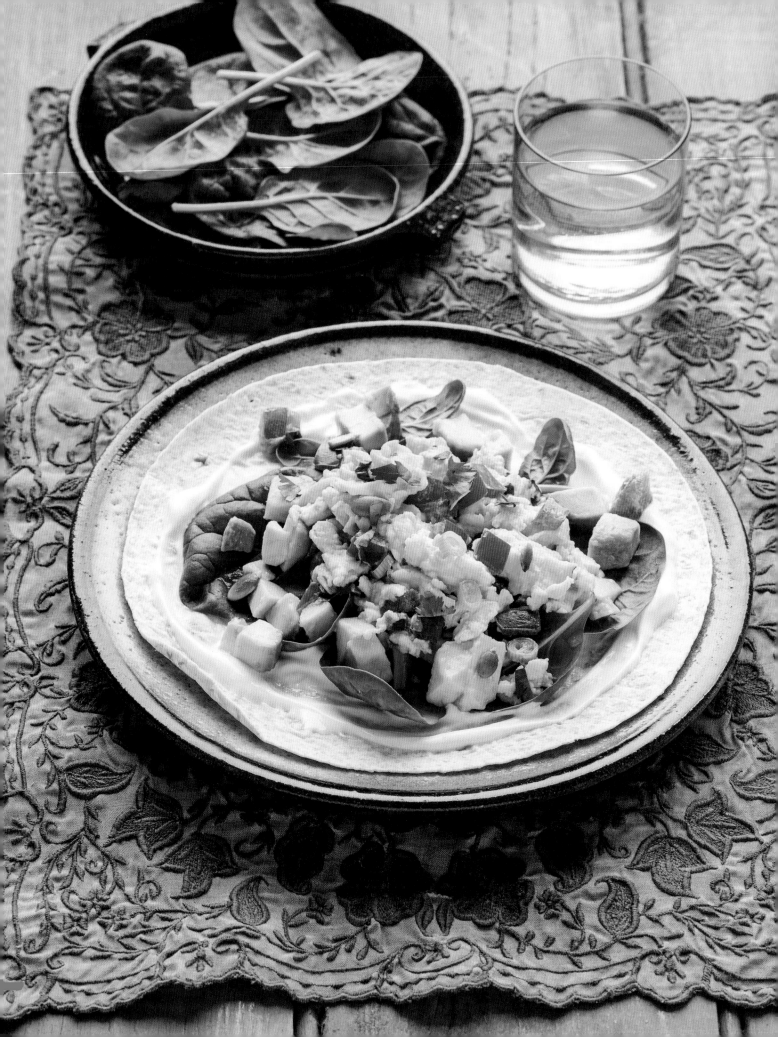

Scrambled egg and spinach tortilla

For a lunchbox or picnic, you can prepare the filling separately and package it up to take with you. Assemble the tortilla just before you're ready to eat it.

PREPARATION **15 MINUTES**
COOKING **5 MINUTES**
SERVES **4**

1 tablespoon (15 ml) olive oil
2 scallions, chopped
8 eggs, lightly beaten
2 small tomatoes, seeded and chopped
2 tablespoons (30 ml) mixed seeds, such as
   sunflower and pumpkin seeds (pepitas)
1 tablespoon (15 ml) chopped fresh
   cilantro leaves
4 whole-wheat flour tortillas, warmed
2 tablespoons (30 ml) low-fat
   Greek-style yogurt
²/₃ cup (30 g) baby spinach leaves
1 avocado, diced

1 Heat the oil in a large frying pan and cook the scallions over medium heat for 3 minutes, until soft.

2 Pour in the eggs and allow to set slightly before gently pushing them around the pan until scrambled and set.

3 Fold the chopped tomatoes, mixed seeds and cilantro into the scrambled eggs.

4 Lay the tortillas on a clean chopping board and divide the yogurt among them. Top with some baby spinach and avocado, and finish with the scrambled egg mixture. Roll up to serve, folding in the bottom to enclose the filling.

It's a nice touch to warm the tortillas if you are serving them at home for breakfast or brunch.

EACH SERVING PROVIDES
455 calories, 20 g protein, 33 g fat (7 g saturated fat),
21 g carbohydrate (4 g sugars), 5 g fiber, 385 mg sodium

Eggs are a great source of choline, a precursor of one of the brain's key neurotransmitters. It is also important in forming cell membranes, which directly affects brain structure and function.

Crab and corn fritters with avocado and tomato salsa

Use well-drained canned corn kernels, thawed frozen corn kernels, or fresh corn in season. If using fresh, cook the cobs until just tender, and let them cool. Stand the cob upright in a large bowl or on a plate, and use a sharp knife to cut off the kernels.

PREPARATION **25 MINUTES**
COOKING **10 MINUTES PER BATCH**
SERVES **4 (MAKES 12 FRITTERS)**

1 cup (160 g) whole-wheat self-rising flour
$1/2$ teaspoon (2 ml) cayenne pepper
2 eggs
$1/4$ cup (50 ml) skim milk
2 cups (250 g) corn kernels
$2/3$ cup (100 g) crumbled low-fat feta
2 tablespoons (30 ml) snipped fresh chives
$1/2$ pound (200 g) crabmeat
$1^1/2$ tablespoons (22 ml) olive oil

Avocado and tomato salsa
2 tomatoes, seeded and diced
1 large avocado, diced
1 tablespoon (15 ml) lemon juice
2 tablespoons (30 ml) chopped fresh
   cilantro leaves

1 Sift the flour and cayenne pepper into a mixing bowl and and add the husks from the sieve. Make a well in the center. Whisk the eggs and milk together, and gently stir into the flour until just combined. Fold in the corn kernels, feta, chives and crabmeat.

2 To make the avocado and tomato salsa, combine the tomatoes, avocado, lemon juice and cilantro.

3 Heat half the olive oil in a large nonstick frying pan over medium–low heat. Drop the batter into the pan, using about $1/4$ cup (50 ml) for each fritter, and spread to 3 inches (8 cm). Cook in batches for 5 minutes on each side, until golden brown and cooked through. Keep warm while you cook the remaining batter to make 12 fritters in total.

4 Arrange three of the fritters on each plate and top with the avocado and tomato salsa.

The fritters can be baked instead of fried. Preheat the oven to 375°F (190°C) and line a large baking pan with parchment paper. Drop the batter onto the pan, using $1/4$ cup (50 ml) batter for each fritter, and spray with olive oil. Bake for 5 minutes, turn, spray with oil and cook for 5 minutes.

If you are using fresh corn, you will need about 2 corn cobs to make 2 cups (250 g) corn kernels.

EACH SERVING (3 FRITTERS) PROVIDES
532 calories, 28 g protein, 29 g fat (7 g saturated fat),
39 g carbohydrate (6 g sugars), 9 g fiber, 904 mg sodium

It's easy to forget that *corn* is a whole grain because it is so succulent and sweet. Corn provides a good amount of protein, B-group vitamins and fiber. *Crabmeat* is a source of lean protein and brain-boosting minerals such as selenium and chromium.

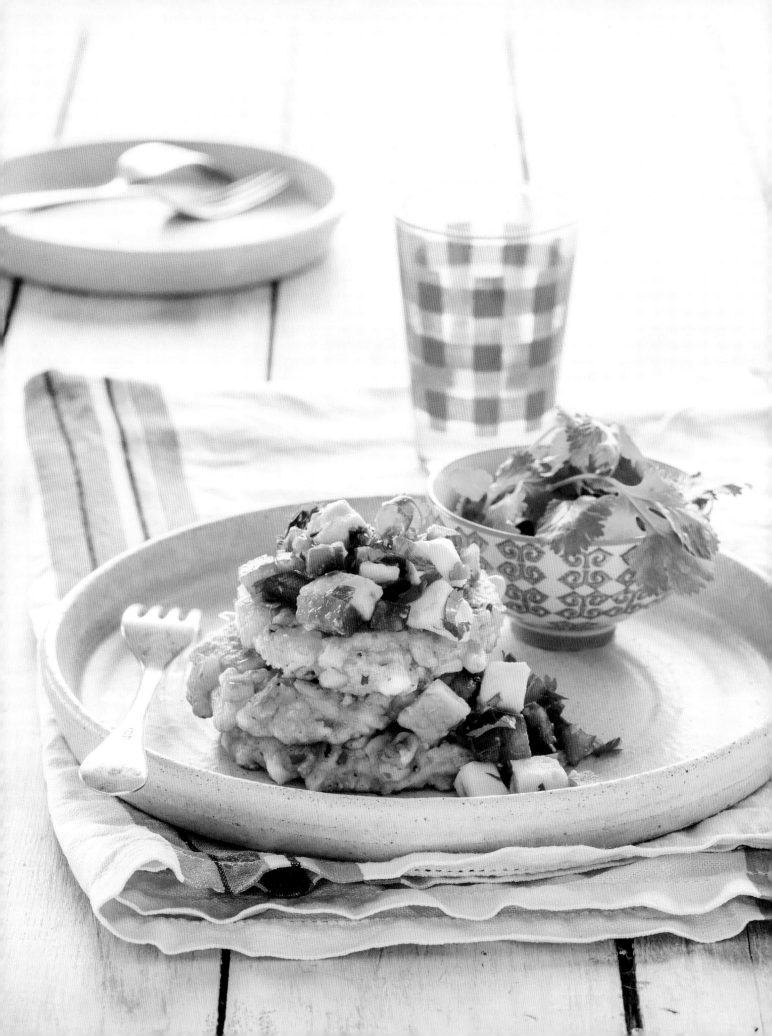

Avocado

Although avocado is actually a fruit, it is an unusual one. Like olives, avocados have a high fat content, making them quite unfruitlike and leading to their use predominantly in savory dishes.

Hass avocados

Although avocados are high in fat, they are a heart-healthy food, as about 20 to 25 percent of their weight is beneficial monounsaturated fat. Substituting saturated fat with healthy monounsaturated fat helps reduce cholesterol levels and the risk of heart attack and stroke.

Avocado contains no cholesterol and it also contains plant sterols (like those that are found in cholesterol-lowering margarines), which help block the absorption of cholesterol from other foods. Because fat is high in energy, it is important for weight control to use avocado instead of other fat sources, rather than adding its calories to your existing dietary intake. Try spreading avocado on bread or toast instead of butter or margarine; using mashed avocado (with a little lemon juice to prevent browning) as a substitute for mayonnaise to moisten sandwich fillings; adding it to salads instead of some of the dressing; or putting avocado chunks on a pizza to replace some of the usual saturated fat cheeses.

Avocado is high in many micronutrients, including folate, niacin and pantothenic acid. Niacin is important for the metabolic processes that deliver energy from food, and symptoms of niacin deficiency include depression, fatigue, memory loss, confusion and poor concentration. Pantothenic acid (formerly known as vitamin B_5) is needed for metabolism of glucose and fat to supply energy. It is also essential for production of the most common neurotransmitter, acetyl choline. The many antioxidants that are found in avocado include lutein and zeaxanthin. These nutrients are important for maintaining healthy vision and are also thought to help protect against macular degeneration, a common cause of age-related vision loss.

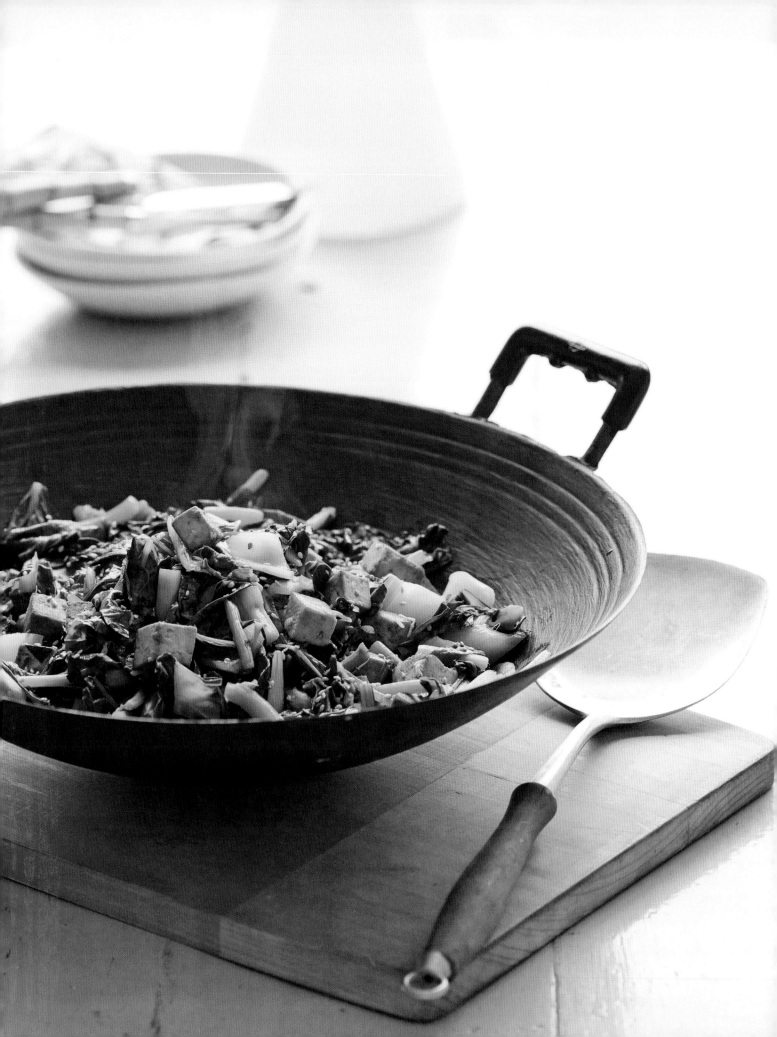

Stir-fried Asian greens and tofu with ginger

You can serve this stir-fry over noodles or rice for a more substantial meal, or omit the tofu and serve as a side dish to meat, fish or chicken. Use any combination of Asian leafy greens, and add some chopped chile with the garlic and ginger if you like it spicy.

PREPARATION **15 MINUTES**
COOKING **10 MINUTES**
SERVES **4**

7 ounces (200 g) firm tofu
2 tablespoons (30 ml) low-sodium
  soy sauce
^{2}/$_3$ pound (300 g) gai lan, trimmed
^{2}/$_3$ pound (300 g) choy sum, trimmed
^{2}/$_3$ pound (300 g) baby bok choy, trimmed
1 tablespoon (15 ml) peanut oil
2 cloves garlic, crushed
2 tablespoons (30 ml) finely grated
  fresh ginger
1 teaspoon (5 ml) sesame oil
2 tablespoons (30 ml) sesame
  seeds, toasted

1   Pat the tofu with paper towels to absorb excess liquid, and cut it into small cubes. Toss with half the soy sauce in a bowl, and set aside until needed, turning occasionally.

2   Cut the gai lan, choy sum and bok choy to separate the stems from the leaves. Cut the stems into 1-inch (2.5-cm) lengths. Roughly shred the leaves.

3   Heat half the peanut oil in a wok over medium–high heat. Stir-fry the tofu cubes for 2 minutes, until lightly browned. Remove from the pan with a slotted spoon and set aside.

4   Heat the remaining peanut oil in the wok and stir-fry the vegetable stems for 2 minutes. Add the crushed garlic and grated ginger, and stir-fry for 1 minute, until the stems are just tender.

5   Add the vegetable leaves, sesame oil and the remaining soy sauce. Stir-fry for 2 minutes, until the leaves are wilted. Return the tofu to the wok and toss until heated through.

6   Serve the vegetables and tofu sprinkled with the toasted sesame seeds.

Gai lan is similar to broccoli but has a longer stalk and a more delicate taste. You can substitute broccoli rabe. Choy sum is related to Napa cabbage, which you can use as a substitute.

EACH SERVING PROVIDES
203 calories, 12 g protein, 13 g fat (2 g saturated fat),
11 g carbohydrate (2 g sugars), 5 g fiber, 422 mg sodium

Cruciferous vegetables, such as the Asian greens used in this recipe, appear to protect heart and brain function. They are also an excellent source of fiber and very low in calories, providing good amounts of vitamins A, C, E and K and many of the B-group vitamins, as well as calcium, potassium and magnesium.

White bean, tomato and anchovy bruschetta

This bruschetta is great for casual entertaining or a snack. It also makes a quick and easy light meal with the addition of a simple green leafy salad.

PREPARATION **20 MINUTES, PLUS 20 MINUTES SOAKING**
COOKING **5 MINUTES**
SERVES **4**

1½ ounce (45 g) can anchovies, drained
milk, for soaking
14½ ounce (400 ml) can cannellini beans,
   rinsed and drained
2 tomatoes, diced
½ small red onion, finely chopped
¼ cup (15 g) firmly packed fresh basil,
   shredded
⅓ cup (7 g) fresh flat-leaf parsley, chopped
2 tablespoons (30 ml) lemon juice
freshly ground black pepper
8 thick slices whole-grain sourdough bread
1 small avocado
2 tablespoons (30 ml) extra virgin olive oil

1   Place the anchovies in a shallow bowl and cover with milk. Set aside for 20 minutes to soak. Drain and pat dry with paper towels, then finely chop.

2   Combine the cannellini beans, tomatoes, onion, basil, parsley, lemon juice and anchovies in a bowl, and season with freshly ground black pepper.

3   Toast the bread, spread it with the avocado and spoon the bean mixture on top. Drizzle with the extra virgin olive oil and serve immediately.

Replace the canned beans with 1½ cups (375 g) cooked beans made from ½ cup (100 g) dried cannellini beans.

EACH SERVING PROVIDES
471 calories, 15 g protein, 22 g fat (4 g saturated fat),
49 g carbohydrate (6 g sugars), 14 g fiber, 461 mg sodium

When looking for *bread* with a low glycemic index (GI), the first choice is a heavy grainy bread. However, sourdough varieties also have a low GI thanks to their slow fermentation process and acid content. They'll keep you feeling full and help maintain a good supply of energy.

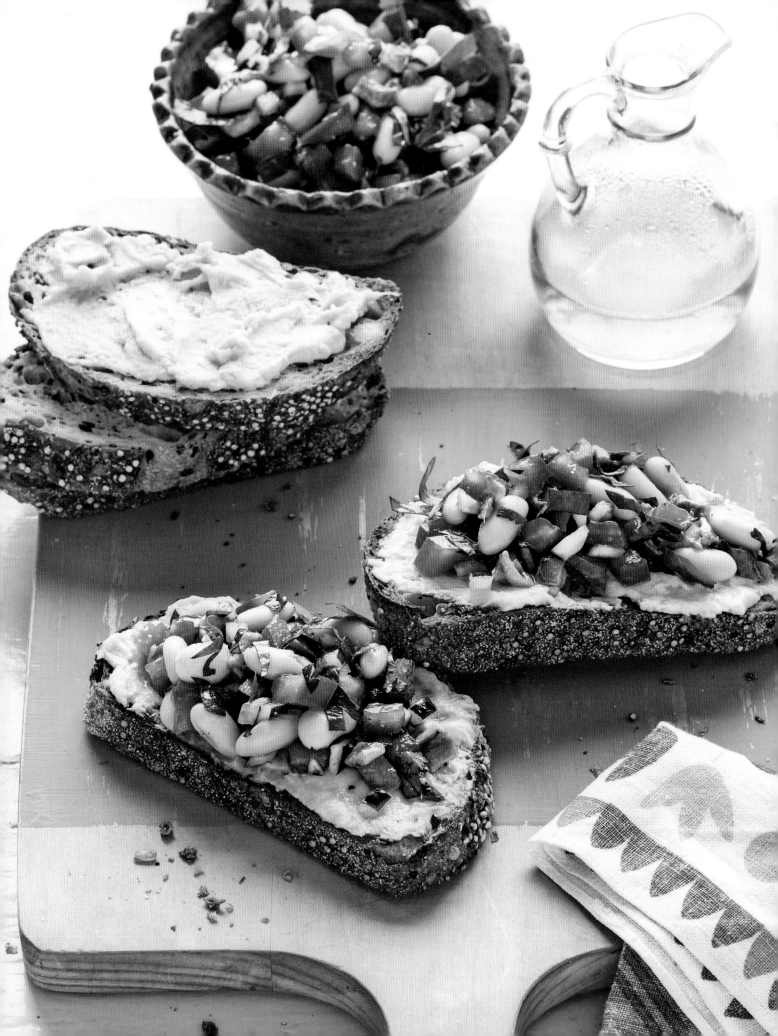

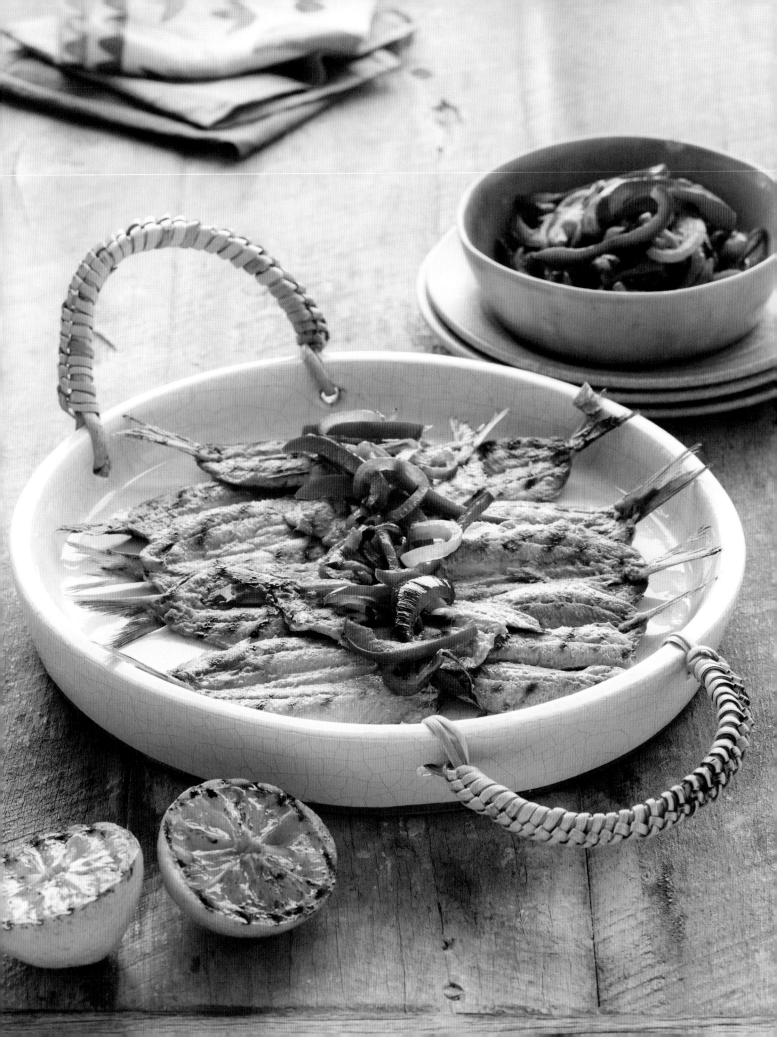

Portuguese-style sardines with peppers and caramelized onions

Fresh sardines evoke the aroma of a Mediterranean summer. This is the way to enjoy them at their best. The butterflied fillets require little preparation and are perfect for the barbecue or pan grilling.

PREPARATION **5 MINUTES**
COOKING **25 MINUTES**
SERVES **4**

2 tablespoons (30 ml) olive oil, plus extra
    for brushing
2 red onions, thinly sliced
1 red pepper, very thinly sliced
2 cloves garlic, crushed
3 sprigs fresh thyme
12 butterflied sardines, about
    2 ounces (60 g) each
1 lemon, halved

1 Heat the olive oil in a large frying pan. Add the onions and cook over medium heat for 10 minutes, until soft and caramelized. Add the peppers, garlic and thyme sprigs, and cook for 5 minutes, until the peppers soften and the mixture is thick and sticky. Remove from the heat.

2 Meanwhile, heat a barbecue grill or grill pan over high heat. Lightly brush the sardines with olive oil, place on the hot grill or pan and cook for 4–5 minutes on each side, until cooked through and marked with grill lines. Lightly brush the cut sides of the lemon halves with olive oil and cook, cut side down, until heated through and charred, about 3 minutes.

3 Arrange the sardines on a platter or individual plates and top with the pepper and caramelized onion mixture. Serve with the grilled lemon halves.

The caramelized onions create the rich sweet flavor of this recipe, so don't be tempted to rush the cooking process. They should be a deep brown color and a very sticky texture.

EACH SERVING PROVIDES
377 calories, 37 g protein, 23 g fat (6 g saturated fat),
4 g carbohydrate (3 g sugars), 2 g fiber, 205 mg sodium

Sardines are a rich source of omega-3 fats, known to improve brain function and even mood. Canned sardines often contain a lot of salt. Using fresh sardines, as in this recipe, helps keep the sodium content low.

Sardine croquettes

These elegant little croquettes are a great way to serve omega-3-rich sardines, especially for anyone not keen on the strong fishy taste that sardines sometimes have. Serve them with a green salad.

PREPARATION **20 MINUTES**
COOKING **10 MINUTES PER BATCH**
SERVES **4 (MAKES 16 CROQUETTES)**

2 large potatoes, about $^2/_3$ pound (300 g), cut into large chunks
1 tablespoon (15 ml) olive or canola oil, plus extra for frying
1 onion, finely chopped
3 cloves garlic, crushed
$^1/_4$ cup (15 g) finely chopped fresh parsley
1 scallion, thinly sliced
1 tablespoon (15 ml) whole-grain mustard
$^1/_2$ teaspoon (2 ml) ground white pepper
1 egg
3 cans sardines, $3^1/_2$ ounces (110 g) each, packed in water, drained
1 cup (80 g) fresh whole-wheat breadcrumbs

1 Cook the potatoes in a saucepan of boiling water for 10 minutes, until tender. Drain and set aside to cool.

2 Heat the oil in a large nonstick frying pan and cook the onion and garlic over medium heat for 5 minutes, until lightly browned.

3 Mash the potatoes with the chopped parsley, scallion, mustard and white pepper. Stir in the onion and garlic, and mix in the egg until well combined. Gently fold in the sardines, keeping them in large pieces rather than breaking up completely.

4 Put the breadcrumbs in a shallow bowl. Using your hands, form the sardine mixture into egg-sized balls, then roll in the breadcrumbs and flatten them slightly.

5   Heat the oil in the cleaned frying pan and cook the croquettes in batches for 5 minutes on each side, until golden and cooked through.

You can also spray the croquettes with oil and bake at 400°F (200°C) for 20 minutes, until golden.

EACH SERVING (4 CROQUETTES) PROVIDES
320 calories, 19 g protein, 18 g fat (3 g saturated fat), 21 g carbohydrate (2 g sugars), 3 g fiber, 176 mg sodium

Sardines are one of the best sources of omega-3 fats, which are beneficial for brain function as well as joints, eyes and the immune system.

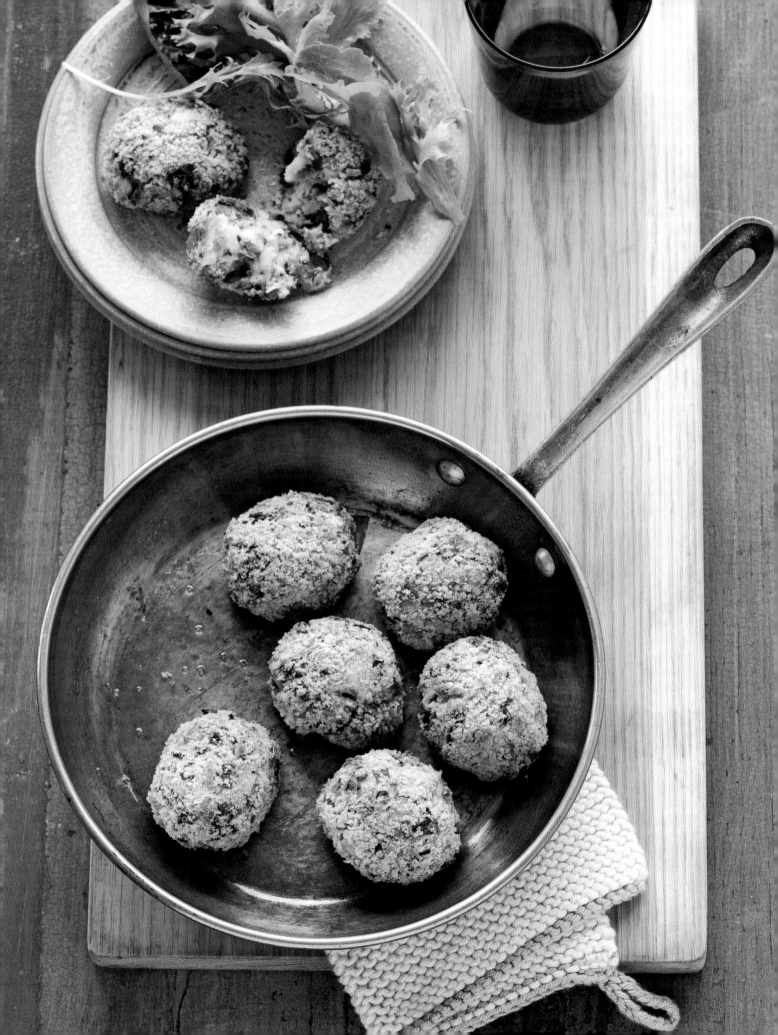

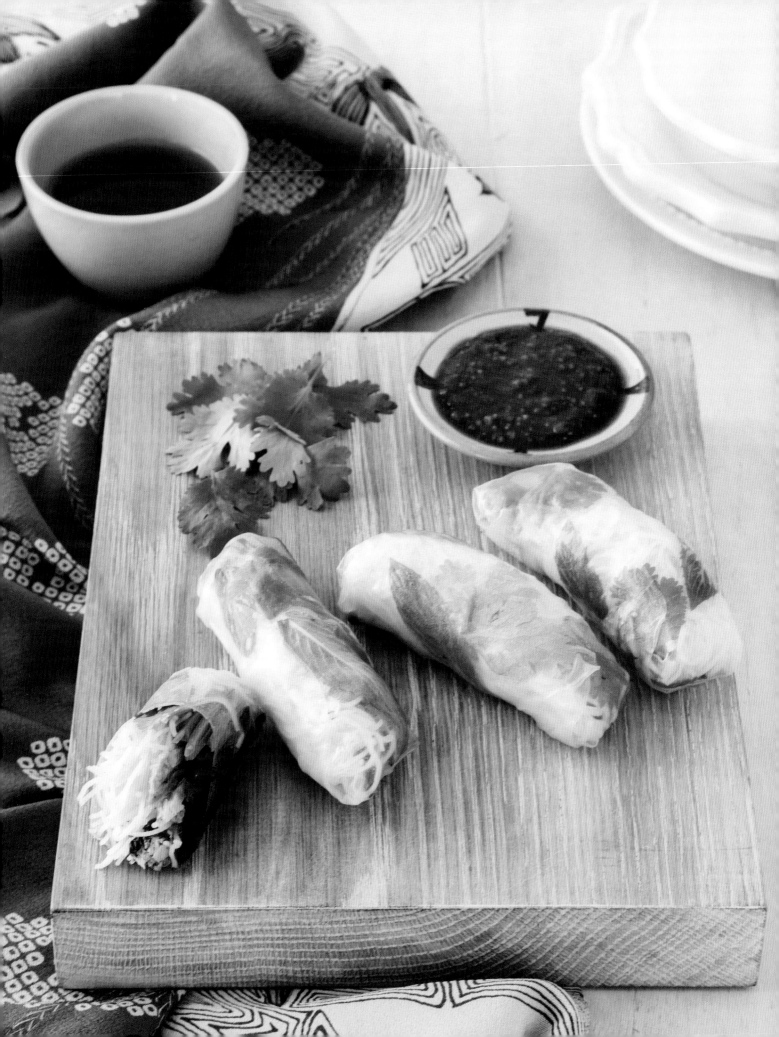

Fresh spring rolls with sardines

Packed with crisp vegetables and herbs, these rolls are a refreshing way to serve sardines and a healthy alternative to deep-fried spring rolls. They are an ideal choice for entertaining as they make great finger food or a light first course.

PREPARATION **35 MINUTES**
MAKES **12**

3$^1/_2$ ounces (100 g) dried rice vermicelli
1 firm, ripe avocado
2 tablespoons (30 ml) lemon or lime juice
12 small (6-inch/15-cm) rice paper wrappers
36 fresh cilantro leaves
24 fresh mint leaves
2 cans sardines, 3$^1/_2$ ounces (110 g) each, drained and flaked
1 carrot, cut into matchsticks
1 small red pepper, cut into matchsticks

Dipping sauce
2 tablespoons (30 ml) hoisin sauce
1 tablespoon (15 ml) low-sodium soy sauce
1 tablespoon (15 ml) creamy peanut butter
1 clove garlic, crushed
$^1/_2$ teaspoon (2 ml) finely chopped red chile

1   Place the noodles in a heatproof bowl and cover with boiling water. Let soak for 5 minutes, then drain in a colander. Rinse under cold water, drain again and squeeze out any remaining water. Using kitchen scissors, cut the noodles into shorter lengths.

2   Slice the avocado and toss it with the lemon or lime juice to prevent it from discoloring.

3   Fill a large shallow dish with very warm water. Working with one rice paper wrapper at a time, dip a wrapper into the water for 1 second, drain off the excess and place on a board. Put three cilantro leaves and two mint leaves in the center of the wrapper. Top with some noodles, some of the avocado, sardines, carrot and pepper.

4   Fold the bottom of the wrapper up over the filling and fold in the sides. Roll up to enclose the filling. Repeat with the remaining wrappers and filling.

5   To make the dipping sauce, mix all the ingredients with 1 tablespoon (15 ml) water in a small bowl.

6   Arrange the spring rolls on a tray so that they are not touching each other. Serve with the dipping sauce.

The wrappers don't need to be completely soft after you dip them in the water, as they will continue to soften.

EACH SERVING (1 SPRING ROLL) PROVIDES
167 calories, 5 g protein, 7 g fat (2 g saturated fat),
20 g carbohydrate (3 g sugars), 2 g fiber, 179 mg sodium

Calcium is important for brain function, and you can get extra calcium by eating the bones of canned sardines and salmon. Green leafy vegetables and herbs also provide some calcium in your diet.

Chicken liver bruschetta with orange zest and green herbs

Chicken livers are rich and creamy—a perfect topping for crunchy toast. Served on its own or with a green salad, this is a great light meal or hearty snack, or you can cut the baguette into bite-sized pieces to make a nutritious appetizer.

PREPARATION 15 MINUTES
COOKING 20 MINUTES
SERVES 4

½ pound chicken livers, about 4 livers
1 tablespoon (15 ml) extra virgin olive oil, plus extra for brushing
1 small red onion or 2–3 shallots, finely chopped
2 tablespoons (30 ml) white wine or low-sodium chicken stock
grated zest of 1 orange
¼ cup (15 g) roughly chopped fresh parsley
freshly ground black pepper
8 slices baguette or other long, thin bread, cut diagonally to make oval slices
1 large clove garlic, halved
arugula, to serve

1   Cut the chicken livers into quarters. Trim and discard any stringy or pale bits.

2   Heat the olive oil in a small frying pan and cook the onion or shallots over medium heat for about 5 minutes, until starting to color. Add the livers and cook, turning often, for 5 minutes. Pour in the wine or stock and cook, stirring, for 2 minutes. Remove from the heat.

3   Stir in the orange zest and parsley, and season with freshly ground black pepper. Transfer the mixture to a blender or food processor and let cool while you prepare the bread.

4   Preheat the broiler to high. Brush both sides of each baguette slice with olive oil. Toast under the grill for 2 minutes on each side, until golden. Rub one side of each slice all over with the cut garlic clove.

5   Using the pulse button, process the liver mixture in short bursts until just combined but still chunky. Spoon onto the baguette slices and serve topped with arugula.

The topping can be blended until smooth with a little olive oil to make a healthy liver pâté. Press the pâté into a ramekin, cover and refrigerate for up to 5 days.

EACH SERVING PROVIDES
235 calories, 12 g protein, 8 g fat (1 g saturated fat), 28 g carbohydrate (3 g sugars), 2 g fiber, 320 mg sodium

Liver is one of the most concentrated sources of brain-boosting nutrients such as zinc and inositol. Here it makes a stylish appetizer or snack combined with antioxidant-rich parsley and tangy orange zest.

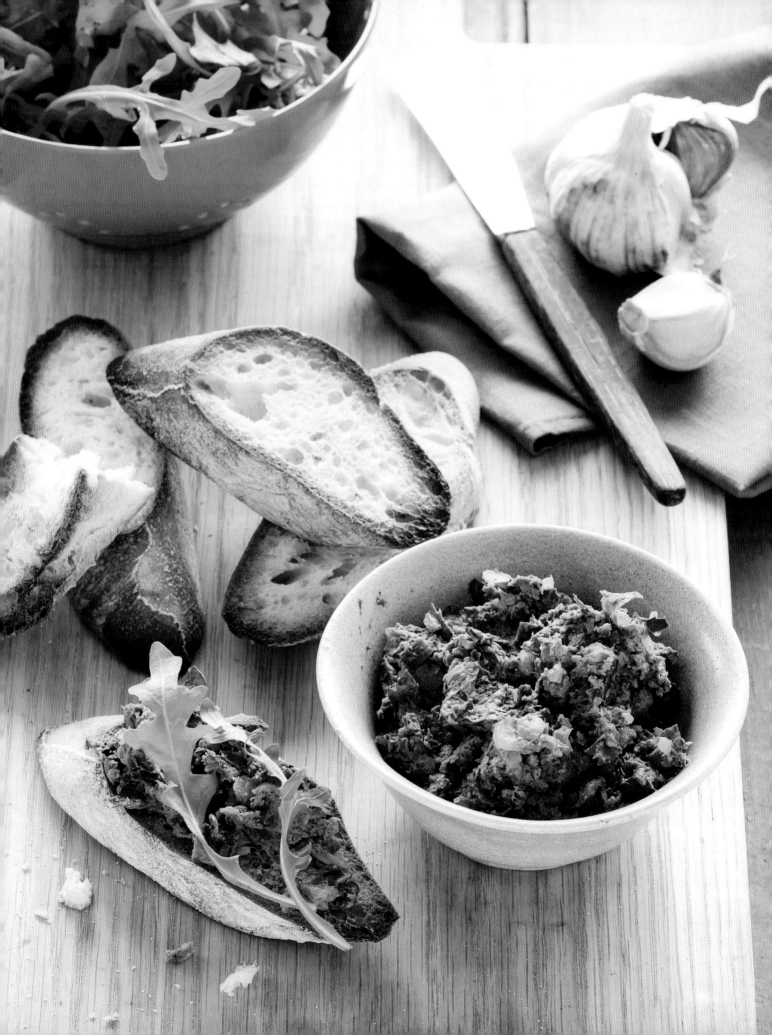

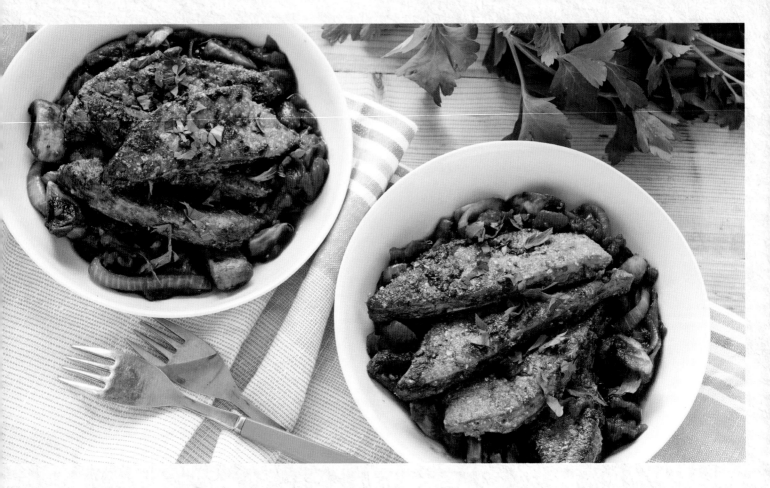

Liver with mushrooms

Tomatoes, mushrooms and caramelized onions combine to
balance the strong flavor of lamb's liver in this dish.

PREPARATION **15 MINUTES**   COOKING **50 MINUTES**   SERVES **4**

2$^1/_2$ tablespoons (37 ml) olive or canola oil
1 large onion, cut into thick rings
4 large mushrooms, roughly chopped
14$^1/_2$ ounce (400 ml) can diced tomatoes
$^1/_2$ cup (30 g) roughly chopped fresh parsley,
   plus extra to serve
1 lamb's liver, about 1 pound (500 g), rinsed
$^1/_4$ cup (35 g) all-purpose flour
freshly ground black pepper

1   Heat 2 tablespoons (30 ml) of the oil in a frying
pan. Gently cook the onion until dark and well
caramelized, about 30 minutes. Add the mushrooms
and stir for 5 minutes, stir in the tomatoes and
simmer for 10 minutes until thick. Stir in the parsley.

2   Trim any stringy bits from the liver, cut on the
diagonal into $^1/_2$-inch (1-cm) slices and pat dry.
Season the flour with freshly ground black pepper.
Toss the liver in the flour until well coated.

3   Heat a large nonstick frying pan and brush with
the remaining oil. Cook the liver over medium heat
for about 3 minutes on each side, until browned.

4   Spoon the mushroom mixture into serving bowls,
top with the liver and sprinkle with the extra parsley.

EACH SERVING PROVIDES

370 calories, 30 g protein, 21 g fat (4 g saturated fat),
15 g carbohydrate (5 g sugars), 3 g fiber, 156 mg sodium

Liver contains all the important nutrients
of meat, in even more concentrated form.
These include vitamins A, D, E, K, B$_{12}$, folate,
and iron, copper and zinc, all nutrients that are
involved in maintaining normal brain function.

Tuna, cucumber and watercress wraps

Wraps are large, thin flatbreads, sometimes sold as lavash or mountain bread. Tortillas can also be used as wraps. Choose a whole-grain or whole-wheat variety for the most health benefits.

PREPARATION **10 MINUTES**   SERVES **2**

2 large whole-grain wraps, about 10 inches
   (26 cm) diameter
1/2 cup (110 g) hummus
2 tablespoons (30 ml) finely chopped red onion
6 ounces (185 g) canned tuna, drained and flaked
1 small cucumber, thinly sliced
1/2 cup (125 g) red cherry tomatoes, quartered
3 cups (90 g) watercress sprigs

1   Spread the bottom half of each wrap with half of the hummus.

2   Arrange the red onion, tuna, cucumber, tomatoes and watercress sprigs on top of the hummus, using half of the ingredients on each wrap. Starting from the bottom, firmly roll up to enclose the filling.

3   Cut each roll in half, and serve immediately.

Watercress can be gritty, so soak it in a sink or large bowl of cold water for 5 minutes, drain and dry it in a salad spinner. Pick off the tender sprigs from the thicker stems. Store the remaining watercress in an airtight bag in the fridge.

EACH SERVING PROVIDES
332 calories, 28 g protein, 13 g fat (3 g saturated fat), 26 g carbohydrate (6 g sugars), 10 g fiber, 498 mg sodium

> Vitamin K is important in controlling blood clotting and inflammation and also appears to reduce damage to brain cells. *Watercress* is an excellent source of vitamin K as well as beneficial minerals and fiber.

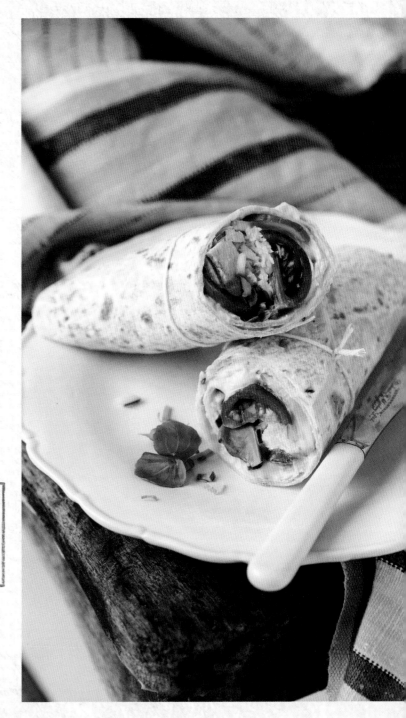

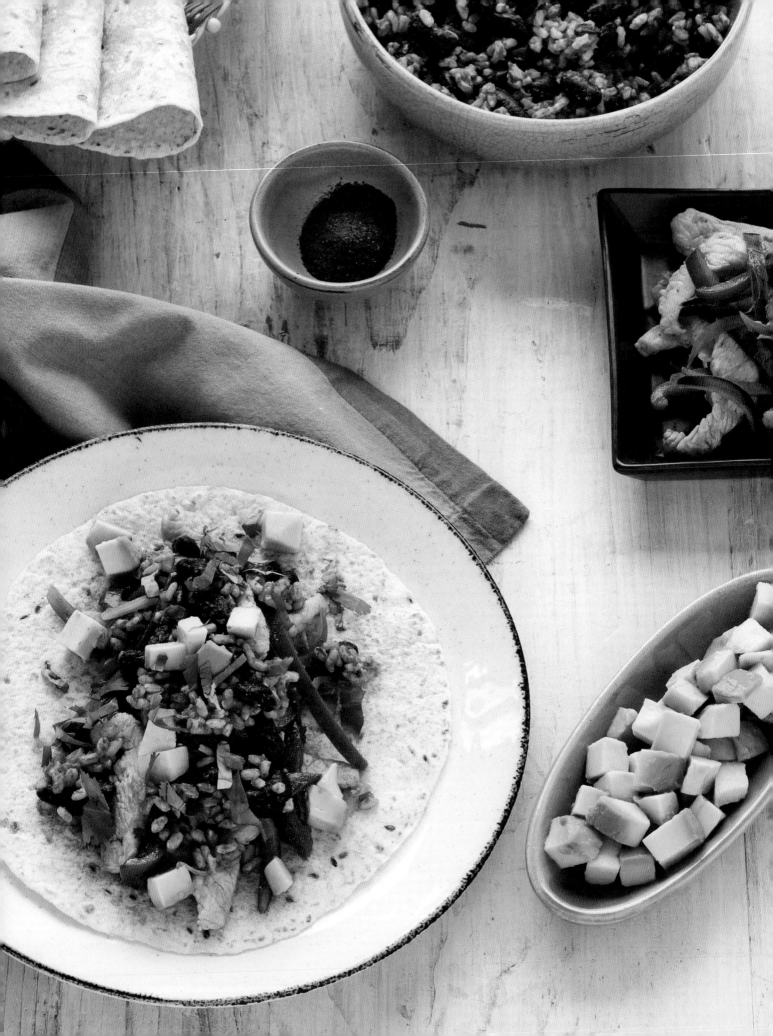

Turkey and bean burritos

Serve the rice and beans, turkey and avocado separately, allowing your guests to assemble their own burritos. The tortillas will stay fresh and each person can create a burrito to suit their taste.

PREPARATION **15 MINUTES**
COOKING **35 MINUTES**
SERVES **4**

½ cup (125 g) long-grain brown rice
8 whole-wheat flour tortillas
15 ounce (425 ml) can red kidney beans,
   rinsed and drained
¼ cup (50 ml) low-sodium chicken stock
1 teaspoon (5 ml) dried cumin
1 teaspoon (5 ml) dried oregano
1 teaspoon (5 ml) smoked paprika
2 tablespoons (30 ml) tomato paste
1 tablespoon (15 ml) olive oil
1 pound (500 g) lean turkey cutlets,
   cut into thin strips
1 red pepper, cut into thin strips
1 red onion, thinly sliced
1 avocado, chopped
1 tablespoon (15 ml) lime juice
2 tablespoons (30 ml) chopped fresh
   cilantro

1   Combine the rice and 1 cup (250 ml) water in a saucepan. Bring to a boil, stir and reduce the heat to low. Cover and simmer for 20 minutes, until all the water is absorbed.

2   Meanwhile, preheat the oven to 350°F (180°C). Wrap the stack of tortillas in foil and bake for 15 minutes, until heated.

3   Combine the rice, kidney beans, stock, cumin, oregano, paprika and tomato paste in a pan, and cook over medium heat for 10 minutes, until the liquid has evaporated.

4   While the rice mixture is cooking, heat the oil in a frying pan and cook the turkey, peppers and onion over medium heat for 10 minutes, until the turkey has browned and the onion has softened.

5   Put the avocado and lime juice in a bowl and gently toss to combine.

6   Serve the warm tortillas topped with the turkey mixture, the rice mixture, a spoonful of avocado and the cilantro.

Replace the canned beans with 2 cups (500 g) cooked beans made from ⅔ cup (140 g) dried red kidney beans.

EACH SERVING PROVIDES
692 calories, 42 g protein, 27 g fat (5 g saturated fat),
74 g carbohydrate (8 g sugars), 11 g fiber, 770 mg sodium

Eating a meal containing *turkey* promotes a feeling of well-being, thanks to its high content of tryptophan, the precursor of the soothing neurotransmitter serotonin.

Beef fajitas with avocado and tomato salsa

The beef is traditionally cooked on a hot steel plate and brought to the table while it is still sizzling. You can cook the fajitas on the barbecue grill. The tortillas can be wrapped in foil and warmed on the grill, too.

PREPARATION **20 MINUTES**
COOKING **20 MINUTES**
SERVES **4**

1 pound (500 g) beef round steak, thinly sliced
1 teaspoon (5 ml) ground cumin
1 teaspoon (5 ml) sweet paprika
juice of 1 lime
12 flour tortillas
1 tablespoon (15 ml) olive oil
1 red onion, thinly sliced
1 small red pepper, thinly sliced
1 small green pepper, thinly sliced
15 ounce (425 ml) can red kidney beans or black beans, rinsed and drained
1 small iceberg lettuce, thinly shredded
½ cup (125 ml) low-fat Greek-style yogurt

Avocado and tomato salsa
1 avocado, chopped
2 tomatoes, chopped
2 scallions, thinly sliced
1 clove garlic, crushed
juice of 1 lime
2 tablespoons (30 ml) chopped fresh cilantro
few drops chili sauce or Tabasco

1 Put the steak in a large bowl. Add the cumin, paprika and lime juice, and toss well to coat the meat in the spices.

2 Preheat the oven to 350°F (180°C). Wrap the stack of tortillas in foil and bake for 15 minutes, until heated.

3 Meanwhile, heat the oil in a large pan and cook the onion over medium heat for 10 minutes, until soft. Add the steak and cook for 5 minutes, until browned.

4 Stir in the peppers and beans, and cook for 5 minutes, until the peppers are soft.

5 To prepare the salsa, combine the avocado, tomatoes, scallions, garlic, lime juice, cilantro and chili sauce or Tabasco sauce in a bowl.

6 Serve the warm tortillas topped with the beef mixture, a little shredded lettuce, the salsa and some yogurt.

Replace the canned beans with 2 cups (500 g) cooked beans made from ⅔ cup (140 g) dried beans, or use a 15 ounce (425 g) can of refried beans. Heat the refried beans in a small saucepan over medium heat for 10 minutes until hot. Cover and keep warm until they are added in Step 4.

EACH SERVING PROVIDES
667 calories, 42 g protein, 31 g fat (9 g saturated fat), 53 g carbohydrate (8 g sugars), 9 g fiber, 548 mg sodium

All *legumes* are good for your heart, boosting circulation to the brain. They also contain resistant starch that lowers the glycemic index (GI) of the meal.

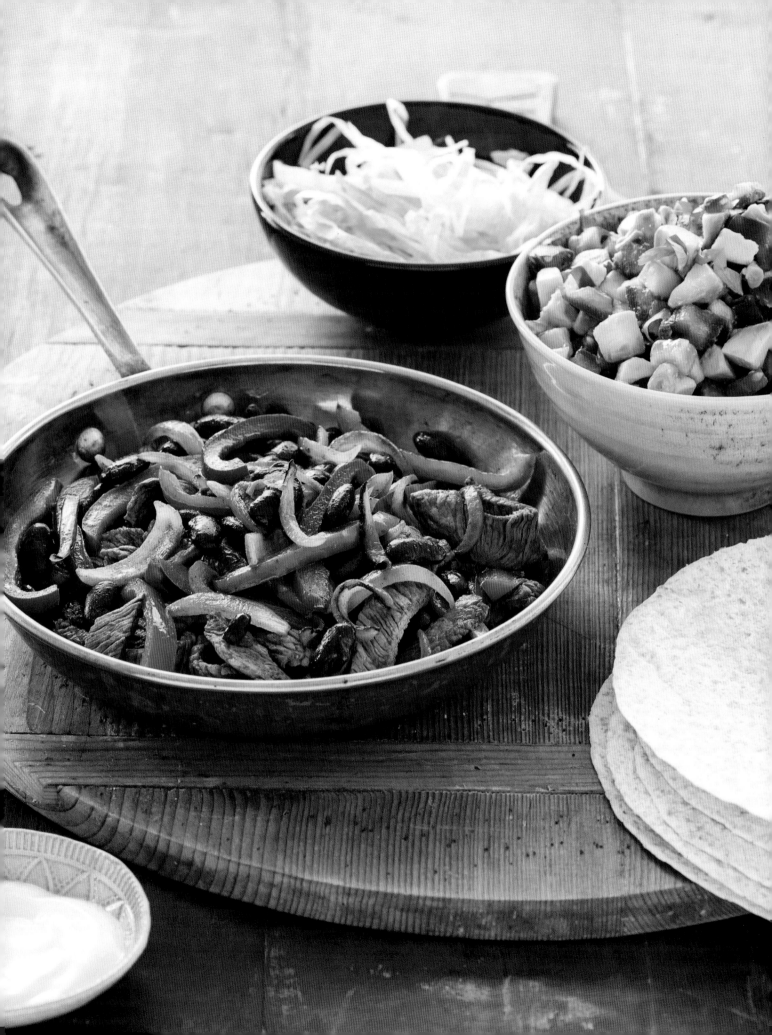

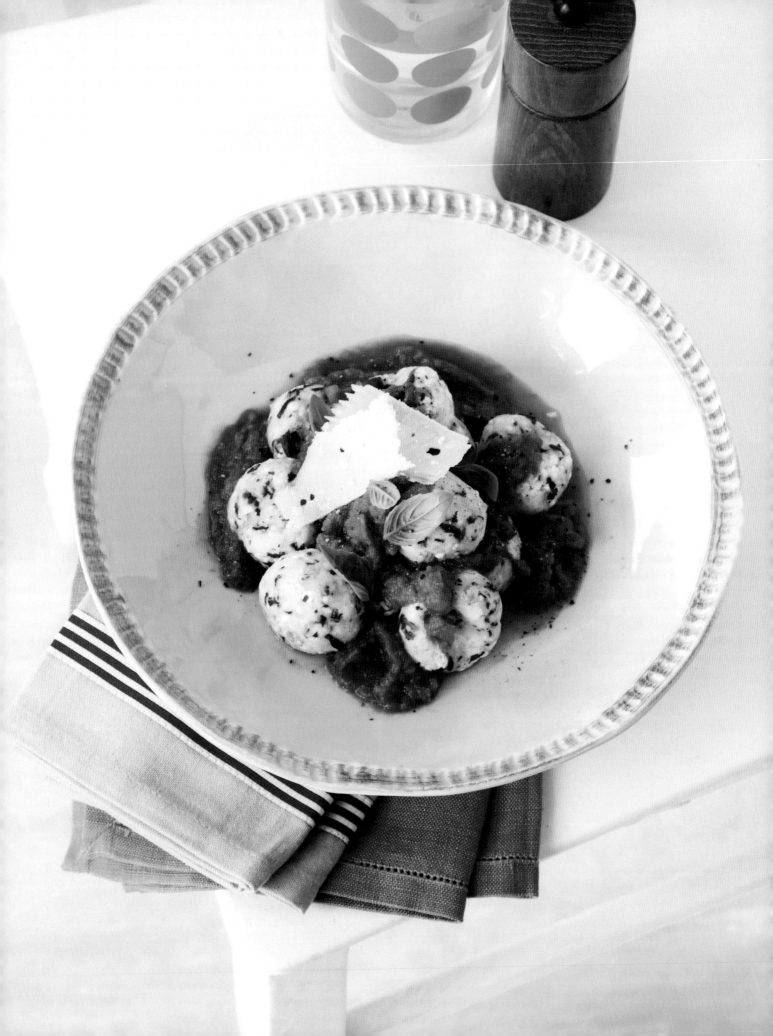

Ricotta and spinach gnocchi with tomato sauce

If you have time, prepare the gnocchi ahead and refrigerate them until needed.

PREPARATION **30 MINUTES, PLUS 20 MINUTES CHILLING**
COOKING **50 MINUTES**
SERVES **4**

1 cup (200 g) spinach, trimmed
1 egg, lightly beaten
$^2/_3$ cup (110 g) whole-wheat all-purpose flour, plus extra for dusting
$^1/_2$ cup (50 g) finely grated parmesan
shaved parmesan, to serve
fresh small basil leaves, to serve
freshly ground black pepper

Ricotta
12 cups (3 L) low-fat milk
2 tablespoons (30 ml) Epsom salts
$^1/_3$ cup (75 ml) white vinegar or lime juice

Tomato sauce
1 tablespoon (15 ml) olive oil
1 onion, finely chopped
5 cloves garlic, crushed
$3^1/_4$ cups (800 g) fresh diced tomatoes, or two $14^1/_2$ ounce (400 ml) cans diced tomatoes

1   To make the ricotta, bring the milk to a boil in a large saucepan. Add the Epsom salts and vinegar or lime juice and quickly stir. Cook over low heat, without stirring, for 10 minutes to allow the ricotta to rise.

2   Line a fine sieve or colander with cheesecloth. Put the spinach in a heatproof bowl and strain the ricotta over the spinach, allowing the hot whey to wilt the spinach. Drain the spinach, and let the ricotta drain and cool.

3   To make the sauce, heat the oil in a large saucepan. Gently sauté the onion for 5–10 minutes, until translucent. Add the garlic and cook, stirring, for 1 minute. Stir in the fresh or canned tomatoes and simmer for 15 minutes, until the sauce is thick. Keep the sauce hot while you make the gnocchi, or reheat it while the gnocchi is in the fridge.

4   Meanwhile, use a food processor or sharp knife to very finely chop the spinach, and squeeze it with your hands to dry it. Combine the chopped spinach with the cooled ricotta and the egg. Add the flour and grated parmesan, and briefly stir until completely mixed.

5   Roll the ricotta mixture into tablespoon-size (15 ml) balls on a lightly floured surface, adding the extra flour if needed. Push with your thumb to slightly flatten the gnocchi. Place on a tray and refrigerate for 20 minutes.

6   Cook the gnocchi in several batches in a large saucepan of boiling water. Remove them with a slotted spoon as they float to the surface. Serve in heated bowls with the hot sauce, topped with some shaved parmesan, basil leaves and freshly ground black pepper.

You can use ready-made ricotta for this dish—you will need about 16 ounces (500 g) dry ricotta, the type sold in a plastic strainer. Avoid using the wet kind sold in tubs.

EACH SERVING PROVIDES
612 calories, 50 g protein, 13 g fat (5 g saturated fat), 75 g carbohydrate (55 g sugars), 8 g fiber, 674 mg sodium

Cutting down on salt helps to control blood pressure and reduce the risk of stroke. By making your own *ricotta*, you can avoid the salt and additives usually found in commercial varieties, and it also gives a better result in recipes requiring a light, dry texture, like this gnocchi dish. Try using lime juice instead of vinegar for extra antioxidants and a burst of tangy flavor.

Farfalle with zucchini and pine nut pesto

PREPARATION **15 MINUTES**
COOKING **15 MINUTES**
SERVES **4**

1 tablespoon (15 ml) olive oil
2 zucchini, halved and thinly sliced on the diagonal
1 clove garlic, thinly sliced
10 ounces (300 g) whole-wheat farfalle
grated parmesan, to serve

Pine nut pesto
1 cup (50 g) firmly packed fresh basil
1 cup (20 g) fresh flat-leaf parsley
1 clove garlic
2 tablespoons (30 ml) pine nuts
1/4 cup (30 g) finely grated parmesan
1/4 cup (50 ml) extra virgin olive oil

1   To make the pine nut pesto, put the basil, parsley, whole garlic clove, pine nuts and parmesan in a food processor, and process until the mixture forms a rough paste. With the motor running, gradually add oil in a slow stream until a smooth paste forms. Set aside while you cook the zucchini and farfalle.

2   Heat the olive oil in a frying pan, add the zucchini and garlic, and cook over medium heat for 5 minutes, until the zucchini is soft and the liquid has evaporated.

3   Meanwhile, cook the farfalle in a large saucepan of boiling water according to the package directions, until al dente. Drain the pasta, reserving about 1/2 cup (125 ml) of the cooking water.

4   Fold the pesto into the warm pasta with the zucchini mixture, thinning the pesto with a little of the pasta cooking water if it is hard to mix. Gently toss to coat the pasta with the pesto.

5   Divide the pasta among four serving bowls and serve topped with grated parmesan.

EACH SERVING PROVIDES
492 calories, 14 g protein, 28 g fat (5 g saturated fat), 47 g carbohydrate (1 g sugars), 10 g fiber, 121 mg sodium

Pine nuts are high in heart- and brain-healthy monounsaturated fatty acids and vitamin E. They are also a good source of manganese, which is part of the body's antioxidant system.

Pasta with tomatoes and almond pesto

PREPARATION **15 MINUTES**
COOKING **15 MINUTES**
SERVES **4**

1 tablespoon (15 ml) olive oil
1 red onion, sliced
1 clove garlic, sliced
1 cup (200 g) yellow cherry tomatoes, halved
1 cup (200 g) red cherry tomatoes, halved
12 ounces (375 g) whole-wheat spaghetti
fresh small basil leaves, to serve
shaved parmesan, to serve

Almond pesto
2 cups (100 g) firmly packed fresh basil
1 clove garlic, chopped
2 tablespoons (30 ml) roasted almonds
1/4 cup (30 g) finely grated parmesan
1/4 cup (50 ml) extra virgin olive oil

1   To make the pesto, put the basil, garlic, almonds and parmesan in a food processor, and process until the mixture forms a rough paste. With the motor running, gradually add oil forming a smooth paste.

2   Heat the oil in a large frying pan. Cook the onion over medium heat for 10 minutes, until just soft. Stir in the garlic and tomatoes, and cook for 5 minutes, until the tomato skins just start to split. Transfer to a bowl and gently crush the tomatoes.

3   Meanwhile, cook the spaghetti in a large saucepan of boiling water according to the package directions, until al dente. Drain the pasta, reserving about 1/2 cup (125 ml) of the cooking water.

4   Add the pesto and half the tomatoes to the pasta, with enough of the pasta cooking water to thin the pesto, and toss well to coat the pasta.

5   Divide the pasta among four bowls and top with the remaining tomatoes, the basil and parmesan.

EACH SERVING PROVIDES
558 calories, 17 g protein, 27 g fat (5 g saturated fat), 61 g carbohydrate (4 g sugars), 13 g fiber, 135 mg sodium

The brain-protective substances found in *tomatoes* and *basil* are easier for your body to absorb when you eat them with a little fat, such as the beneficial fats in the olive oil and almonds.

With its low glycemic index, whole-wheat pasta is a perfect brain food, supplying long-lasting fuel to keep you going all day.

Left: Farfalle with zucchini and pine nut pesto
Right: Pasta with tomatoes and almond pesto

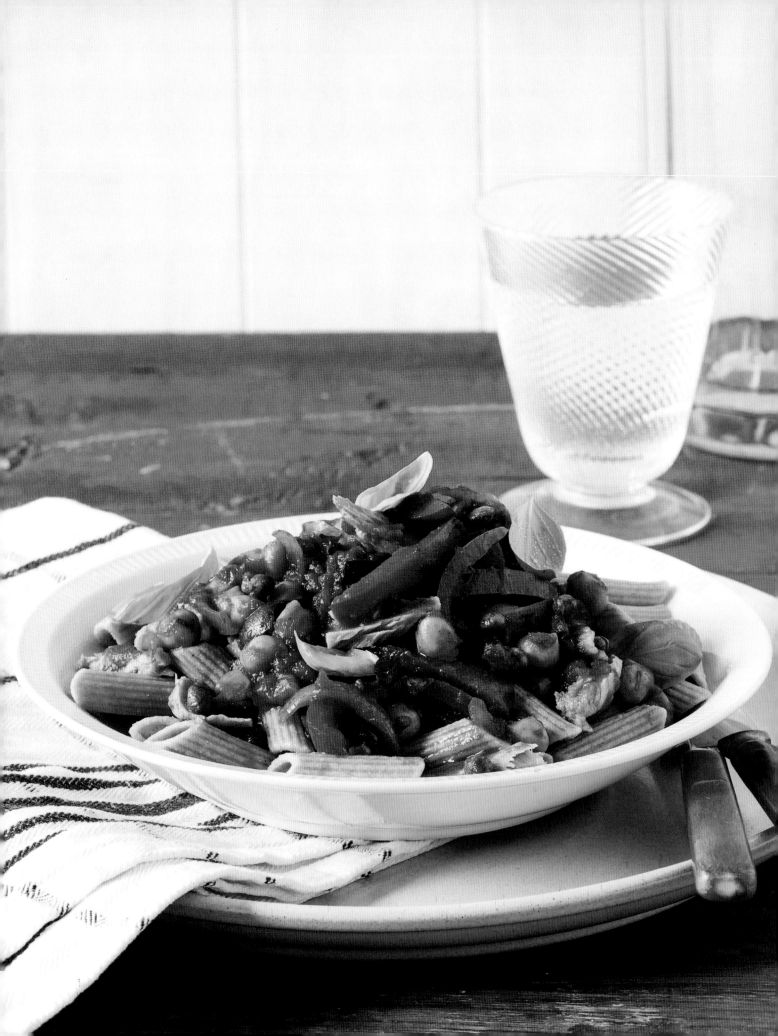

Penne with tuna, tomatoes and chickpeas

This recipe uses pantry staples for a quick weeknight dish. Try not to stir the pasta sauce too much while it's cooking—you want the tuna in large chunks, rather than broken up into small flakes.

PREPARATION **15 MINUTES**
COOKING **40 MINUTES**
SERVES **4**

1 tablespoon (15 ml) olive oil
1 red onion, thinly sliced
1 clove garlic, crushed
1 red chile, seeded and thinly sliced
1 teaspoon (5 ml) ground cinnamon
8 kalamata olives, pitted and chopped
14^1/$_2$ ounce (400 ml) can diced tomatoes
15 ounce (425 ml) can chickpeas, rinsed
  and drained
14^1/$_2$ ounce (400 g) can tuna in water, drained
1 red pepper, thinly sliced
2 tablespoons (30 ml) capers, rinsed and
  squeezed dry
grated zest and juice of 1 lemon
14 ounces (400 g) whole-wheat penne
2 tablespoons (30 ml) fresh basil

1   Heat the oil in a large frying pan and cook the onion over medium heat for 10 minutes, until soft and golden. Stir in the garlic, chile, cinnamon and olives. Cook for 2 minutes, until the cinnamon is fragrant.

2   Add the tomatoes, chickpeas, tuna, pepper, capers, lemon zest and 1 cup (250 ml) water. Bring to a boil, reduce the heat and simmer for 20 minutes, until reduced and thickened slightly. Stir in the lemon juice.

3   While the sauce is cooking, cook the penne in a large saucepan of boiling water following the package directions, until al dente. Drain the penne, reserving 1 cup (250 ml) of the cooking water.

4   Thin the sauce with the cooking water, return to a boil and cook over high heat for 5 minutes.

5   Serve the pasta topped with the sauce and garnished with basil leaves.

This sauce freezes well and also makes a good filling for cannelloni tubes.

Replace the canned chickpeas with 2 cups (500 g) cooked chickpeas made from ^{2}/$_3$ cup (140 g) dried chickpeas.

EACH SERVING PROVIDES
574 calories, 38 g protein, 12 g fat (2 g saturated fat), 77 g carbohydrate (7 g sugars), 15 g fiber, 447 mg sodium

Pasta has a low glycemic index (GI), so the energy is released slowly for a long-lasting supply. It gives your body, especially your brain, the energy it needs to function. The GI of whole-wheat pasta is even lower than white pasta.

Tomatoes

Botanically, tomatoes are classified as a fruit, but in addition to their sweetness and acid they contain natural glutamates, which create the savory "umami" taste commonly used to enhance the flavors of dishes and salads.

Clockwise from bottom left: vine-ripened tomatoes, grape kumatoes, yellow cherry tomatoes, small red cherry tomatoes, green heirloom tomato, baby plum tomatoes on the vine, kumatoes, oxheart heirloom tomatoes (in large bowl), medley mix (in bowl)

There is a simple rule to choosing the most nutritious fruits and vegetables: Choose the most colorful ones, as these usually have the highest concentrations of antioxidants, found in the brightly colored pigments of fresh produce. Many of the red, orange and yellow colors in fruits and vegetables are from carotenoids, which are precursors of vitamin A. Although tomatoes do contain some carotenoids, they get their gorgeous red color from an altogether different substance, lycopene. Lycopene is not a precursor of vitamin A, but a powerful antioxidant in its own right—some studies have shown that it has twice the antioxidant activity of beta-carotene. Unlike many antioxidants, cooking and processing does not destroy lycopene. Instead, the cooking and processing actually help to release lycopene from the tomato cells and also convert it to a form that is more easily absorbed by the body. This means that the tomatoes used in soups and sauces, and tomato paste and sun-dried tomatoes, are better sources of lycopene than raw

tomatoes. And since it is fat-soluble, lycopene is also much better absorbed when it is served with a healthy fat such as olive oil, nuts, seeds or avocado.

Another beneficial substance that can be found in tomatoes is uridine. Uridine appears to be an essential part of the process by which choline contributes to repairing the brain cell membranes, and together uridine and choline are being investigated in research examining how to reduce the loss of brain function as a result of aging. Foods that are high in uridine include tomatoes, yeast, liver and broccoli, but it is thought that very little of the uridine eaten in these foods is actually absorbed into the body. This may make it more important to make sure you eat enough of these good uridine sources.

Tomatoes are also very high in vitamin C. As well as being another part of the body's antioxidant system, vitamin C is essential for maintaining healthy blood vessels, making it important for the supply of blood to the brain. Tomatoes also provide good amounts of fiber and B-group vitamins, including thiamine, niacin, vitamin B_6 and folate.

Spaghetti with radicchio and tuna

Bitter greens such as radicchio and Belgian endive are good for the brain in many different ways. In this recipe, the rich flavors of sun-dried tomatoes and tuna help to balance the bitterness of the greens so that everyone can enjoy their benefits.

PREPARATION **10 MINUTES, PLUS 1 HOUR SOAKING**
COOKING **20 MINUTES**
SERVES **4**

$^3/_4$ cup (75 g) dry sun-dried tomatoes, or about $^1/_2$ cup (125 g) moist sun-dried tomatoes
2 tablespoons (30 ml) olive or canola oil
1 red onion, halved and thinly sliced
2 cloves garlic, crushed
2 cups (60 g) radicchio or Belgian endive leaves, torn into bite-sized pieces
5 ounces (150 g) whole-wheat spaghetti, linguine or fettucine
$^1/_4$ cup (7 g) chopped fresh flat-leaf parsley
14$^1/_2$ ounce (400 ml) can chunk light tuna, packed in water, drained

1 If you are using dry sun-dried tomatoes, place them in a heatproof bowl and cover with boiling water. Soak for at least 1 hour and drain well. Cut the soaked or moist sun-dried tomatoes into $^1/_2$-inch (1 cm) pieces.

2 Heat the oil in a large saucepan and cook the onion over low heat for 10 minutes, until starting to color. Add the garlic and cook for 1 minute. Add the chopped sun-dried tomatoes and cook for 2 minutes. Add the radicchio or endive. Stir for about 3 minutes, until the leaves are wilted and the stems have softened.

3 While the sauce is cooking, cook the pasta in a large saucepan of boiling water following package directions, until al dente. Drain the pasta.

4 Stir half the parsley into the sauce, then stir into the pasta until well combined. Fold in the tuna, mixing gently so it stays in chunks. Serve the pasta sprinkled with the remaining parsley.

EACH SERVING PROVIDES
356 calories, 28 g protein, 13 g fat (2 g saturated fat), 32 g carbohydrate (7 g sugars), 7 g fiber, 92 mg sodium

Radicchio is a member of the chicory family. It is a good source of fiber and is particularly high in many different antioxidants, including polyphenols, which protect brain cells from damage.

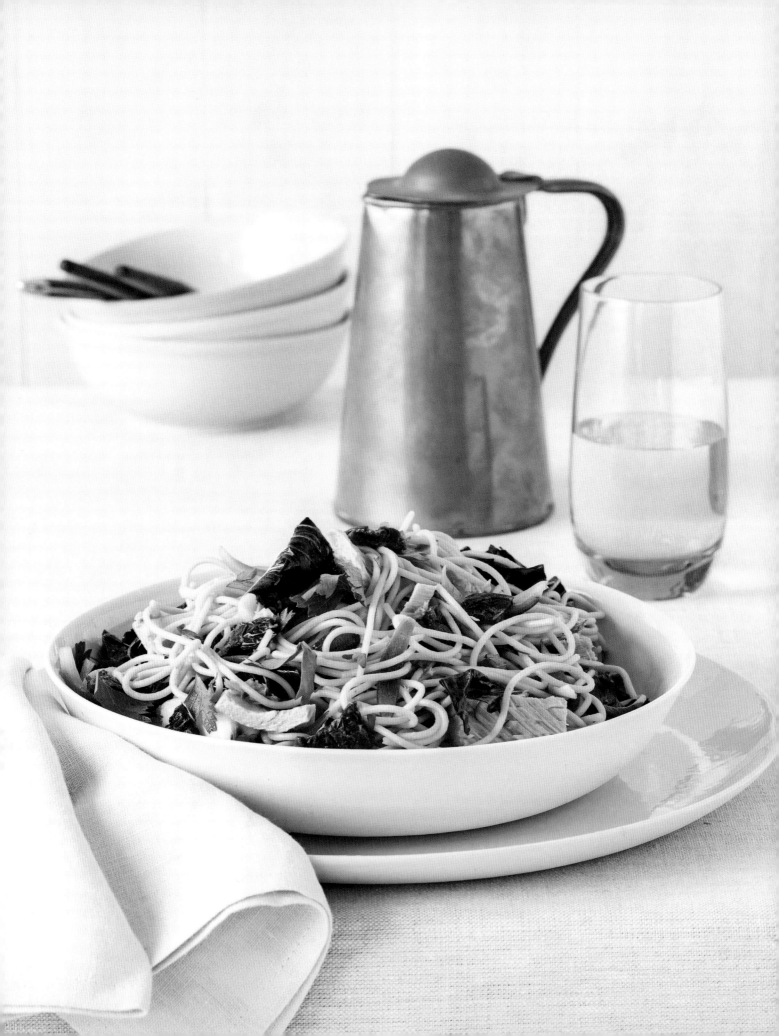

Super side dishes

Vegetables become superstars in these spectacular side dishes. Each recipe harnesses the natural flavors of the vegetables so they become tasty and healthy accompaniments to any meal, adding a wide variety of powerful brain-boosting nutrients.

Japanese-style spinach with soy and sesame

1 pound (500 g) spinach, trimmed
1/4 cup (40 g) sesame seeds, toasted
1 teaspoon (5 ml) superfine sugar
1 tablespoon (15 ml) low-sodium soy sauce
2 tablespoons (30 ml) low-sodium chicken stock, boiling hot

Put the spinach in a metal colander over a saucepan of simmering water, cover and steam for 5 minutes, until bright green and tender. Transfer to a bowl of ice water and cool. Drain and squeeze any excess liquid from the spinach. Cut the spinach into 4-inch (10-cm) lengths. Using a mortar and pestle, grind the toasted sesame seeds just until the seeds break open, being careful not to grind them into a paste. Transfer the ground sesame seeds to a bowl, add sugar, soy sauce, hot stock, and stir until the sugar dissolves. Pour the dressing over the spinach and serve.

SERVES 4

Baked cauliflower with turmeric

1 tablespoon (15 ml) coconut oil
1 teaspoon (5 ml) ground turmeric
1/2 teaspoon (2 ml) ground cumin
1/2 teaspoon (2 ml) ground coriander
1 pound (500 g) cauliflower, cut into florets
freshly ground black pepper
chopped fresh cilantro, to garnish

Preheat the oven to 425°F (220°C). Combine the coconut oil and spices in a large bowl. Add the cauliflower and toss to coat. Spread the cauliflower in a baking pan. Season with freshly ground black pepper. Bake, tossing occasionally, for 30 minutes, until the cauliflower is browned and tender. Serve garnished with cilantro.

SERVES 4

Roasted radishes

1 1/2 cups (350 g) red and pink radishes, halved
1 tablespoon (15 ml) olive oil
freshly ground black pepper
1 teaspoon (5 ml) fresh rosemary

Preheat the oven to 425°F (220°C). Toss the radishes with the olive oil, pepper and rosemary in a large bowl. Spread in a baking dish in a single layer. Bake, stirring occasionally, for about 25 minutes, until the radishes are crisp on the outside and soft inside. Serve warm.

SERVES 4

Brussels sprouts are a member of the cruciferous brassica family of vegetables, all great sources of antioxidants that prevent heart disease and stroke, and appear to help protect brain function.

Butternut squash and *sweet potatoes* are high in beta-carotene, the precursor of vitamin A, which is essential for healthy eyesight and immune function.

Sesame seeds are a great source of manganese, copper and magnesium, for brain function.

Broccoli has the highest content of carotenoids among cruciferous vegetables, and is an excellent source of lutein—two substances important for healthy eyesight.

Glazed baby brussels sprouts

20 baby brussels sprouts, about 10 ounces (300 g) total, stems trimmed
2 tablespoons (30 ml) extra virgin olive oil
1 tablespoon (15 ml) balsamic vinegar or molasses
freshly ground black pepper

Preheat the oven to 425°F (220°C). Put the sprouts in a baking dish that holds them snugly. Drizzle with the olive oil and toss to coat. Bake for 30 minutes, turning frequently, until dark brown and very tender. Drizzle with the vinegar or molasses, toss to coat, and sprinkle with freshly ground black pepper.

SERVES 4

Roasted lemon broccoli with almonds

$1^{2}/_{3}$ cups (400 g) broccoli florets
1 tablespoon (15 ml) olive oil
2 teaspoons (10 ml) finely grated lemon zest
2 tablespoons (30 ml) slivered almonds

Preheat the oven to 350°F (180°C). Line a baking pan with parchment paper. Spread the broccoli in the pan. Combine the oil and lemon zest in a small bowl. Drizzle over the broccoli and toss to coat. Bake the broccoli for 20 minutes, until lightly browned and just tender. Meanwhile, bake the almonds in a small baking pan for 3 minutes, until golden. Transfer to a plate to cool. Serve the broccoli sprinkled with the almonds.

SERVES 4

Mashed sweet potatoes and butternut squash with sage

$^{2}/_{3}$ pound (300 g) sweet potatoes, roughly chopped
$^{3}/_{4}$ pound (400 g) butternut squash, roughly chopped
$^{1}/_{4}$ cup (50 ml) low-fat milk
2 teaspoons (10 ml) finely chopped fresh sage
freshly ground black pepper

Put the sweet potatoes and squash in a steamer over a saucepan of boiling water and cook for 15 minutes, until very tender. Drain the water from the pan and put the vegetables in the pan. Set the pan over low heat to evaporate the excess liquid. Remove the pan from the heat and use a potato masher to mash the vegetables until almost smooth. Beat in the milk and chopped sage using a wooden spoon. Season with freshly ground black pepper.

SERVES 4

From left: Glazed baby brussels sprouts; Roasted radishes; Mashed sweet potatoes and butternut squash with sage

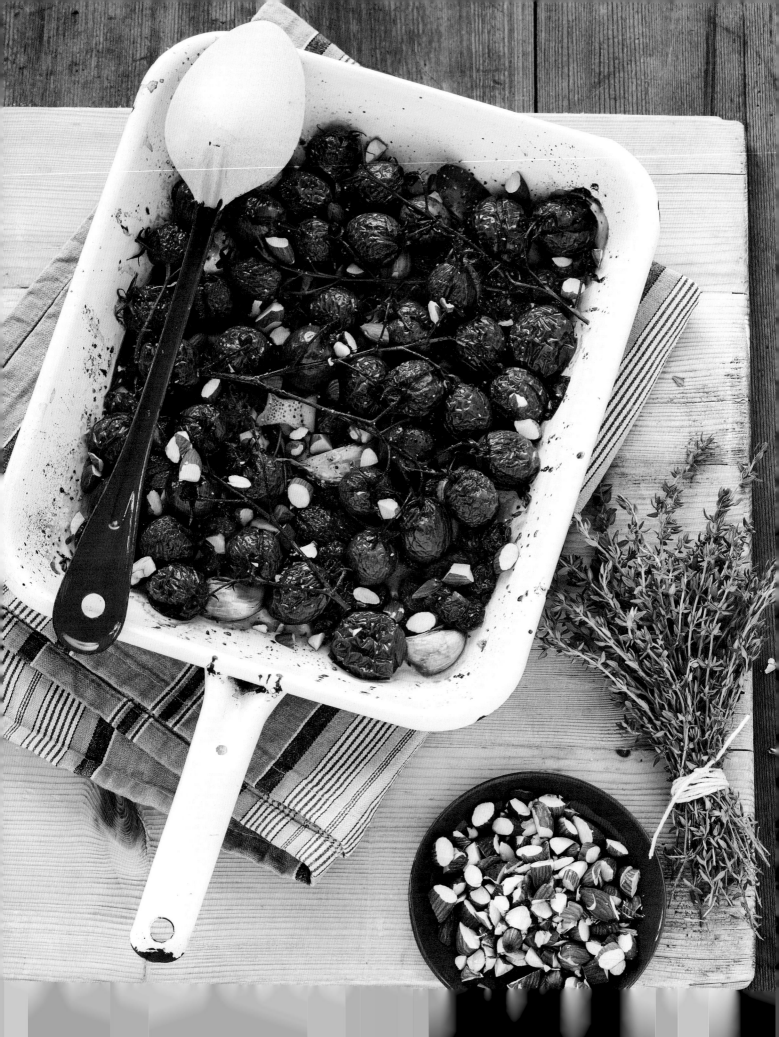

Glazed tomatoes with raisins, almonds and garlic

The humble tomato takes a starring role in this spectacular rustic dish that combines the flavors of herbs, lemon and garlic to create a great accompaniment to roasted meats.

PREPARATION **10 MINUTES, PLUS OVERNIGHT SOAKING**
COOKING **30 MINUTES**
SERVES **4 AS A SIDE DISH**

½ cup (65 g) large golden raisins
4 long sprigs fresh oregano
4 long sprigs fresh thyme
4 bay leaves
1 lemon
8 cloves garlic, unpeeled
2 tablespoons (30 ml) extra virgin olive oil
1 tablespoon (15 ml) molasses or
    maple syrup
freshly ground black pepper
1 pound (500 g) small tomatoes on the vine,
    such as cherry or baby plum tomatoes
¼ cup (60 g) raw almonds, roughly chopped

1 Soak the raisins in boiling water for at least 2 hours, preferably overnight.

2 Preheat the oven to 425°F (220°C).

3 Arrange the oregano, thyme and bay leaves in a shallow roasting pan to make a nest for the tomatoes. Using a small, sharp knife, cut off the lemon rind in strips and add to the pan. Juice the lemon and set aside.

4 Using the flat side of a large knife, lightly crush the garlic cloves so that the skins split. Scatter the garlic over the herb mixture. Drain the raisins and arrange over the garlic.

5 In a large bowl, combine the lemon juice, olive oil and molasses or maple syrup with a generous grinding of black pepper. Gently toss the tomatoes in the dressing until they are well coated, and arrange in the roasting pan. Pour the remaining dressing over the top.

6 Bake the tomatoes for 30 minutes, until they are split and softened, occasionally basting with the cooking juices. Serve sprinkled with the chopped almonds.

EACH SERVING PROVIDES
264 calories, 5 g protein, 18 g fat (2 g saturated fat),
23 g carbohydrate (20 g sugars), 6 g fiber, 26 mg sodium

Tomatoes contain powerful antioxidants that may help to protect against dementia. Cooking the tomatoes makes these antioxidants much more available for your body to absorb.

Baked stuffed peppers with herbed ricotta and tomato

This colorful dish celebrates the ripe flavors of summer with a combination of peppers, tomatoes, garlic and basil. Serve it as a side dish, or add whole-grain bread for a lovely light meal.

PREPARATION **10 MINUTES**
COOKING **30 MINUTES**
SERVES **6 AS A SIDE DISH**

6 baby red peppers, or 3 large red peppers,
   about 1 pound (500 g) total
4 cloves garlic, crushed
6 red cherry tomatoes, halved
1/3 cup (75 ml) extra virgin olive oil
1 cup (200 g) dry ricotta
1/4 cup (25 g) finely grated parmesan,
   plus extra to serve
2 large sprigs fresh basil (about 16 leaves),
   finely chopped
freshly ground black pepper

1   Preheat the oven to 300°F (150°C).

2   Remove the cores and seeds from the peppers. Arrange the peppers in an ovenproof dish and sprinkle the garlic inside.

3   Fit two tomato halves inside each pepper, with the cut surfaces facing upwards. Drizzle with the olive oil.

4   Put the ricotta in a bowl, add the parmesan and basil, and mix until well combined. Divide the mixture among the peppers, pressing it on top of the tomato halves.

5   Bake the peppers for 20 minutes, and sprinkle the tops with the extra parmesan and some freshly ground black pepper. Bake for another 10 minutes, until the tops are golden. Serve immediately.

If you are using large peppers, cut each pepper in half lengthwise so that the halves lie flat, cutting right through the stem. Remove the core and seeds, leaving the stem intact.

Use ready-made dry ricotta or use one-half of the ricotta recipe on page 129. Avoid using the wet ricotta sold in tubs.

Serve the peppers with some crusty whole-grain bread for mopping up the juices.

EACH SERVING PROVIDES
197 calories, 6 g protein, 17 g fat (5 g saturated fat),
5 g carbohydrate (4 g sugars), 2 g fiber, 117 mg sodium

Plants from the *basil* family have been used for centuries in herbal remedies thought to enhance brain function. Basil is now known to contain powerful antioxidants that can reduce inflammation and improve blood flow to the brain.

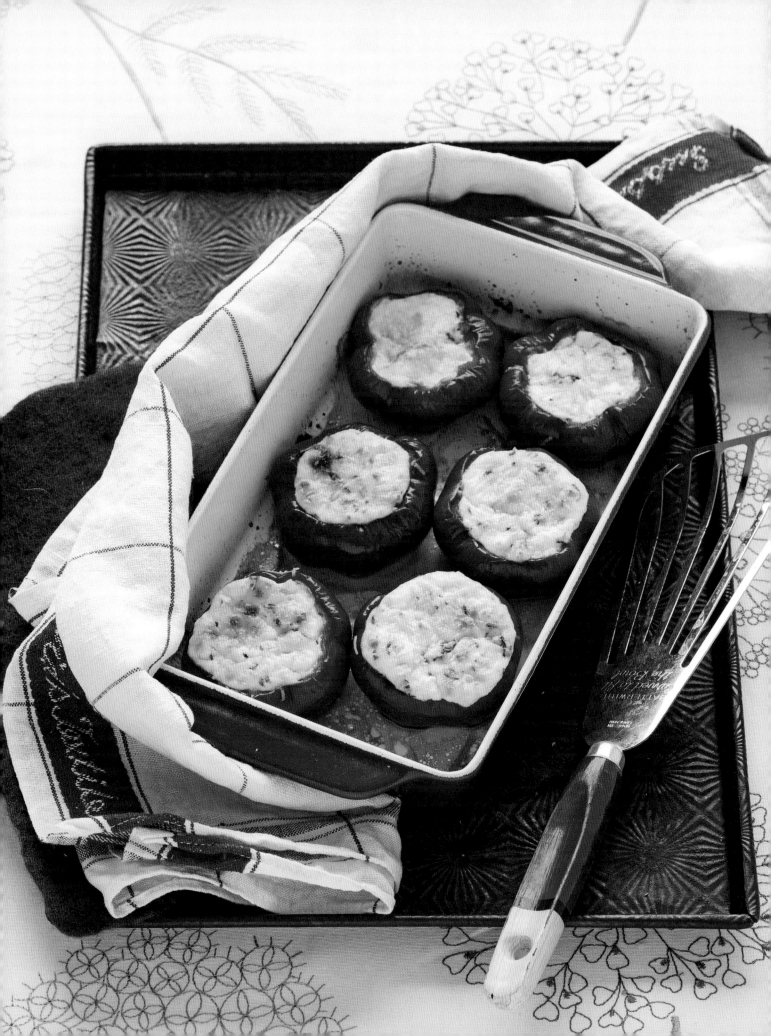

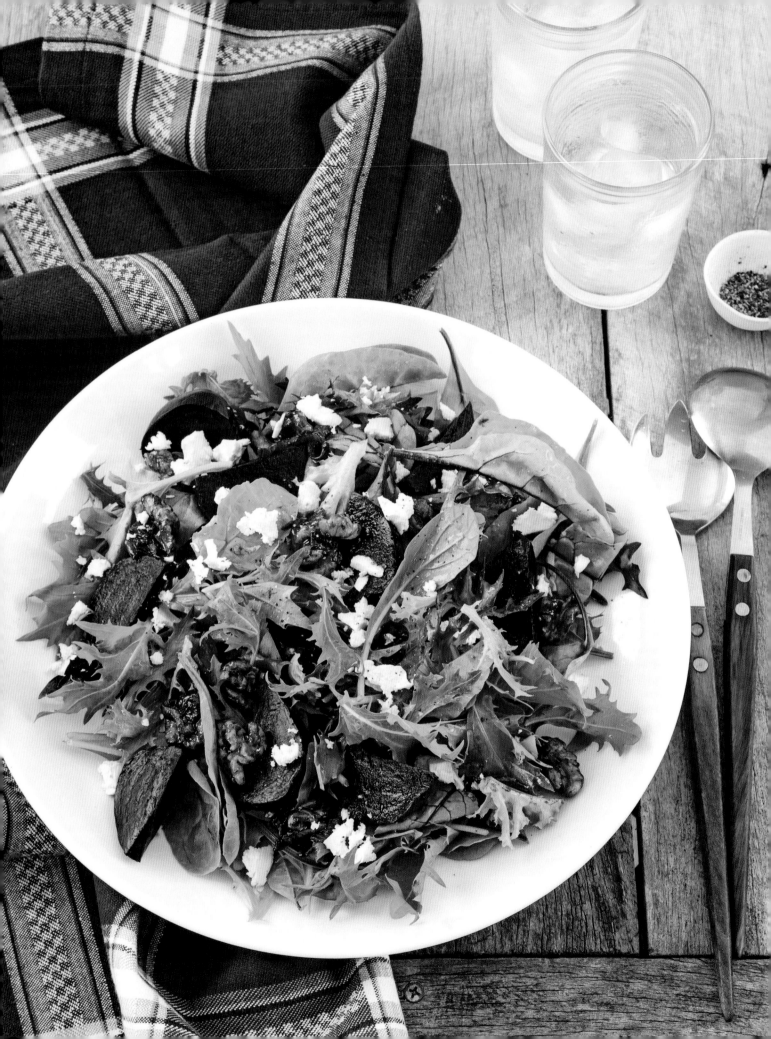

Baked beets with balsamic-glazed shallots, walnuts and feta

Beets become succulently sweet when slowly roasted in the oven. In this salad, roasted beets are combined with caramelized shallots, crunchy walnuts and creamy feta.

PREPARATION **10 MINUTES**
COOKING **1 HOUR**
SERVES **4 AS A SIDE DISH**

6 small red or yellow beets, about ³/₄ pound (400 g) total
¹/₂ cup (50 g) walnut halves
1 tablespoon (15 ml) olive oil
4 shallots, peeled and sliced
¹/₄ cup (50 ml) balsamic vinegar
1 tablespoon (15 ml) brown sugar
2 cups (about 80 g) mixed salad leaves
²/₃ cup (100 g) crumbled low-fat feta
freshly ground black pepper

1 Preheat the oven to 400°F (200°C). Wrap the beets in foil and bake for 1 hour, until tender.

2 Meanwhile, toast the walnuts in a dry saucepan, stirring constantly, until lightly browned all over. Transfer to a plate and set aside.

3 Add the oil to the saucepan and gently cook the shallots over low heat, stirring occasionally, for 15–20 minutes, until dark brown and caramelized. Add the vinegar and brown sugar, and bring to a boil. Stir in the walnuts to coat them with the balsamic glaze.

4 Peel the cooled beets (the skins should just slip off) and cut them into halves or quarters. Combine the beets with the shallot and walnut mixture.

5 Serve the salad greens on a large platter, topped with the beet mixture. Pour any balsamic glaze remaining in the pan over the salad. Sprinkle the crumbled feta on top and season with freshly ground black pepper.

EACH SERVING PROVIDES
262 calories, 11 g protein, 17 g fat (4 g saturated fat), 16 g carbohydrate (16 g sugars), 4 g fiber, 360 mg sodium

Beets are considered one of nature's brain superfoods, providing a rich source of vitamins and minerals, with high levels of antioxidants and natural nitrates that improve performance and blood flow to the brain.

Quinoa pilaf with almonds and sesame seeds

Quinoa is a nutritious, high-protein seed grain. Here it's used to make a warm pilaf that's great on its own, as a salad or used as an accompaniment to curries and stews.

PREPARATION **10 MINUTES**   COOKING **35 MINUTES**   SERVES **4 AS A SIDE DISH**

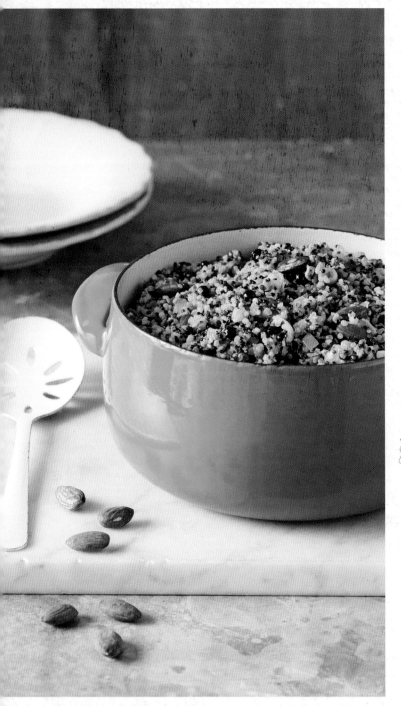

1 cup (200 g) quinoa
$^1/_4$ cup (40 g) sesame seeds
2 tablespoons (30 ml) canola or olive oil
1 small onion, finely chopped
2 cloves garlic, crushed
2 cups (500 ml) low-sodium vegetable stock
$^1/_4$ cup (35 g) currants
$^2/_3$ cup (100 g) raw almonds
1 scallion, sliced

1   Put the quinoa in a fine sieve and rinse under cold water; let drain.

2   Toast the sesame seeds in a large, dry saucepan, stirring constantly until they are golden all over. Remove from the pan and set aside.

3   Add the oil to the pan and cook the onion over low heat for 10 minutes, until just colored. Add the garlic and cook for another 3–4 minutes, until just starting to color.

4   Stir in the quinoa, stock, currants, almonds and toasted sesame seeds, and bring to a boil. Cover, reduce the heat to low and simmer for 15 minutes, until the quinoa is tender.

5   Stir the scallion into the pilaf and serve.

This pilaf looks gorgeous made with a mixture of white, red and black quinoa.

EACH SERVING PROVIDES
468 calories, 14 g protein, 31 g fat (6 g saturated fat), 33 g carbohydrate (5 g sugars), 7 g fiber, 520 mg sodium

Healthy fats from nuts, seeds and grains help maintain the brain's blood supply. *Quinoa* is known as the "super grain" because it provides complete protein, and it is higher in unsaturated fat and lower in carbohydrate than other grains.

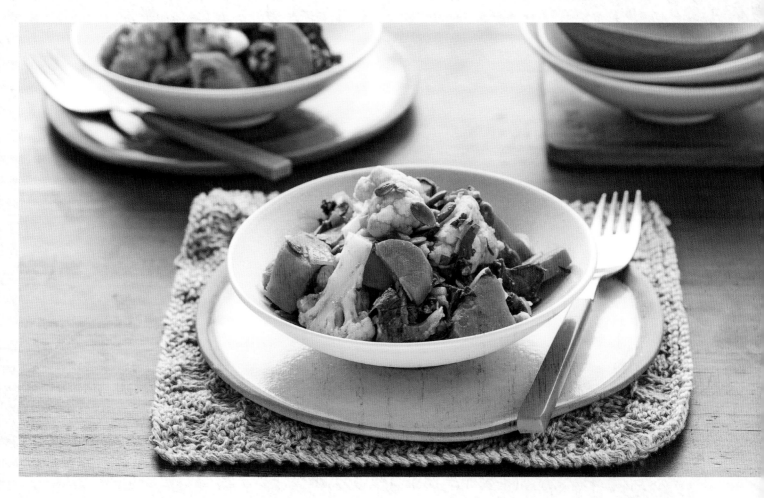

Spiced vegetable medley

The warm and aromatic cardamom seeds add a delicate hint of spice to the tender vegetables. Serve sprinkled with toasted pumpkin seeds.

PREPARATION **20 MINUTES**   COOKING **25 MINUTES**   SERVES **4 AS A SIDE DISH**

2 tablespoons (30 ml) olive or canola oil
1 onion, chopped
1 celery stalk, sliced
2 carrots, halved and sliced
4 cloves garlic, crushed
seeds from 10 green cardamom pods
1 tablespoon (15 ml) ground coriander
$^1/_2$ pound (250 g) sweet potatoes, chopped
$^1/_2$ cup (125 g) cauliflower florets,
   cut into quarters
$^1/_2$ cup (125 g) spinach, shredded
finely grated zest of 1 lemon
$^2/_3$ cup (30 g) chopped fresh cilantro leaves

1   Heat the oil in a large saucepan over medium–high heat. Add the onion, celery, carrots, garlic and cardamom seeds. Stir, cover and cook for 3 minutes. Sprinkle in the ground coriander. Cover and cook for 3 minutes.

2   Add the sweet potatoes and $^3/_4$ cup (175 ml) boiling water, cover and bring to a boil. Reduce the heat and simmer for 10 minutes. Add the cauliflower and cook for 8 minutes, until all the vegetables are tender.

3   Add the spinach and cook, stirring, for 1 minute, until the spinach has wilted. Stir in the lemon zest and chopped cilantro, and serve hot.

EACH SERVING PROVIDES

165 calories, 4 g protein, 10 g fat (1 g saturated fat), 16 g carbohydrate (7 g sugars), 6 g fiber, 48 mg sodium

Spinach contains colorful carotenoids named lutein, zeaxanthin and beta-carotene that are great for eye health and brain function.

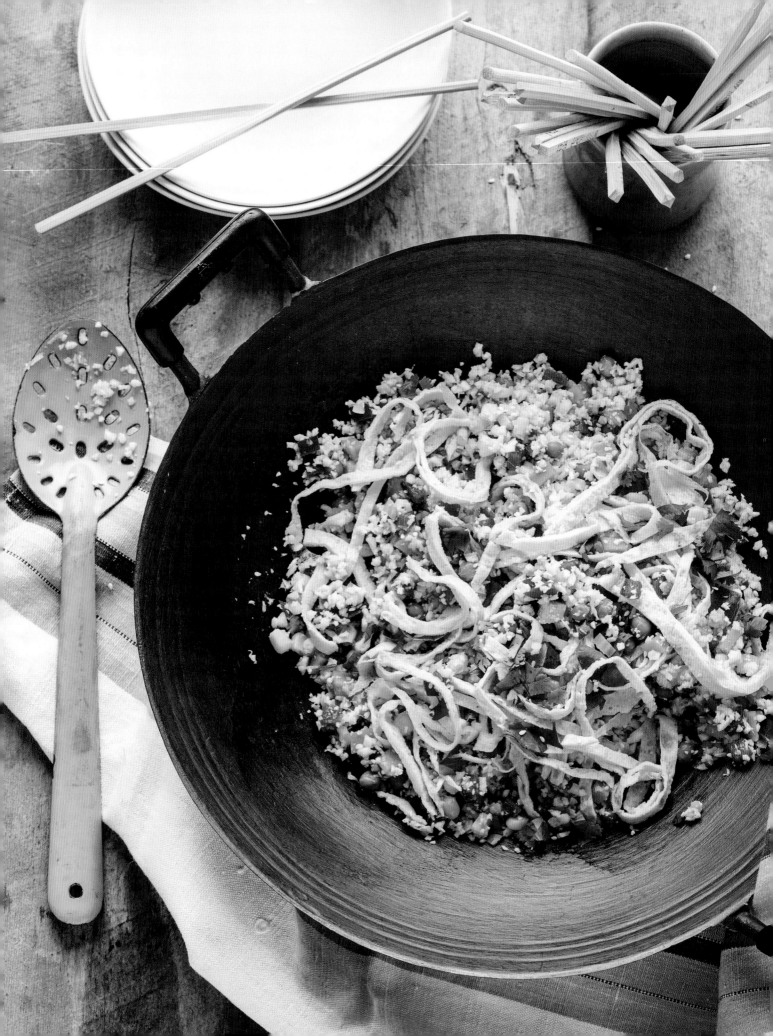

Cauliflower fried rice

No rice is used in this dish—the cauliflower is cut to resemble grains of rice. If you don't have a food processor, use a sharp knife to shave the cauliflower into thin slices, then chop it into rice-sized pieces.

PREPARATION **15 MINUTES**
COOKING **15 MINUTES**
SERVES **4 AS A SIDE DISH**

²/₃ pound (300 g) cauliflower, cut into florets
2 tablespoons (15 ml) rice bran oil
2 eggs, lightly beaten
2 scallions, thinly sliced
1 tablespoon (15 ml) grated fresh ginger
1 celery stalk, diced
1 red pepper, diced
2 carrots, diced
²/₃ cup (100 g) peas
¹/₂ cup (100 g) corn kernels
¹/₂ cup (125 ml) low-sodium chicken stock
1 tablespoon (15 ml) low-sodium soy sauce
few drops of sesame oil
2 tablespoons (30 ml) chopped fresh
    cilantro leaves
2 tablespoons (30 ml) toasted sesame seeds

1   Put the cauliflower in a food processor. Using the pulse button, process in short bursts to chop the cauliflower into small pieces, roughly the size of rice.

2   Heat half the oil in a wok over medium heat, add the eggs and swirl to coat the base of the wok. Cook until set around the edges, then turn and cook the other side. Transfer the omelet to a plate to cool slightly, and cut into thin strips.

3   Heat the remaining oil in the wok and add the scallions, ginger, celery, pepper and carrots. Stir-fry for 5 minutes, until the carrots are just soft. Add the peas, corn, cauliflower, stock, soy sauce and sesame oil. Stir-fry for 5 minutes, until the cauliflower is soft.

4   Remove the wok from the heat and fold in the omelet strips, cilantro and toasted sesame seeds.

Use canola or peanut oil if you don't have rice bran oil.

EACH SERVING PROVIDES
221 calories, 10 g protein, 15 g fat (3 g saturated fat),
12 g carbohydrate (6 g sugars), 6 g fiber, 336 mg sodium

Cauliflower is an excellent source of vitamin K, a key part of the body's anti-inflammatory system. Vitamin K acts in the body's early response to inflammation, protecting the brain and cardiovascular system from damage.

Brain-boosting dips

These nutritious dips feature great flavors with a fraction of the fat, salt and preservatives often found in store-bought dips. Serve them with cut-up fresh vegetables or with oven-baked wedges of whole-wheat pitas or corn tortillas.

Edamame bean dip

1 cup (165 g) shelled edamame
$^{1}/_{2}$ cup (130 g) silken tofu
$2^{1}/_{2}$ teaspoons (12 ml) soy sauce
$1^{1}/_{2}$ teaspoons (7 ml) sesame oil
$^{1}/_{2}$ teaspoon (2 ml) wasabi

Cook the edamame in a saucepan of boiling water for 5 minutes. Drain and rinse under cold running water, then drain well. Put the edamame and tofu in a food processor and process until combined. Add the soy sauce, sesame oil and wasabi, and process until well combined and almost smooth, occasionally stopping to scrape down the side of the bowl. Transfer to a small serving bowl.

SERVES 4 (MAKES 1 CUP/250 g)

Chunky avocado and tomato dip

1 large avocado
1 tablespoon (15 ml) lime juice
2 tomatoes, seeded and diced
2 scallions, thinly sliced
2 tablespoons (30 ml) roughly chopped
  fresh cilantro leaves
pinch of cayenne pepper

Cut the avocado in half and remove the pit. Dice the flesh and immediately toss with the lime juice. Add the tomatoes, scallions, chopped cilantro and cayenne pepper. Gently toss to combine. Serve the dip immediately.

SERVES 6 (MAKES $2^{1}/_{2}$ CUPS/625 g)

Beet hummus

5 baby beets, about 1 pound (500 g) total
$^{1}/_{2}$ teaspoon (2 ml) ground cumin
15 ounce (425 ml) can chickpeas, rinsed, drained
2 cloves garlic, chopped
2 tablespoons (30 ml) tahini
2–3 tablespoons (30–45 ml) lemon juice, to taste

Scrub the beets and trim the stems to 1 inch (2.5 cm). Place in a large saucepan of boiling water and cook, partially covered, for 40 minutes, until very tender when pierced with a skewer. Drain and let cool slightly. When cool enough to handle, slip off the skins from the beets. Roughly chop the flesh and place in a food processor. Toast the cumin in a small, dry frying pan over medium heat, stirring, for 1 minute, until fragrant. Add the chickpeas, garlic, tahini, lemon juice and cumin to the food processor, and process until smooth and well combined. Transfer to a serving bowl. Cover and refrigerate until ready to serve.

SERVES 6 (MAKES $2^{1}/_{2}$ CUPS/625 g)

Asparagus guacamole

1 pound (500 g) asparagus spears, trimmed and
    chopped into small pieces
1 small brown (yellow) onion, chopped
1 clove garlic, halved
1 tablespoon (15 ml) lemon juice
1 large tomato, seeded and finely chopped
2 tablespoons (30 ml) low-fat mayonnaise
1 tablespoon (15 ml) finely chopped fresh
    cilantro or parsley
$1/4$ teaspoon (1 ml) chili powder
4 drops chili sauce or Tabasco
freshly ground black pepper

Pour $3/4$ inch (2 cm) of water into a saucepan and add
the asparagus. Bring to a boil, reduce the heat, cover
and simmer for 3–5 minutes, until tender. Drain the
asparagus and transfer to a food processor, along
with the onion, garlic and lemon juice. Process
until smooth, adding 2 tablespoons (30 ml) water if
needed. Combine the tomato, mayonnaise, cilantro
or parsley, chili powder and chili sauce or Tabasco in
a bowl. Stir in the asparagus mixture until blended.
Season with freshly ground black pepper. Cover and
refrigerate until ready to serve. Stir the guacamole
before serving.

SERVES 6 (MAKES 2$1/2$ CUPS/625 g)

The phytoestrogens in *soy foods* appear to
have beneficial effects on heart health and brain
function. *Asparagus* is an excellent source of
folate, fiber and antioxidants important for heart
and brain health. Because asparagus contains
no fat, asparagus guacamole is a low-calorie
alternative to the avocado version.
Beets and *chickpeas* are both good
sources of folate, which the brain and blood
need for normal functioning. Folate deficiency
causes forgetfulness and insomnia. Folate is also
found in *avocado* and *cilantro*. *Avocado* is a
good source of vitamins C and E, essential
parts of the body's antioxidant system.

From left: Beet hummus; Edamame bean dip;
Chunky avocado and tomato dip

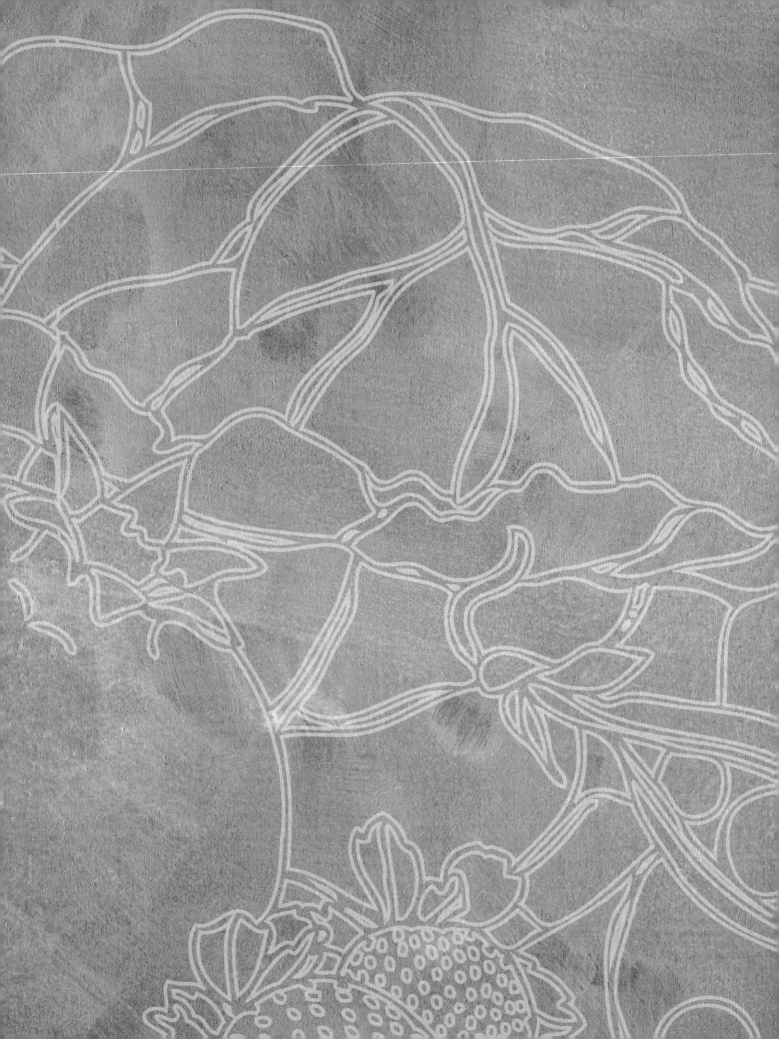

Mind-improving main dishes

Balance protein foods with the best of nature's brain-friendly ingredients.

Sesame-crusted kidney bean burgers

This is a vegetarian version of a classic that even confirmed meat lovers will enjoy. The patties are coated with sesame seeds instead of breadcrumbs for extra crunch and nutritional benefits.

PREPARATION **15 MINUTES**
COOKING **25 MINUTES**
SERVES **4**

1 tablespoon (15 ml) canola or olive oil
1 onion, finely chopped
1 small carrot, grated
3 cloves garlic, crushed
1 tablespoon (15 ml) ground cumin
2 teaspoons (10 ml) paprika
15 ounce (425 ml) can red kidney beans, rinsed and drained
$^1\!/_2$ cup (80 g) sesame seeds
4 whole-grain burger buns, toasted
lettuce, sliced beets, sliced tomatoes and sliced red onions, to serve

1   Preheat the oven to 350°F (180°C). Line a baking pan with parchment paper.

2   Heat the oil in a frying pan and cook the onion and carrot over medium heat for 3–4 minutes, until soft. Add the garlic and spices, and cook, stirring, for 1 minute. Transfer to a large bowl and let cool.

3   Add the kidney beans to the cooled onion mixture and roughly mash them with a potato masher. Shape the mixture into four patties.

4   Spread the sesame seeds on a plate. Roll the patties in the sesame seeds, gently pressing them on. Put the patties on the prepared pan and bake for 20 minutes, until heated through and the sesame seeds are lightly golden.

5   Serve each patty on a toasted bun with the lettuce, beets, tomato and red onion.

Replace the canned beans with 2 cups (500 g) cooked beans made from $^2\!/_3$ cup (140 g) dried red kidney beans.

EACH SERVING PROVIDES
377 calories, 16 g protein, 16 g fat (2 g saturated fat), 43 g carbohydrate (5 g sugars), 12 g fiber, 601 mg sodium

As well as being a good source of healthy fats, *sesame seeds* are rich in zinc, a mineral with essential roles in learning, memory and brain development.

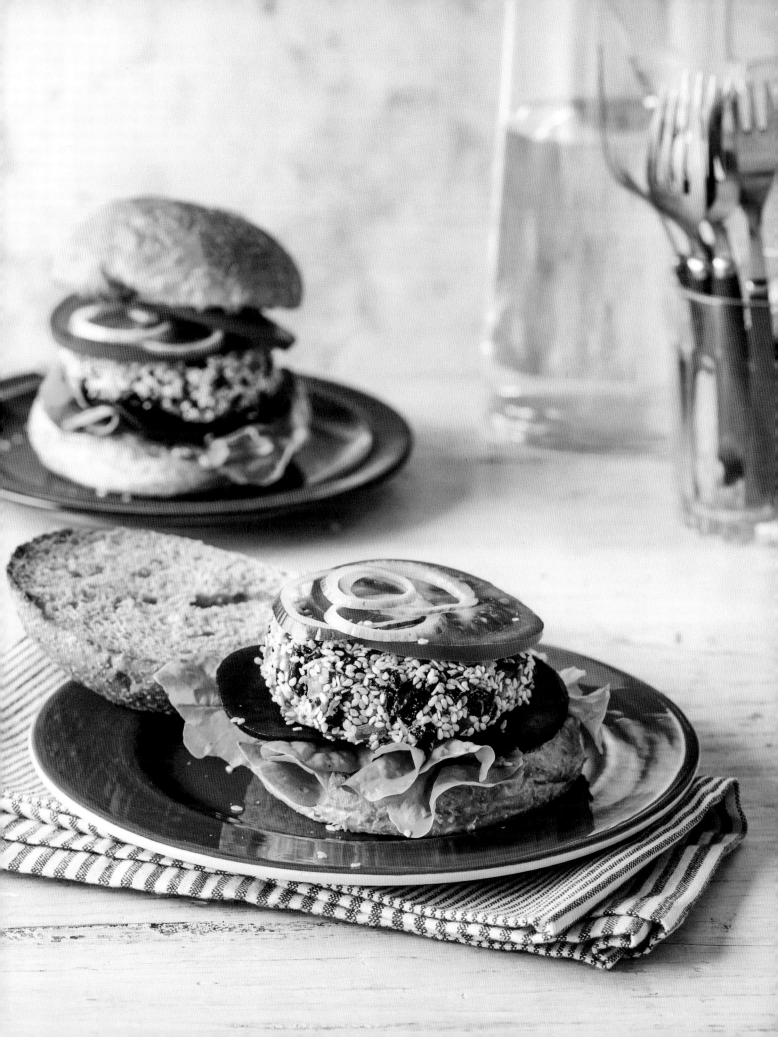

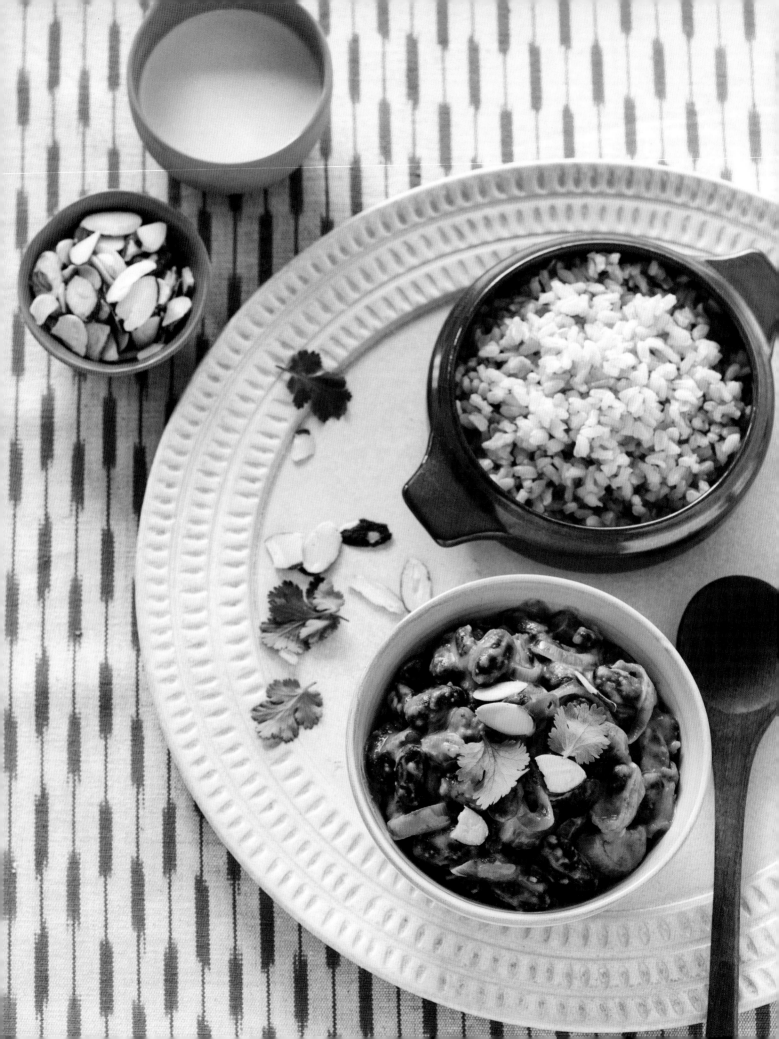

Kidney bean curry

This curry is fragrant with South Indian spices and creamy coconut milk. You can use any legume for this recipe, including other dried beans, chickpeas or lentils. Serve the curry with brown rice and steamed greens to round out the meal.

PREPARATION **15 MINUTES, PLUS OVERNIGHT SOAKING**
COOKING **1 HOUR 20 MINUTES**
SERVES **4**

$2/3$ cup (140 g) dried red kidney beans
1 tablespoon (15 ml) canola or olive oil
4 shallots, peeled and sliced
1 cinnamon stick
4 cardamom pods, crushed
4 cloves, ground
1-inch (2.5-cm) piece fresh turmeric, grated
2-inch (5-cm) piece fresh ginger, grated
1 long green chile, thinly sliced on
   the diagonal
10 curry leaves (optional)
1 cup (250 ml) low-sodium vegetable stock
$1/2$ cup (125 ml) low-fat coconut milk
8 sprigs fresh cilantro, roughly chopped
$1/4$ cup (40 g) raw almonds, sliced

1   Soak the kidney beans in cold water overnight, or for at least 5 hours. Drain and cook in plenty of fresh water for about 1 hour, until just tender. Drain and set aside.

2   Heat the oil in a large frying pan and cook the shallots over low heat for 10 minutes, until golden and translucent. Add the cinnamon stick, cardamom pods, cloves, turmeric, ginger and chile. Cook, stirring occasionally, for 5 minutes, until fragrant.

3   Add the curry leaves, if using, stock, coconut milk and kidney beans. Simmer for about 5 minutes, until thickened.

4   Serve the curry topped with the cilantro and almonds.

Replace the dried beans with a 15 ounce (425 ml) can red kidney beans, and omit step 1.

You can replace the whole spices with ground spices: Use 2 large pinches of ground cardamom, a large pinch of ground cloves and 2 teaspoons (10 ml) of ground turmeric.

EACH SERVING PROVIDES
266 calories, 11 g protein, 15 g fat (5 g saturated fat), 18 g carbohydrate (4 g sugars), 10 g fiber, 281 mg sodium

Curcumin, the active component that makes turmeric yellow, is thought to protect against some types of dementia, helping to maintain normal brain function.

Lentil moussaka

We have transformed the classic moussaka to make a vegetarian version that is lower in fat. Spinach isn't a traditional ingredient, but we've added it for extra goodness.

PREPARATION **30 MINUTES**
COOKING **1 HOUR 30 MINUTES**
SERVES **6**

1 tablespoon (15 ml) olive oil
1 onion, chopped
2 cloves garlic, crushed
14$\frac{1}{2}$ ounce (400 ml) can diced tomatoes
4 cups (1 L) low-sodium vegetable stock
2 cups (370 g) dried brown or French-style
  puy lentils, rinsed and drained
1 teaspoon (5 ml) dried oregano
$\frac{1}{2}$ teaspoon (2 ml) ground allspice
$\frac{1}{4}$ teaspoon (1 ml) ground cinnamon
2 large eggplants, about 1$\frac{2}{3}$ pounds (800 g)
  total, cut into $\frac{1}{2}$ inch (1-cm) slices
olive oil spray
$\frac{2}{3}$ pound (350 g) spinach
2 tablespoons (30 ml) tomato paste
freshly ground black pepper
2 cups (500 ml) low-fat Greek-style yogurt
2 eggs
$\frac{1}{4}$ cup (30 g) grated low-fat cheddar
paprika, for dusting

1 Heat the oil in a large saucepan. Cook the onion over medium heat, stirring occasionally, for 5 minutes, until soft and golden. Add the garlic and cook, stirring, for 30 seconds.

2 Stir in the diced tomatoes, stock, lentils, oregano, allspice and cinnamon, cover and bring to a boil. Reduce the heat to medium–low, cover and cook, stirring occasionally, for 55 minutes, until the lentils are tender.

3 Meanwhile, heat a large, heavy-bottom frying pan over medium heat. Spray the eggplant with olive oil and cook in batches for 2 minutes on each side, until softened and lightly golden. Set aside to cool.

4 Preheat the oven to 400°F (200°C). Lightly grease an 8 x 11 x 2$\frac{1}{2}$ inch (20 x 28 x 6 cm) baking dish.

5 Cut the spinach leaves from the stems; discard the stems. Thoroughly wash and dry the leaves, roughly chop them and add to the lentils with the tomato paste. Stir until the spinach has wilted. Season with freshly ground black pepper.

6 Use half the eggplant to make a layer on the bottom of the prepared dish, with the slices slightly overlapping. Spread half the lentil mixture over the eggplant. Repeat with the remaining eggplant and lentils.

7 Whisk the yogurt and eggs together, and spread over the lentils. Sprinkle with the cheese and lightly dust with paprika. Bake for 30 minutes, until the topping is set and lightly golden. Let stand for 15 minutes before serving.

EACH SERVING PROVIDES
405 calories, 30 g protein, 12 g fat (4 g saturated fat),
46 g carbohydrate (18 g sugars), 15 g fiber, 980 mg sodium

Lentils easily replace part or all of the ground beef in many family favorites, adding nutritients and fiber, and also reducing the fat and the cost.

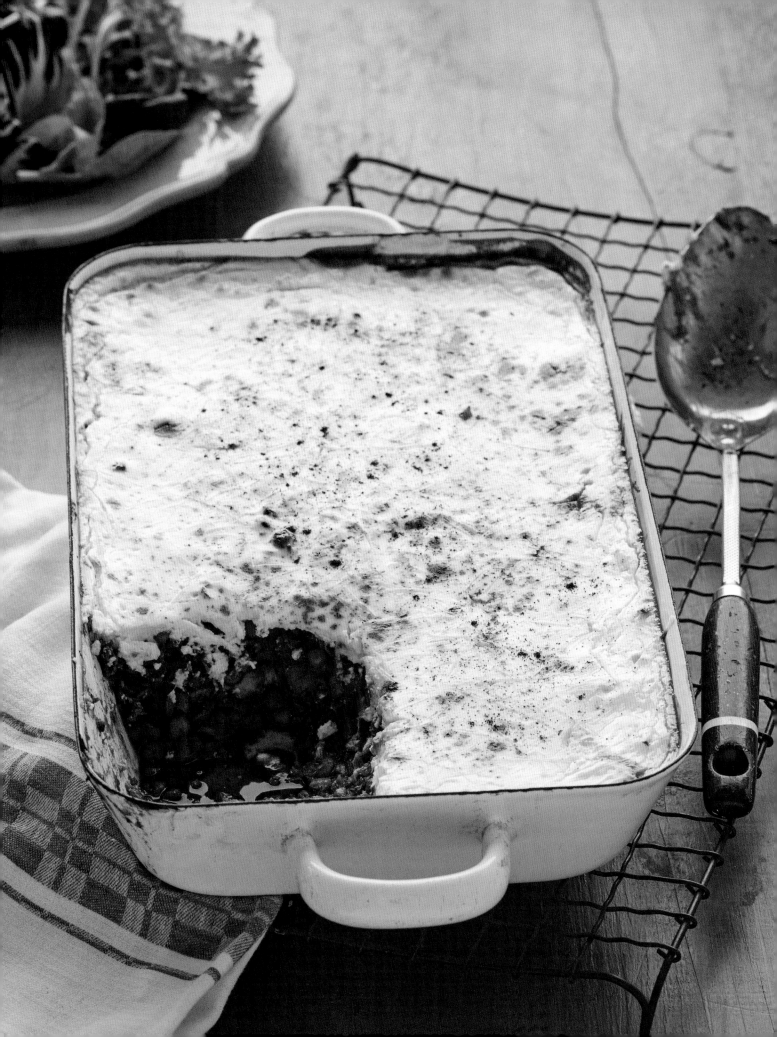

Whole grains

Whole grains appear to protect against cardiac disease and some cancers, and this is thought to be due to their high content of fiber, antioxidants and beneficial fats.

The outside layer of a grain—the bran and the germ—are removed during processing to make white rice and white flour. Whole grains still have this outside layer, which contains most of the fiber and many of the nutrients, and these are missing when whole grains are refined into white flour. For example, the bran and germ contain almost 90 percent of a grain's thiamine, which is lost during milling. Thiamine is needed for the body to metabolize carbohydrate, fat and protein to produce energy. It is essential for neurotransmission, and the effects of thiamine deficiency include neurological problems and brain damage. Processing also removes half of the grain's selenium and folate, three-quarters of the zinc, and 80 percent of the niacin.

Unprocessed grains contain significantly higher amounts of protective plant substances, such as phytoestrogens, which help to modify inflammation, maintain digestive function and keep cholesterol levels low for a healthy cardiovascular system to fuel the brain. By avoiding processed white grains and flours, and using whole-grain and whole-wheat products, you can boost your intake of important vitamins, minerals and antioxidants, as well as beneficial fats found in bran and wheat germ. Whole-grain foods include brown rice, wheatberries, rolled oats, multigrained and/or seeded bread, popcorn and quinoa. To buy whole-grain foods, look for the word "whole" in the ingredients list of cereal grain products. Watch out for products that have been colored brown and those that say "wheat flour," which just means white flour.

Clockwise from bottom left: freekeh, fine brown bulgur, rolled oats, red quinoa, popping corn, pearl barley, cornmeal or polenta, white quinoa, brown rice, black quinoa

You can also increase the whole-grain content of your diet by substituting whole-wheat flour for some of the white flour in recipes. Not all recipes are suitable for this: For example, delicate pastries, light airy cakes and some sauces can become heavy or gluey from the extra fiber of whole-wheat flour. However, whole-wheat flour works well in many cookies, puddings, pastas and fruity or nutty cakes. You may need to experiment to find the ideal proportions. Try swapping half of the white flour for whole-wheat flour in the recipe—you can decide to use more (or less) whole-wheat flour in the recipe next time. You may also need to increase the liquid part of the recipe, as the fiber in the whole-wheat flour will absorb more moisture than white flour.

Recently there has been debate about whether we should be following a very low carbohydrate diet in order to minimize the risk of dementia. The theory behind this suggestion is that increased blood glucose levels promote inflammatory changes in the brain, increasing the risk of cell damage and dementia. It would then stand to reason that minimizing blood glucose levels by avoiding carbohydrate should minimize dementia risk. However, epidemiologists point to studies of populations following plant-based diets that have a very low dementia risk while consuming quite large amounts of carbohydrate. The key seems to be controlling blood glucose levels by eating foods with a low glycemic index (GI), and plenty of plant foods. In general, whole-grain foods have a lower GI than refined foods, and they also provide other beneficial substances that decrease the risk of dementia. Instead of completely avoiding carbohydrate foods, enjoy more whole-grain foods while avoiding processed carbohydrates.

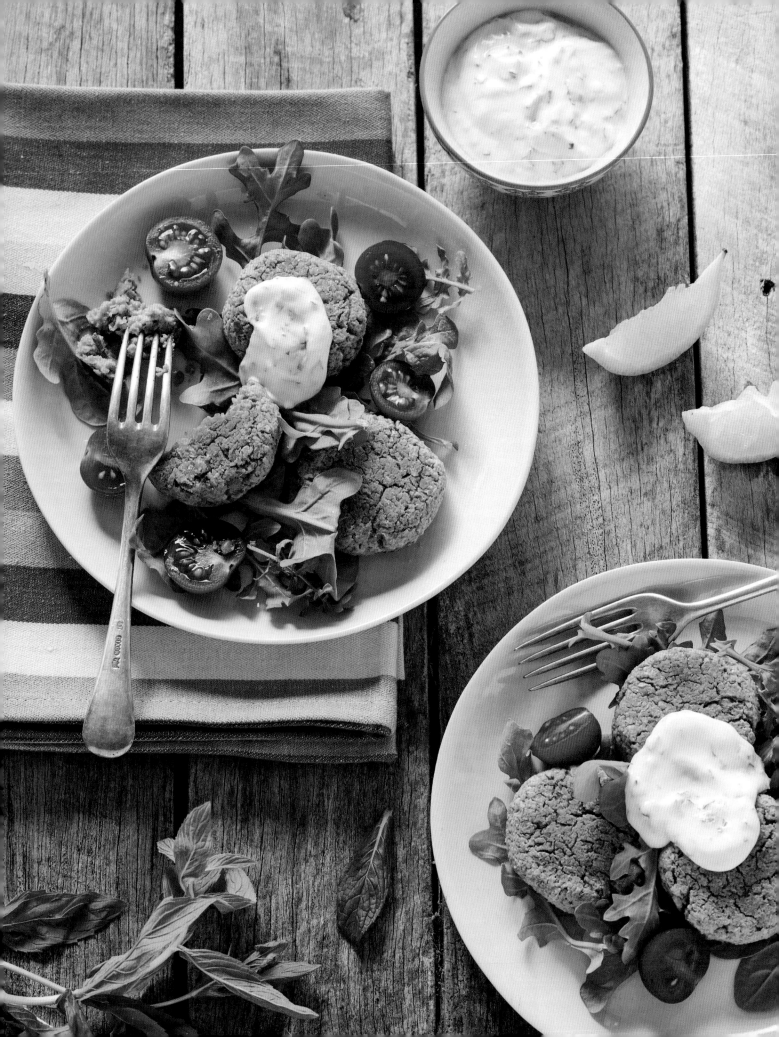

Oven-baked chickpea patties

These delicately spiced patties are very versatile. Serve them with a salad or couscous for a main meal, put them on a whole-grain bun for a burger, or shape them into bite-sized rounds to make healthy finger food or lunchbox snacks.

PREPARATION **20 MINUTES**
COOKING **25 MINUTES**
SERVES **4 (MAKES 12)**

3 teaspoons (15 ml) olive oil
4 scallions, thinly sliced
2 cloves garlic, crushed
1 teaspoon (5 ml) ground cumin
1 teaspoon (5 ml) ground coriander
$\frac{1}{2}$ teaspoon (2 ml) ground turmeric
2 cans chickpeas, 15 ounces (425 ml) each, rinsed and drained
$\frac{1}{4}$ cup (65 g) tahini
olive oil spray
$\frac{1}{3}$ cup (75 ml) low-fat Greek-style yogurt
2 tablespoons (30 ml) fresh mint leaves, finely chopped
$\frac{1}{4}$ cup (60 g) baby arugula
1 cup (250 g) red cherry tomatoes, halved
lemon wedges, to serve

1   Preheat the oven to 400°F (200°C). Lightly oil a large baking pan.

2   Heat the olive oil in a small frying pan. Cook the scallions over medium–low heat for 3 minutes, until soft. Stir in the garlic and spices, and cook for 30 seconds, until fragrant. Set aside.

3   Put the chickpeas, spice mixture and tahini in a food processor. Process until combined and almost smooth, occasionally stopping and scraping down the side of the bowl with a spatula. Shape the mixture into 12 patties.

4   Arrange the patties on the prepared pan. Spray with olive oil and bake, turning once, for 20 minutes, until golden brown.

5   Combine the yogurt and mint in a small bowl.

6   Divide the arugula and tomatoes among serving plates and add the patties. Serve with a dollop of mint yogurt, and lemon wedges for squeezing.

Replace the canned chickpeas with 4 cups (1 kg) cooked chickpeas made from 1$\frac{1}{3}$ cups (300 g) dried chickpeas.

EACH SERVING (3 PATTIES) PROVIDES
304 calories, 14 g protein, 18 g fat (3 g saturated fat),
22 g carbohydrate (5 g sugars), 10 g fiber, 356 mg sodium

Chickpeas make this a high-protein, high-fiber dish, with a low glycemic index for long-lasting brain fuel. Adding tahini and yogurt helps to make a complete protein.

Thai-style mussels with chile and basil

The flavors of lemongrass, basil, chile and coconut milk come together in this quick and easy recipe. If you want a more substantial meal, serve the mussels with steamed brown rice and a crunchy Thai-style green salad.

PREPARATION **15 MINUTES**
COOKING **15 MINUTES**
SERVES **4**

4 pounds (2 kg) mussels
1 tablespoon (15 ml) canola oil
1/4 cup (75 g) shallots, finely chopped
2 cloves garlic, finely chopped
1 small red chile, seeded and
    finely chopped
1 lemongrass stem, white part only,
    thinly sliced
1 cup (250 ml) low-sodium fish or
    vegetable stock
1/2 cup (125 ml) low-fat coconut milk
1/4 cup (15 g) firmly packed fresh
    basil, shredded
lime wedges, to serve

1 Scrub the mussels and pull out the beards. Discard any broken mussels, or open ones that don't close when tapped. Rinse well and set aside.

2 Heat the oil in a large saucepan over medium heat. Cook the shallots, garlic, chile and lemongrass, stirring, for about 5 minutes, until soft and fragrant.

3 Stir in the stock and bring to a simmer. Add the mussels, cover and cook for 5 minutes. Discard any mussels that don't open. Stir in the coconut milk.

4 Transfer the mussels and liquid to a serving dish and sprinkle with the basil. Serve with the lime wedges.

For an authentic flavor, use Thai basil if you can find it in an Asian food store, but regular basil is fine.

EACH SERVING PROVIDES
183 calories, 14 g protein, 10 g fat (4 g saturated fat),
9 g carbohydrate (2 g sugars), <1 g fiber, 751 mg sodium

A great example of sustainable seafood, *mussels* are one of the best-known food sources of zinc, which helps maintain your immune system. They are also high in manganese, which aids in optimal brain functioning.

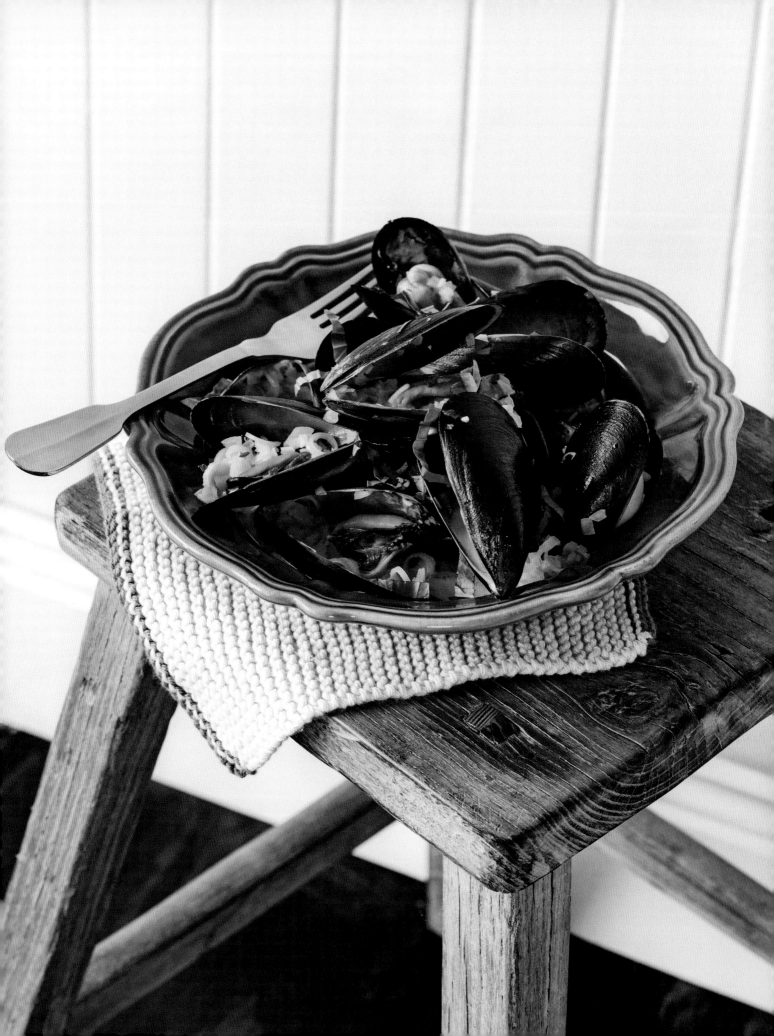

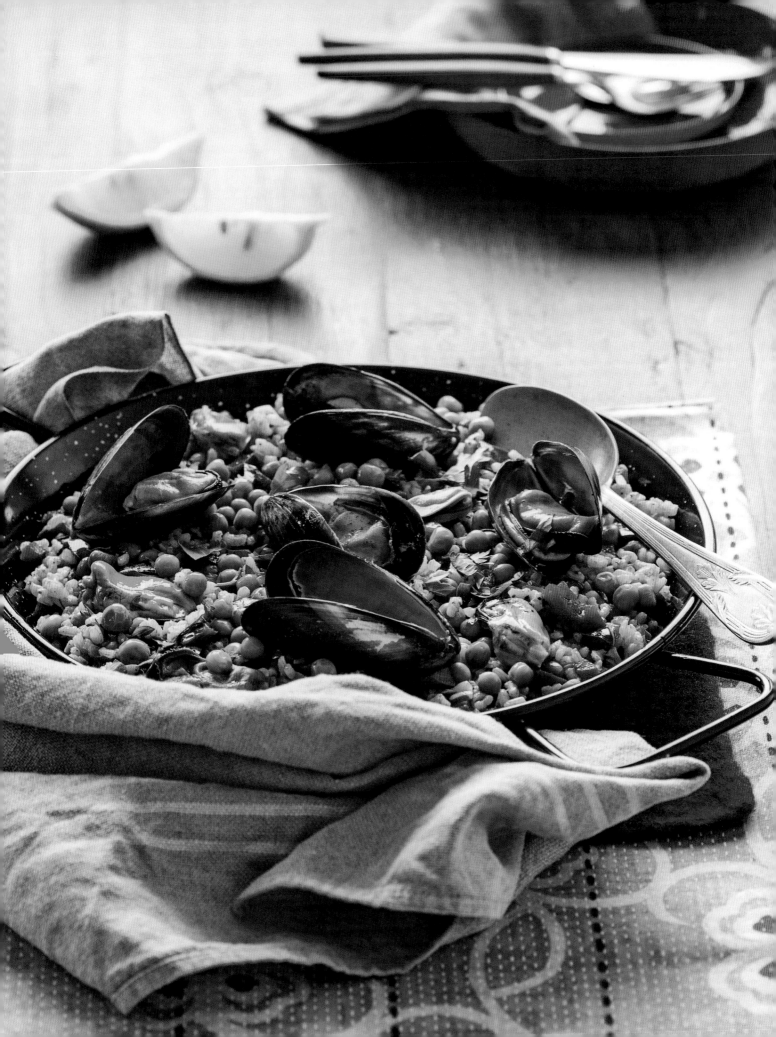

Brown rice paella with mussels and peppers

Paella is usually made with specific varieties of polished white rice that cook quickly and create a lovely texture but lack the fiber and nutrients found in brown rice. This brown rice paella has the traditional flavors of paella, but is more nutritious.

PREPARATION **20 MINUTES, PLUS 10 MINUTES STANDING**
COOKING **1 HOUR 45 MINUTES**
SERVES **6**

2 pounds (1 kg) mussels
$^1/_3$ cup (75 ml) extra virgin olive oil
1 red onion, diced
2 large red peppers, cut into short, thin strips
4 cloves garlic, crushed
1 teaspoon (5 ml) fennel seeds
1 teaspoon (5 ml) smoked paprika
3 cups (750 ml) low-sodium chicken stock
1$^1/_4$ cups (275 g) short-grain brown rice
1 cup (250 ml) white wine
large pinch of saffron threads
1 cup (155 g) peas
chopped fresh parsley, to serve
1 lemon, cut into wedges, to serve

1   Scrub the mussels and pull out the beards. Discard any broken mussels, or open ones that don't close when tapped. Rinse well and set aside.

2   Heat the oil in a 12-inch (30-cm) paella pan or a large, heavy-bottom frying pan. Cook the onion over medium heat for 5 minutes, until starting to color. Add the peppers and cook for 3 minutes. Add the garlic, fennel seeds and paprika, and cook over low heat for 2 minutes. Meanwhile, pour the stock into a saucepan and bring to a boil.

3   Stir the rice into the onion mixture until well coated. Add the wine, saffron and 2 cups (500 ml) of the hot stock, and bring to a boil.

4   Lay the mussels on top of the rice so that their openings are horizontal. As they open, transfer them to a heatproof bowl and set aside. Reduce the heat and simmer for 1 hour, stirring every 15 minutes and rotating the pan so that the paella cooks evenly. Stir in the remaining stock as needed to keep the mixture just barely wet.

5   Continue to cook the paella over low heat, rotating the pan but without any further stirring, until the rice is tender and the remaining liquid has evaporated, up to 30 minutes.

6   Scatter the peas over the top of the rice, remove the pan from the heat and tightly cover with a lid or foil. Let stand for 10 minutes before adding the mussels and sprinkling with the parsley. Serve with the lemon wedges.

You can replace the wine with extra stock. If preferred, remove some mussels from their shells and add to the paella. Reserve some in their shells for garnish. Discard any mussels that don't open when cooked.

You can use any combination of seafood, lean meats and vegetables in a paella. We use *mussels* here due to their excellent nutritional profile, rich in brain-boosting vitamin B$_{12}$ as well as healthy fats and zinc.

EACH SERVING PROVIDES
380 calories, 12 g protein, 14 g fat (2 g saturated fat), 44 g carbohydrate (5 g sugars), 4 g fiber, 568 mg sodium

Grilled salmon with sautéed greens

A simple bed of greens with a hint of lemon and garlic makes a
perfect complement to the salmon in this quick and easy dish.
Add a whole-grain side dish or bread to make a complete meal.

PREPARATION **15 MINUTES**
COOKING **10 MINUTES**
SERVES **4**

4 boneless, skinless salmon fillets,
  about 5 ounces (150 g) each
1¹/₂ tablespoons (22 ml) olive oil
2 large cloves garlic, crushed
²/₃ cup (150 g) cabbage, finely shredded
1 cup (about 200 g) kale, stems trimmed,
  finely shredded
1 cup (about 250 g) Swiss chard,
  stems trimmed, finely shredded
2 teaspoons (10 ml) toasted sesame seeds
lemon wedges, to serve

1 Preheat a grill pan over medium–high heat. Brush the
salmon fillets with 2 teaspoons (10 ml) of the olive oil and
cook for 3 minutes. Turn and cook for another 2 minutes,
until just cooked through. Transfer to a plate and let rest.

2 Heat the remaining olive oil in a large saucepan, add
the garlic and cook over medium heat for 30 seconds, until
fragrant. Add the cabbage, kale and Swiss chard, and cook,
tossing, for about 3 minutes, until wilted and tender.

3 Divide the greens among four serving plates, top with
the salmon and sprinkle with the sesame seeds. Serve the
lemon wedges on the side for squeezing.

Make sure the kale and chard are well washed. The best way
to do this is to submerge the trimmed leaves in a large bowl (or
clean sink) of cold water. Swish with your hand, and let stand
for 10 minutes. Any grit will fall to the bottom of the bowl. Drain
the leaves, and dry thoroughly in a salad spinner to remove any
remaining water.

It is easy to overcook fish, leaving it dry. Remove the fish from
the pan when it is still slightly translucent in the middle—it will
continue to cook for another 5–10 minutes, and be perfect by
the time you serve it.

EACH SERVING PROVIDES
324 calories, 33 g protein, 19 g fat (4 g saturated fat),
7 g carbohydrate (2 g sugars), 4 g fiber, 222 mg sodium

Cabbage and *kale* are members of the cruciferous
family of vegetables, which includes broccoli,
cauliflower, bok choy and brussels sprouts. These
vegetables are great sources of sulforaphane, a powerful
anti-inflammatory substance thought to protect against
degenerative conditions, such as dementia.

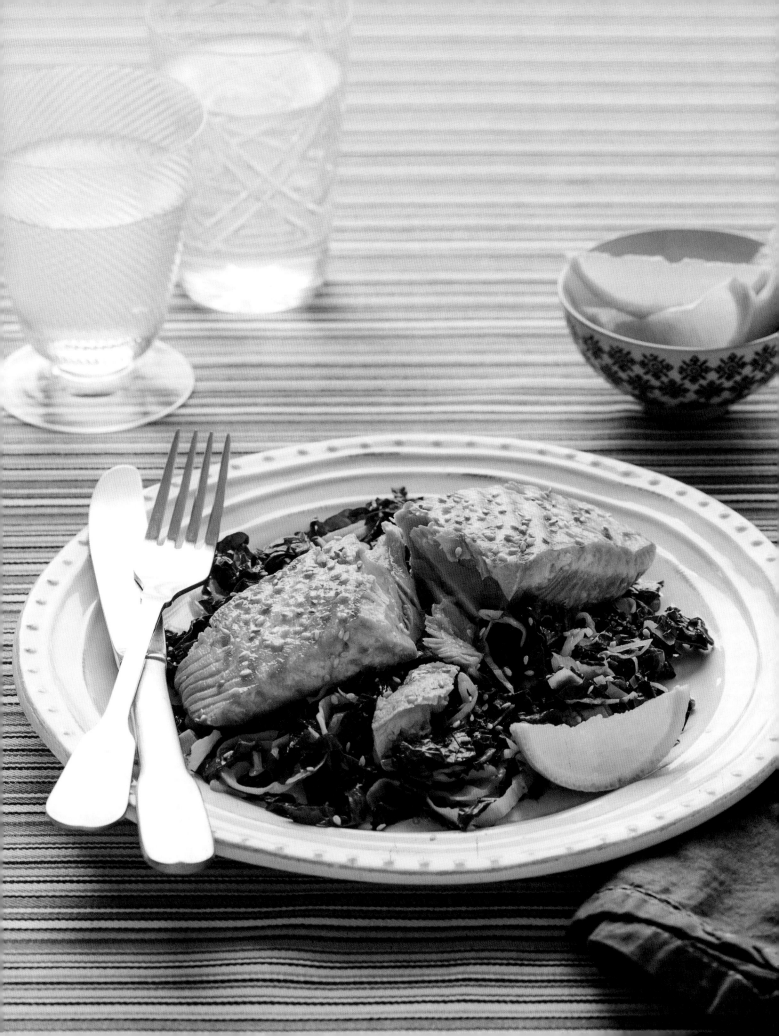

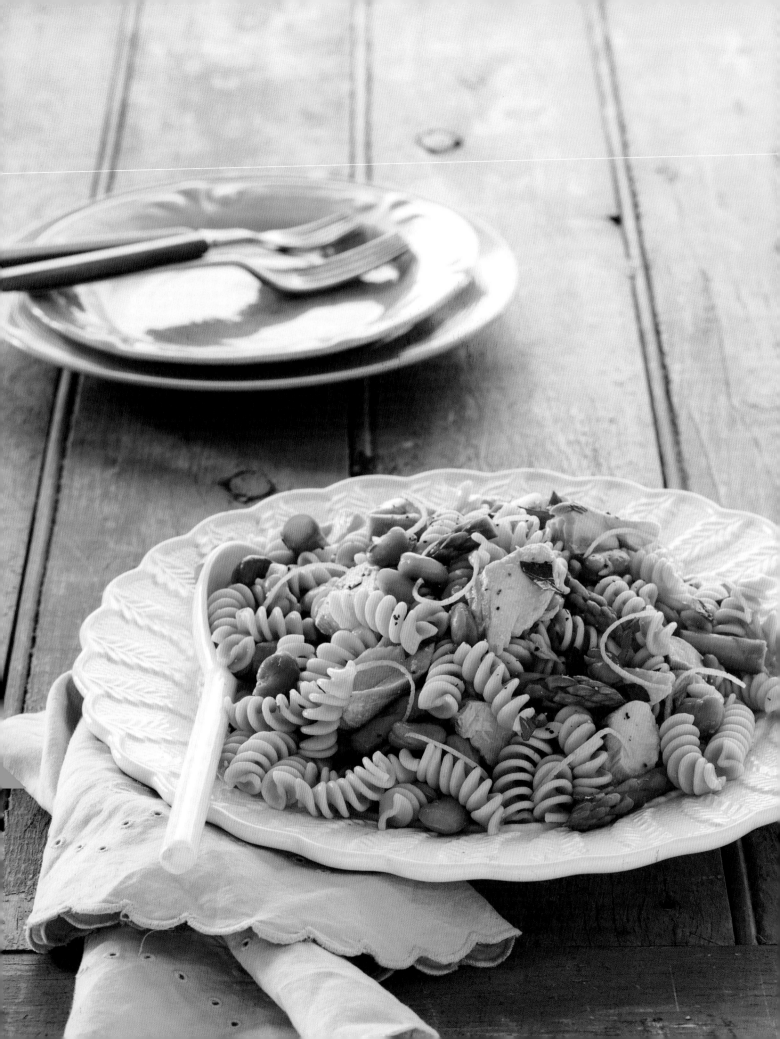

Salmon, fava bean and asparagus fusilli

This dish celebrates spring with the color and nutrients of fresh, seasonal asparagus and fava beans. It is equally good served as a warm main dish or as a cold salad.

PREPARATION **15 MINUTES**
COOKING **15 MINUTES**
SERVES **4**

12 ounces (350 g) whole-wheat fusilli
6 asparagus spears, trimmed and cut into short lengths
1¼ cups (280 g) peeled fava beans
¾ pound (400 g) boneless, skinless salmon fillets
3 teaspoons (15 ml) finely grated lemon zest
1 tablespoon (15 ml) lemon juice
1 tablespoon (15 ml) extra virgin olive oil
⅓ cup (10 g) fresh flat-leaf parsley, chopped
freshly ground black pepper

1 Cook the fusilli in a large saucepan of boiling water according to the package directions, until al dente, adding the asparagus and fava beans for the last 2 minutes of cooking. Drain the pasta and vegetables, and return them to the pan.

2 Meanwhile, half-fill a deep frying pan with water and bring to a simmer. Add the salmon and return to a simmer. Cover and gently poach for 10 minutes, until the salmon is just cooked through. Use a slotted spoon to transfer it to a plate. Allow the salmon to cool slightly, then use a fork to break it into large flakes.

3 Stir the lemon zest, lemon juice and olive oil into the pasta and vegetables. Toss to combine. Add the salmon and parsley, season with freshly ground black pepper and toss to combine.

If you are using fresh fava beans, you will need about 1 pound (500 g) fava bean pods. You can also use frozen fava beans—thaw them before using.

To peel fava beans, make a small slit at one end with your thumbnail and slip the bean from the skin. Smaller beans may not need to be peeled.

EACH SERVING PROVIDES
505 calories, 36 g protein, 16 g fat (2 g saturated fat), 55 g carbohydrate (1 g sugars), 14 g fiber, 72 mg sodium

Fava beans are high in protein and heart-protective fiber. They are combined here with the omega-3 fats in the salmon for a dish that promotes a good blood supply for the brain.

Herb-crusted salmon with spinach salad

PREPARATION **10 MINUTES**
COOKING **15 MINUTES**
SERVES **4**

3 slices whole-wheat bread
1 cup (60 g) fresh parsley
2 tablespoons (30 ml) olive oil
4 skinless salmon fillets, about
   6 ounces (175 g) each
freshly ground black pepper
2 tablespoons (30 ml) whole-grain mustard
1/4 cup (50 ml) lemon juice
2/3 cup (150 g) baby spinach leaves
1/2 red onion, thinly sliced

1   Preheat the oven to 450°F (230°C). Line a baking pan with foil.

2   Combine the bread, parsley and 1 tablespoon (15 ml) of the oil in a food processor. Pulse in short bursts until coarse crumbs form.

3   Place the salmon fillets on the prepared pan and sprinkle with freshly ground black pepper. Spread the top of each fillet with 2 teaspoons (10 ml) of the mustard. Sprinkle the crumb mixture on top of the mustard, gently pressing to help it stick. Bake for 12 minutes, until the salmon is opaque.

4   Meanwhile, in a large bowl, combine the lemon juice with the remaining olive oil, and season with black pepper. Add the spinach and onion, and toss to combine.

5   Serve the hot salmon with the spinach salad or a salad of mixed lettuce leaves, blanched broccoli, shredded carrot and thinly sliced red onion.

EACH SERVING PROVIDES
390 calories, 38 g protein, 22 g fat (4 g saturated fat), 7 g carbohydrate (2 g sugars), 4 g fiber, 170 mg sodium

> In this recipe, *salmon*, high in omega-3 fats, is baked with a parsley crust, combining the benefits of the fish oil with the antioxidants from the herbs.

Salmon with grapes and pepitas

PREPARATION **10 MINUTES**
COOKING **20 MINUTES**
SERVES **4**

4 salmon cutlets
1 cup (250 g) red grapes
2 cloves garlic, thinly sliced
1 leek, white part only, thinly sliced
1 teaspoon (5 ml) grated lemon zest
2 tablespoons (30 ml) pepitas (pumpkin seeds)
1/3 cup (75 ml) verjuice or low-sodium chicken stock
8 sprigs fresh thyme

1   Preheat the oven to 400°F (200°C).

2   Cut four 8-inch (20-cm) squares of parchment paper. Place a salmon cutlet, skin side down, in the center of each sheet of parchment paper.

3   Put the grapes, garlic, leek, lemon zest, pepitas and verjuice or stock in a bowl and mix to combine.

4   Spoon the grape mixture over the salmon, top with the thyme sprigs and fold in the edges of the paper to enclose the salmon. Place the parcels on a large baking pan and bake for 20 minutes, until the salmon is tender.

5   Transfer the salmon parcels to four plates or a platter and serve with a whole-grain side dish, such as pearl barley, and with steamed green beans and pattypan squash.

EACH SERVING PROVIDES
295 calories, 32 g protein, 14 g fat (3 g saturated fat), 12 g carbohydrate (11 g sugars), 2 g fiber, 75 mg sodium

Verjuice is the sour liquid obtained from unripe grapes or crabapples and is used in cooking to impart tartness to a recipe. It can be difficult to find (try specialty grocery stores or ordering online); you can use lemon juice or white wine vinegar instead.

> *Grapes* and *verjuice* are high in two powerful antioxidants, quercetin and resveratrol, associated with a reduction in the effects of aging on the brain.

Left: Herb-crusted salmon with spinach salad
Right: Salmon with grapes and pepitas

Salmon is one of the richest known sources of omega-3 fatty acids, essential for normal brain development and a stable mood.

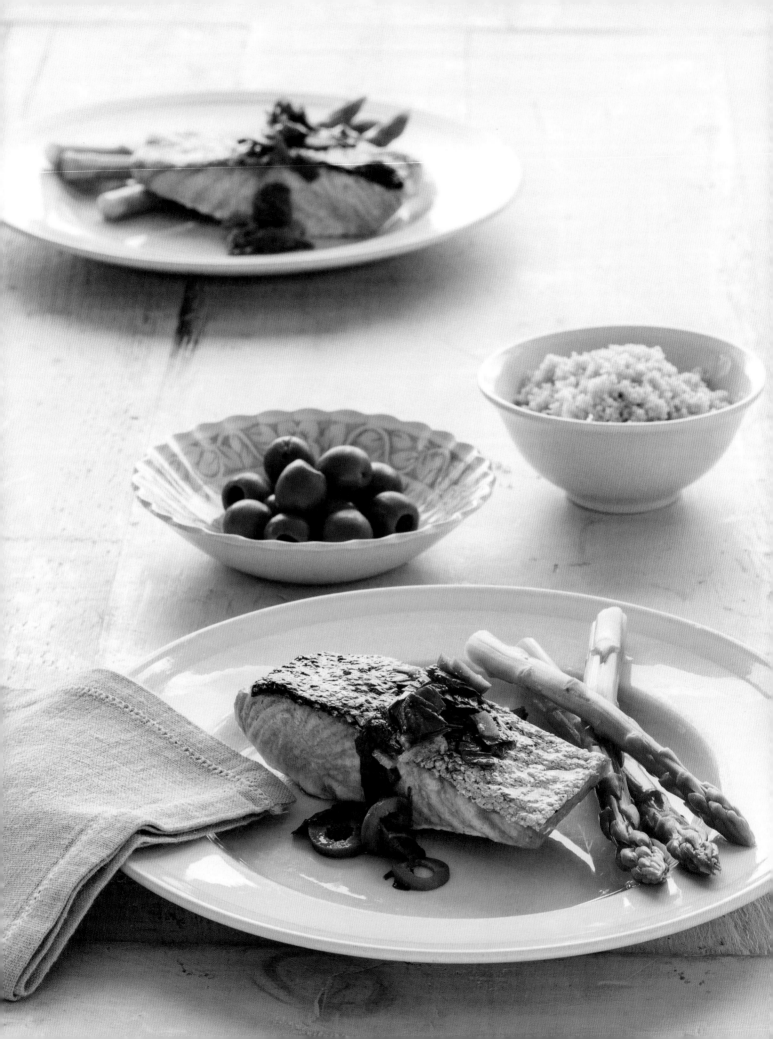

Salmon with preserved lemon and green olives

This simple dish showcases the versatility of preserved lemon, and is a lovely way to add more fish to your diet. The olives and lemon are a perfect foil for the richness of the salmon.

PREPARATION **15 MINUTES**
COOKING **15 MINUTES**
SERVES **4**

4 salmon fillets, about $^{1}/_{4}$ pound (125 g) each
freshly cracked black pepper

Preserved lemon dressing
$^{1}/_{2}$ cup (15 g) roughly chopped fresh mint
8 Sicilian green olives, pitted and sliced
1 clove garlic, chopped
$^{1}/_{2}$ teaspoon (2 ml) ground allspice
1 teaspoon (5 ml) ground cumin
1 tablespoon (15 ml) finely chopped
   preserved lemon rind
2 tablespoons (30 ml) lemon juice
2 tablespoons (30 ml) extra virgin olive oil

1   Preheat the broiler to medium–high. Line a broiler pan with a sheet of lightly oiled foil.

2   Season the salmon with cracked black pepper and place on the pan, skin side down. Broil the salmon, turning once, for 15 minutes, or cooked to your liking.

3   Meanwhile, to make the dressing, put the mint, olives, garlic, allspice, cumin, preserved lemon, lemon juice and olive oil in a bowl, and mix to combine.

4   Place the salmon on four serving plates and spoon the dressing over the top. Serve with steamed asparagus and couscous.

Discard the flesh of the preserved lemon and use only the rind. Remove as much of the white pith from the rind as possible before chopping.

EACH SERVING PROVIDES
277 calories, 26 g protein, 19 g fat (3 g saturated fat), 2 g carbohydrate (<1 g sugars), <1 g fiber, 277 mg sodium

Olives and *preserved lemon* are both high-sodium foods, so the amounts used in this recipe are limited. Feel free to increase the amounts of the herbs and spices to taste, however, as all of these are high in brain-boosting antioxidants.

Black bean and salmon tostadas

Yogurt replaces sour cream in this healthier version of Mexican tostadas. For a main meal, serve them with steamed brown rice and extra tomato, avocado, onion and lettuce.

PREPARATION **20 MINUTES**
COOKING **10 MINUTES**
SERVES **4**

4 corn tortillas
olive oil spray
$1/2$ pound (200 g) boneless, skinless
   salmon fillets
Mexican chili powder, for sprinkling
15 ounce (425 ml) can black beans, rinsed
   and drained
2 tomatoes, seeded and chopped
1 avocado, diced
$1/2$ red onion, finely chopped
2 tablespoons (30 ml) chopped fresh
   cilantro leaves
2 tablespoons (30 ml) lime juice
4 iceberg lettuce leaves, shredded
$1/4$ cup (50 ml) low-fat Greek-style yogurt

1   Preheat the oven to 375°F (190°C). Spray the tortillas with olive oil and place on two baking pans. Bake for 8–10 minutes, turning halfway through, until the tortillas are lightly golden and starting to crisp (they will crisp more on cooling). Transfer to a wire rack to cool.

2   Meanwhile, heat a frying pan over medium–high heat. Spray the salmon with olive oil and lightly sprinkle with the Mexican chili powder. Cook for 3 minutes, then turn and cook for 2 minutes, until the salmon is just cooked through. Transfer to a plate to cool.

3   Combine the black beans, tomatoes, avocado, onion, cilantro and lime juice in a bowl. Use a fork to flake the salmon, and add to the bowl. Gently fold together.

4   Place the tortillas on four serving plates and top with the lettuce. Spoon the salmon and bean mixture over the lettuce, and serve with a dollop of yogurt.

Mexican chili powder is a spice mix made from paprika, chile, cumin, oregano, pepper and garlic. If unavailable, use your favorite chili powder or spice mix, but avoid brands with added salt.

Replace the canned black beans with 2 cups (500 g) cooked beans made from $2/3$ cup (140 g) dried beans.

EACH SERVING PROVIDES
347 calories, 18 g protein, 19 g fat (4 g saturated fat),
23 g carbohydrate (4 g sugars), 7 g fiber, 306 mg sodium

Studies of people with depression have found reduced levels of *inositol* in their brains. Inositol is important in maintaining cell membrane structure and appears to work with choline to nourish the brain. Legumes and citrus fruits both provide inositol and are combined in this Mexican-style recipe with a variety of other good antioxidant sources.

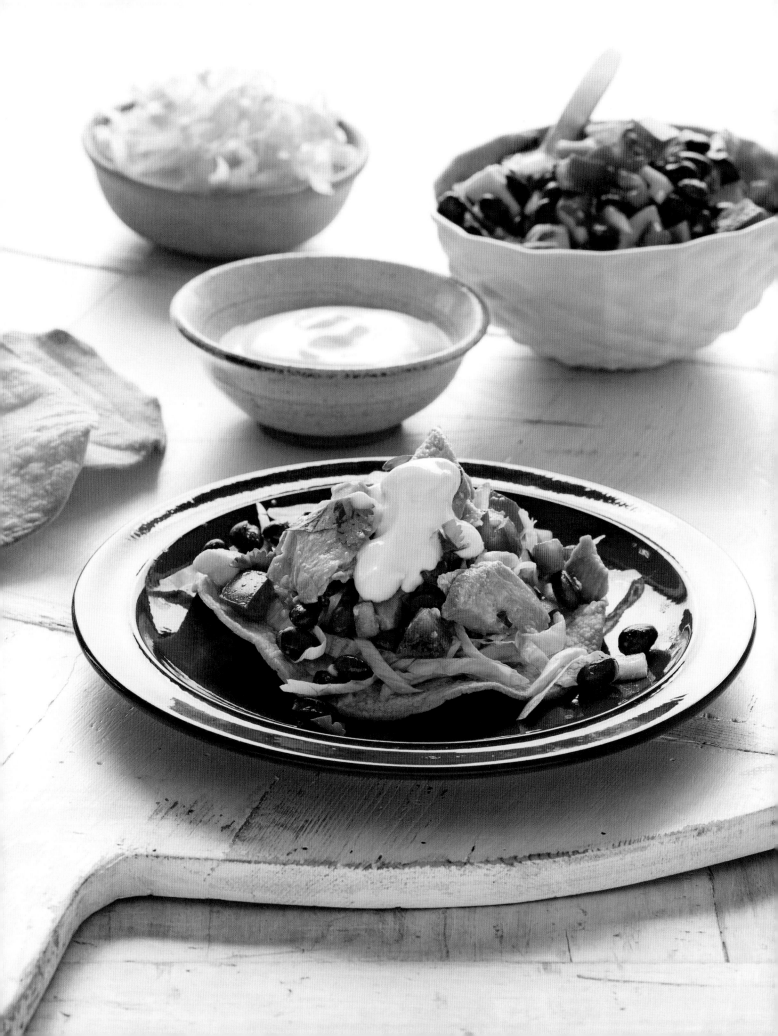

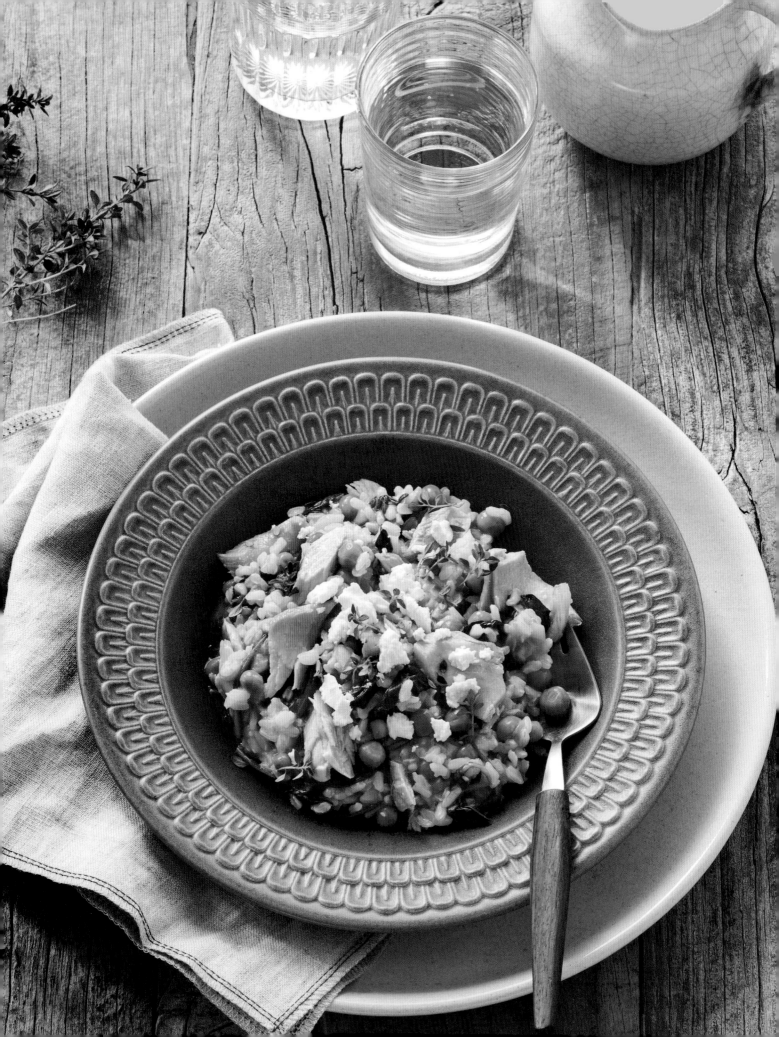

Brown rice risotto with salmon, lemon thyme and feta

Brown rice provides a different texture from the classic risotto, and adds extra nutrients and fiber. Partially cooking the rice first cuts down on the time it would normally take to continuously stir the risotto.

PREPARATION **15 MINUTES**
COOKING **45 MINUTES**
SERVES **4**

1 cup (220 g) short- or medium-grain brown rice
1³⁄₄ cups (425 ml) low-sodium vegetable stock
1 tablespoon (15 ml) olive oil
4 scallions, thinly sliced
2 cloves garlic, crushed
1 cup (155 g) frozen peas
4 boneless, skinless salmon fillets, about ¹⁄₃ pound (150 g) each
1¹⁄₃ cups (60 g) baby spinach leaves
2 teaspoons (10 ml) fresh lemon thyme leaves
¹⁄₂ cup (80 g) crumbled low-fat feta
freshly ground black pepper

1   Preheat the oven to 325°F (160°C). Line a baking pan with parchment paper.

2   Bring a large saucepan of water to a boil. Add the rice and cook for 20 minutes, until almost tender. Drain well.

3   Heat the stock in a small saucepan. Keep hot over very low heat without boiling.

4   Heat the olive oil in a large saucepan over medium heat. Cook the scallions and garlic, stirring, for 2 minutes, until soft. Add the partially cooked rice and stir to coat in the oil. Pour in the hot stock one ladleful at a time, stirring constantly until the stock has been absorbed. Add the peas with the last ladleful of stock. It will take about 20 minutes to add all the stock and cook the rice.

5   Meanwhile, place the salmon on the prepared pan and bake for 15 minutes.

6   Add the spinach to the risotto and stir until wilted and heated through. Remove from the heat. Flake the salmon and fold into the risotto with half the lemon thyme.

7   Spoon the risotto into four bowls and serve sprinkled with the feta, remaining lemon thyme and some freshly ground black pepper.

If you can't find lemon thyme, use regular thyme, and add 1 teaspoon (5 ml) finely grated lemon zest with the thyme.

Whole grains such as brown rice are a key source of energy and fuel for the brain and are packed with nutrients that are important for cardiovascular health. The nutrients, such as fiber, selenium and magnesium, are most concentrated on the outer surface of each grain—the part removed during processing.

EACH SERVING PROVIDES
541 calories, 42 g protein, 20 g fat (5 g saturated fat), 48 g carbohydrate (4 g sugars), 4 g fiber, 743 mg sodium

Fish

Oily fish are the best known source of omega-3 fats. While your body is able to take some of the fats you eat and convert them to other fats, omega-3 fats are "essential fatty acids"—a type that the body cannot make.

We completely rely on dietary sources for the important omega-3 fats. These essential fatty acids are required for normal brain and eye development during infancy and childhood, but they are also needed for optimal brain function in adulthood, and a deficiency or an imbalance of these fats results in an impaired brain performance. The high proportion of fat in the brain's structure means that the fats we eat can have a direct effect on brain function. In the case of omega-3 fats, this means flexible, more responsive cell membranes.

Omega-3 fats also promote the development of new neurons and they are are important in the formation of neurotransmitters. Omega-3 fatty acids seem to play a role in mood and behavior, perhaps by being involved in the body's anti-inflammatory system. Research has found that higher blood levels of omega-3 fats correlate with a lower incidence of depression. Soothing inflammation may also be important in preventing premature aging of the entire body, but particularly of the brain.

Fish is a great protein source. Like poultry, it provides less iron and zinc than red meat, but is still an excellent meat replacement. For good heart health, the American Heart Association recommends eating two 3½ ounce (100 g) servings of oily fish every week, as a substitute for meat. The protein in fish provides a variety of essential amino acids including tryptophan, which is the precursor to feel-good serotonin. As with other flesh foods, it is easy to overcook fish, rendering it dry and tasteless. You can help to lock in moisture by using whole fish instead of fillets, and by using moist cooking methods such as braising, steaming, and wrapping in foil, pastry or banana leaves. Another useful tip is to remove fish from the heat when the center is still slightly translucent. The fish will continue to cook for another 5 to 10 minutes, so it will be perfectly cooked by the time you serve it.

You may have heard worrying reports about fish being high in mercury, which is toxic to the brain. However, health experts say the benefits of eating fish greatly exceed the potential risks.

Still, it is a good idea to take steps to minimize your intake of toxic contaminants by carefully choosing your fish. Species with high levels of mercury are generally the large or very long-lived ones that consume large amounts of other fish and gradually concentrate toxins over time. The U.S. Food and Drug Administration advises pregnant women and children to avoid species of fish that are known to have high levels of mercury, such as shark, swordfish, king mackerel, marlin, orange roughy and tilefish. Other adults should limit their weekly intake of these fish species and check local advisories about the safety of fish caught by family and friends in local lakes, rivers and coastal areas.

While we obtain most of our vitamin D from sunlight, people become more reliant on dietary sources if they do not go out in the sun, or if for religious or modesty reasons they cover up most of their skin. Some fish are a good source of vitamin D, which can be very valuable in such situations. Fish are also a good source of iodine, which is needed for normal brain development and essential for the myelin layer that protects the neurons. Without iodine, a growing child will experience intellectual impairment. When you eat canned fish such as salmon that contains small bones, don't throw them away—they are a great source of calcium, which is important to the entire nervous system as it is used in making nerve signals.

Fish is also a good source of pyridoxine (vitamin B_6), which is required for the synthesis of neurotransmitters including noradrenaline, serotonin and dopamine. Depression, insomnia and confusion are all symptoms of vitamin B_6 deficiency. Vitamin B_{12} comes only from animal foods, including fish, and works with folate to maintain the myelin that protects the nerves. As well as being important in the production of neurotransmitters, vitamin B_{12} helps reduce inflammatory homocysteine levels, which are thought to damage blood vessels and contribute to an increased risk of dementia and stroke.

Clockwise from far left: rainbow trout, sardines, ocean trout, tuna, salmon

Trout baked in grape leaves

Grape leaves are available from delicatessens or the deli counter in large supermarkets. They come in large packs, so divide them into smaller packages and freeze them.

PREPARATION **10 MINUTES**
COOKING **30 MINUTES**
SERVES **4**

4 rainbow trout, about ³/₄ pound (400 g) each, cleaned and scaled
2 lemons, thinly sliced
1 onion, sliced
2 tablespoons (30 ml) fresh flat-leaf parsley, roughly chopped
16 grape leaves
1 tablespoon (15 ml) olive oil
²/₃ pound (300 g) red cherry tomatoes on the vine
lemon wedges, to serve

Raisin couscous
¹/₂ cup (100 g) couscous
1 tablespoon (15 ml) raisins, roughly chopped
¹/₂ teaspoon (2 ml) ground allspice
²/₃ cup (150 ml) low-sodium chicken stock, boiling hot
2 tablespoons (30 ml) toasted pine nuts
2 tablespoons (30 ml) chopped fresh flat-leaf parsley
2 tablespoons (30 ml) chopped fresh dill

1 Preheat the oven to 400°F (200°C). Line a large baking pan with parchment paper.

2 Pat the inside cavity and skin of the fish dry with paper towels. Place a few slices of the lemon with the onion and parsley inside the cavity of each fish. Arrange the rest of the lemon slices over the top of the fish.

3 Wrap the fish in the grape leaves, enclosing the lemon slices, and drizzle with the olive oil. Arrange the fish and tomatoes on the prepared pan.

4 Bake the fish for 25–30 minutes, depending on the size, until the fish is tender and comes away easily from the bone when tested with a flat-bladed knife.

5 Meanwhile, prepare the couscous. Put the couscous, raisins and allspice in a heatproof bowl, add the boiling stock and let stand for 5 minutes, until all the liquid has been absorbed. Fluff up the couscous with a fork to separate the grains. Add the pine nuts, parsley and dill, and mix to combine.

6 Serve the fish with the couscous and lemon wedges.

EACH SERVING PROVIDES
362 calories, 46 g protein, 13 g fat (2 g saturated fat), 13 g carbohydrate (6 g sugars), 4 g fiber, 573 mg sodium

Red wine, like red grapes, contains the antioxidant resveratrol, which is thought to protect the brain and heart from aging. *Grape leaves* are another good source, which combines this brain-protective substance with the benefits of green leafy vegetables.

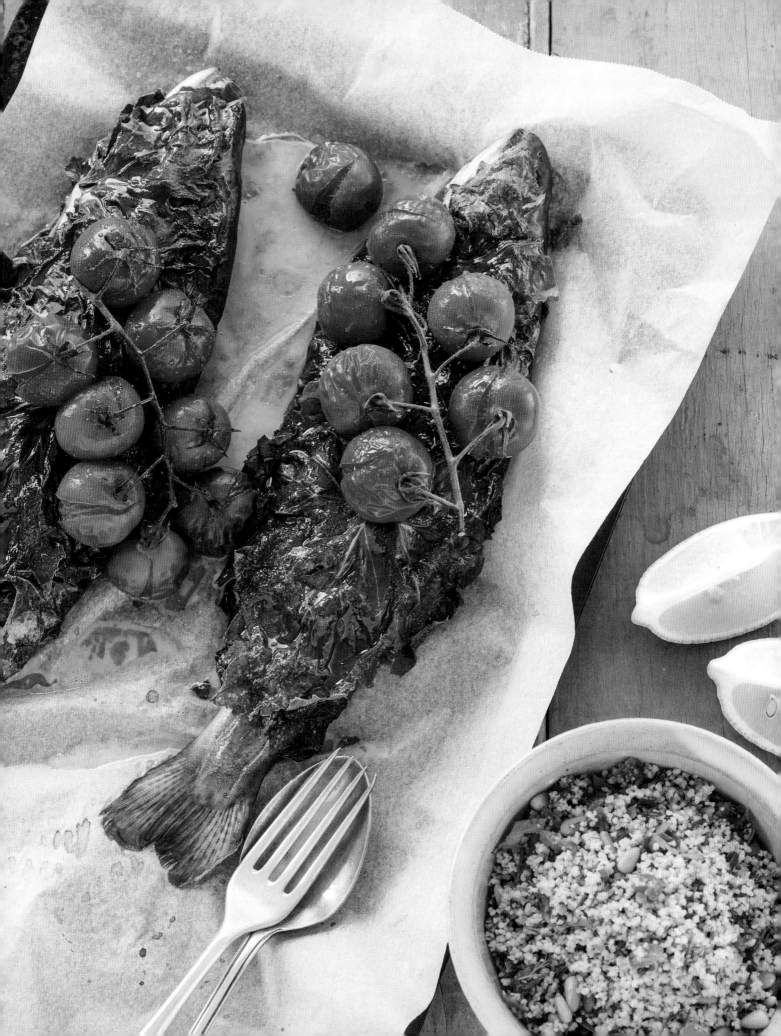

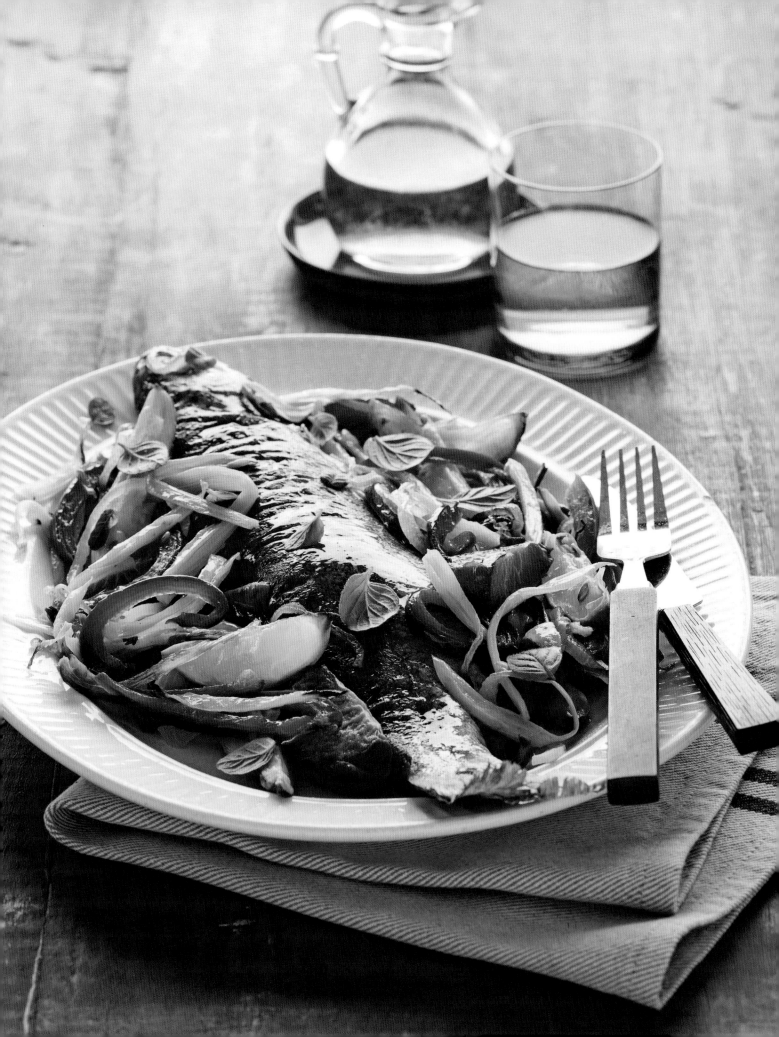

Roasted trout on rainbow vegetables

Trout stuffed with lemon and herbs is served with a rainbow of roasted vegetables. If whole trout aren't available, you can use boned and butterflied trout. Thyme, lemon thyme or dill can be used in place of the oregano.

PREPARATION **20 MINUTES**
COOKING **40 MINUTES**
SERVES **4**

2 lemons
1 red pepper, cut into thin strips
1 green pepper, cut into thin strips
2 vine-ripened tomatoes, cut into wedges
1/2 pound (250 g) fingerling potatoes,
  scrubbed and quartered lengthwise
1 red onion, cut into thin wedges
1 bulb fennel, cut into thin strips,
  fronds reserved
2 tablespoons (30 ml) olive oil
4 small rainbow or brown trout, about
  3/4 pound (400 g) each, cleaned and scaled
8 sprigs fresh oregano, plus extra leaves
  for garnishing

1   Preheat the oven to 400°F (200°C).

2   Slice one lemon and set aside. Cut the other lemon into thin wedges. Put the lemon wedges, peppers, tomatoes, potatoes, onion, fennel and some of the reserved fronds on a large baking pan. Drizzle with half the olive oil and gently toss to coat. Bake the vegetables for 20 minutes.

3   Meanwhile, rinse the trout and pat dry with paper towels. Place a few of the lemon slices and 2 sprigs of oregano inside the cavity of each fish. Brush the fish with the remaining oil.

4   Gently toss the vegetables, arrange the fish on top and bake for 20 minutes, until the fish flakes away from the bone when tested with the tip of a knife.

5   Divide the vegetables among four plates, top with the fish and serve garnished with oregano leaves.

EACH SERVING PROVIDES
363 calories, 46 g protein, 13 g fat (2 g saturated fat),
14 g carbohydrate (7 g sugars), 6 g fiber, 181 mg sodium

A member of the celery family, *fennel* is a good source of manganese, which is essential for normal brain function. It also provides good amounts of immune-boosting zinc.

Fish fillets with oat crumb topping

Lemony fish fillets are given a crunchy baked crumb topping that helps lock in the moisture. Serve the fish with a salad or some steamed seasonal vegetables.

PREPARATION **15 MINUTES**
COOKING **15 MINUTES**
SERVES **4**

$^1/_2$ cup (50 g) rolled oats
$^1/_2$ cup (80 g) whole-wheat all-purpose flour
$^1/_4$ cup (15 g) chopped fresh parsley
finely grated zest and juice of 1 lemon
freshly ground black pepper
$^1/_4$ cup (70 g) olive or canola oil spread
1 pound (500 g) firm white fish fillets, bones removed
$^1/_2$ cup (125 ml) low-sodium fish or chicken stock

1   Preheat the oven to 400°F (200°C).

2   In a blender or food processor, combine the oats, flour, parsley, lemon zest and some freshly ground black pepper. Blend until the oats are coarsely ground. Add the olive oil spread and blend until the mixture just comes together.

3   Arrange the fish in a single layer, skin side down, in a shallow 4 cup (1 L) ovenproof dish that fits the fillets snugly. Pour in the stock and lemon juice, and top with the crumb topping, spreading it evenly over the fish.

4   Bake for 15 minutes, until the topping is well-browned and the fish is just cooked through. Serve hot.

For more crunch, leave some of the rolled oats whole, or add some nuts to the mixture.

EACH SERVING PROVIDES
327 calories, 30 g protein, 14 g fat (4 g saturated fat), 20 g carbohydrate (<1 g sugars), 4 g fiber, 192 mg sodium

Oats contain a soluble fiber that works to reduce cholesterol levels, clearing the way for better circulation to the brain. The crumb topping has a low glycemic index, due to the whole-grain flour and oats.

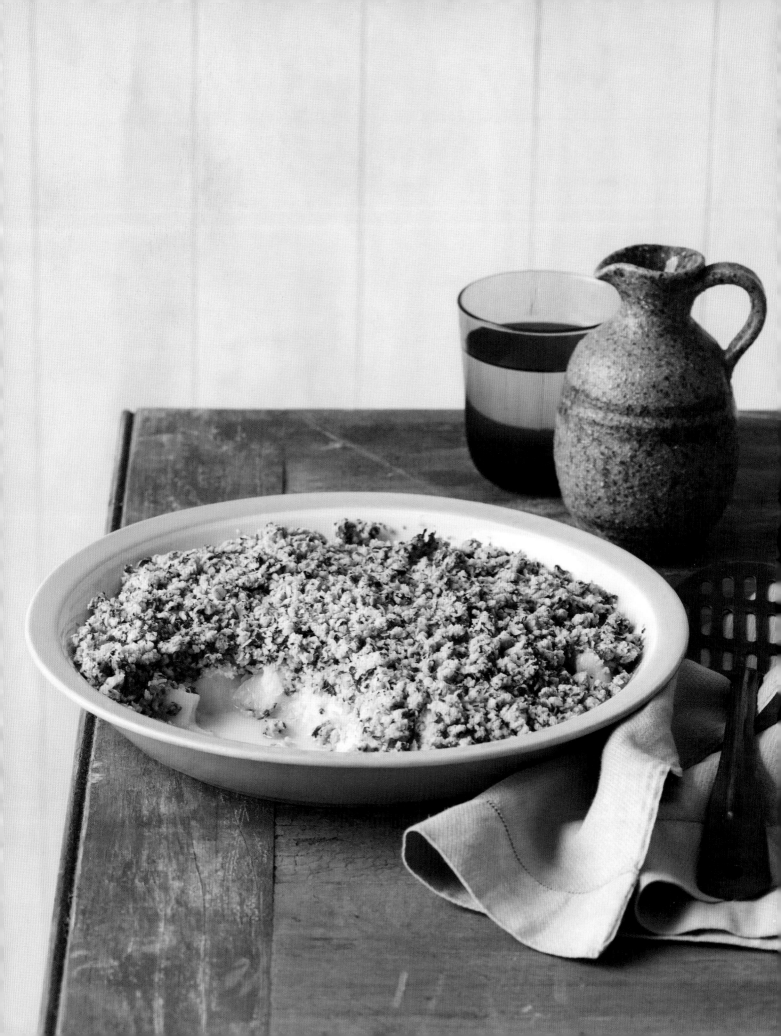

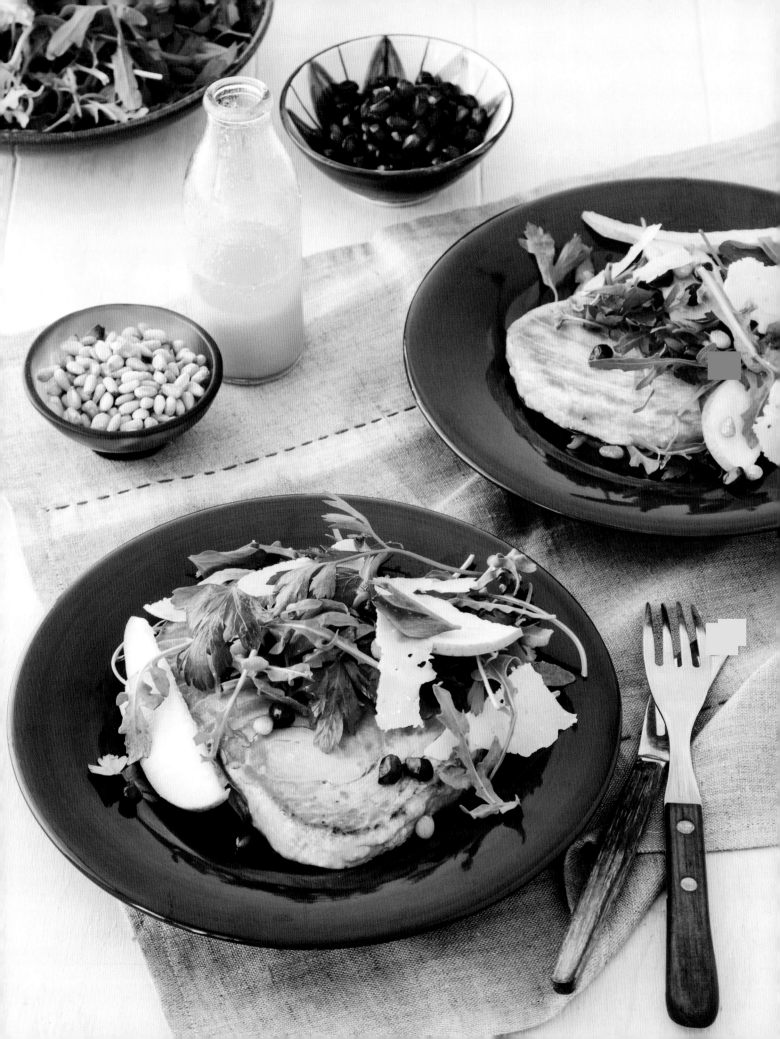

Tuna with parsley and pomegranate salad

Fresh tuna steaks are pan-fried and served with a crisp salad of parsley, wild arugula, pear, pomegranate seeds and toasted pine nuts—a perfect accompaniment to the fish.

PREPARATION **15 MINUTES**
COOKING **5 MINUTES**
SERVES **4**

1 tablespoon (15 ml) olive oil
4 tuna steaks, about 6 ounces (180 g) each
1½ cups (50 g) wild arugula
½ cup (10 g) fresh flat-leaf parsley
1 green pear, thinly sliced
½ cup (50 g) pomegranate seeds
¼ cup (50 g) shaved parmesan
2 tablespoons (30 ml) toasted pine nuts

Dressing
2 tablespoons (30 ml) extra virgin olive oil
1 tablespoon (15 ml) white balsamic vinegar
1 teaspoon (5 ml) maple syrup
grated zest and juice of 1 lemon
1 teaspoon (5 ml) dijon mustard
1 clove garlic, crushed

1   To make the dressing, whisk the extra virgin olive oil, vinegar, maple syrup, lemon zest, lemon juice, mustard and garlic in a bowl until combined.

2   Heat the oil in a large frying pan and cook the tuna over medium–high heat for 2 minutes on each side, until done to your liking.

3   Put the arugula, parsley, pear, pomegranate seeds and parmesan in a bowl, drizzle with the dressing and gently toss to combine.

4   Serve the tuna topped with the salad and dressing, and the toasted pine nuts.

It is important to dress the salad just before serving.

Compared to the standard arugula found in salad leaf mixes, wild arugula has a slightly rougher texture and a more deeply serrated leaf, and its flavor is stronger and a little more peppery. If you can't find the wild kind, standard arugula will do nicely.

EACH SERVING PROVIDES
546 calories, 52 g protein, 33 g fat (9 g saturated fat),
10 g carbohydrate (8 g sugars), 2 g fiber, 294 mg sodium

The concentrated antioxidants that are found in *pomegranates* strengthen your immune system, improve blood circulation and reduce inflammation, promoting optimal brain function.

Fish and broccoli bake

This low-fat baked pasta features fish, broccoli, peas, corn and pasta in a creamy sauce, topped with grated parmesan. Let your choice of vegetables change this dish with the seasons.

PREPARATION **10 MINUTES**
COOKING **50 MINUTES**
SERVES **4**

8 ounces (200 g) whole-wheat penne
2½ cups (600 ml) low-fat milk
1 pound (500 g) boneless white fish fillets, such as cod, snapper, mahi mahi or tilapia
1 bay leaf
2 tablespoons (30 ml) olive oil
1 onion, thinly sliced
¼ cup (35 g) all-purpose flour
1 tablespoon (15 ml) whole-grain mustard
1 teaspoon (5 ml) curry powder
1 cup (200 g) corn kernels
⅔ cup (100 g) frozen peas
1 cup (200 g) broccoli small florets
2 tablespoons (30 ml) chopped fresh mixed herbs, such as dill, parsley and chives
½ cup (50 g) finely grated parmesan

1   Preheat the oven to 400°F (200°C).

2   Cook the penne in a large saucepan of boiling water according to the package directions, until al dente. Drain well and set aside.

3   Meanwhile, pour the milk into a large frying pan. Add the fish and bay leaf. Cook over medium heat for 15 minutes, until the fish flakes when tested with the tip of a knife. Using a slotted spoon, remove the fish from the pan. Discard the bay leaf and reserve the milk. Allow the fish to cool slightly before breaking it into large pieces.

4   Heat the oil in the cleaned frying pan over medium heat. Cook the onion for 10 minutes, until golden. Stir in the flour, mustard and curry powder, and cook, stirring, for 2 minutes, until the flour is smooth and golden. Remove from the heat and gradually stir in the reserved milk. Return to the heat and cook, stirring constantly, until the sauce boils and thickens.

5   Stir in the corn, peas, broccoli, chopped herbs and half the parmesan, and cook for 5 minutes. Stir in the pasta until well combined.

6   Preheat the broiler to high. Pour the pasta mixture into an 8 cup (2 L) ovenproof dish. Sprinkle the remaining parmesan on the top. Broil for 5–10 minutes, until the top is crisp and golden brown. Serve hot.

It is important to cook the flour until golden when you are making the white sauce—uncooked flour can spoil the flavor of a sauce. It is easier to add the milk to the sauce off the heat; this will help to prevent the sauce from becoming lumpy.

Avoid broccoli with yellow flowers blossoming—this is a sign they're past their peak freshness. The stalks and stems should be firm but tender, and the leaves should have a vibrant color and not be wilted.

EACH SERVING PROVIDES
595 calories, 51 g protein, 18 g fat (5 g saturated fat), 58 g carbohydrate (12 g sugars), 11 g fiber, 397 mg sodium

Broccoli is a member of the cruciferous vegetable family, rich in antioxidants and a variety of other special substances thought to protect against degenerative conditions such as dementia.

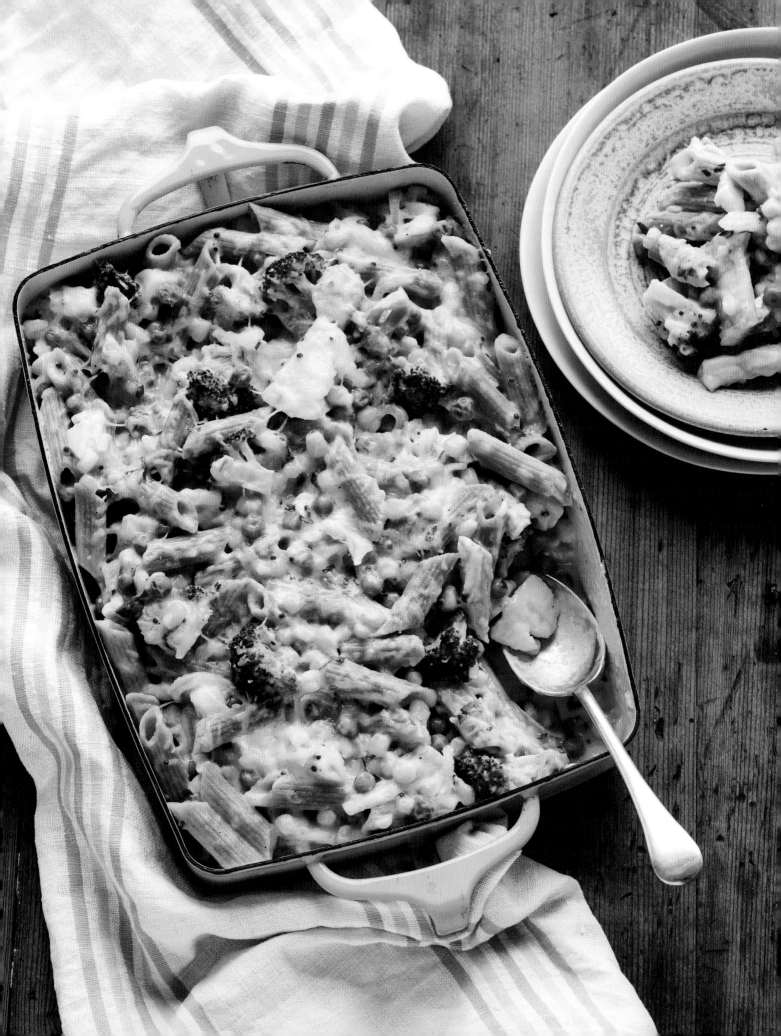

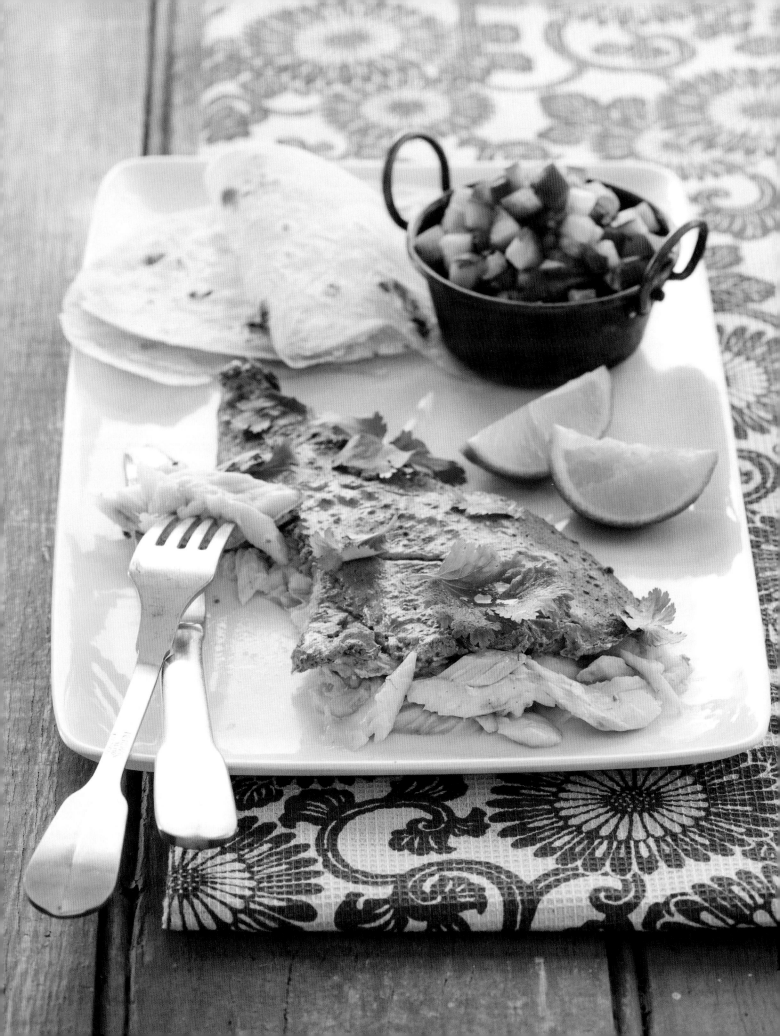

Indian-style tandoori whole fish

The Indian clay oven, or tandoor, lends its name to this method of marinating and roasting that keeps food succulent and full of flavor. Serve the fish with chapattis and a tomato and cucumber salad.

PREPARATION **10 MINUTES, PLUS 2 HOURS MARINATING**
COOKING **40 MINUTES**
SERVES **4**

2 whole snapper, about 1½ pounds
   (700 g) each, or 1 large whole fish, about
   (3–4 pounds (1.5–2 kg), cleaned and scaled
1 cup (250 ml) low-fat plain yogurt
4 cloves garlic, crushed
1 tablespoon (15 ml) paprika
1-inch (2.5-cm) piece fresh turmeric, grated,
   or 1 tablespoon (15 ml) ground turmeric
1-inch (2.5-cm) piece fresh ginger, grated
2 teaspoons (10 ml) cardamom pods, ground
2 teaspoons (10 ml) fenugreek seeds, ground
2 teaspoons (10 ml) coriander seeds, ground
2 teaspoons (10 ml) cumin seeds, ground
juice of 1 lemon or lime, to serve
fresh cilantro sprigs, to serve

1   Place the fish in a nonreactive ovenproof dish with a lid. Cut five or six deep slits in the flesh of the fish on each side, angling inwards towards the fish head.

2   Combine the yogurt, garlic and spices, and spread over both sides of the fish, pressing the mixture into the slits and inside the cavity. Cover and refrigerate for 2 hours.

3   Preheat the oven to 350°F (180°C).

4   If using 2 fish, bake for 30 minutes, until cooked through. If using 1 large fish, bake for 40 minutes, turning it over after 20 minutes and spooning any fallen tandoori mix back on top of the fish.

5   Squeeze lemon or lime juice evenly over the fish before serving, and scatter with cilantro sprigs.

You can make this dish using small individual whole fish or fillets if preferred. If you do this, halve the marinating time, otherwise the acids in the yogurt can start to "cook" the fish flesh, leaving it tough after baking.

EACH SERVING PROVIDES
356 calories, 65 g protein, 6 g fat (2 g saturated fat),
10 g carbohydrate (4 g sugars), 3 g fiber, 301 mg sodium

> The characteristic aroma of curry powder is dominated by *fenugreek*, which has been used as an anti-inflammatory in traditional medicine for thousands of years. The seeds are high in brain-boosting minerals as well as soluble fiber.

Pan-fried swordfish with grapefruit and avocado salsa

It may be quick and easy to make, but this dish will impress your guests with its colorful, refreshing salsa. Serve the swordfish with salad greens and crusty bread for a light, balanced meal.

PREPARATION **20 MINUTES**
COOKING **5 MINUTES**
SERVES **4**

4 swordfish fillets, about $\frac{1}{3}$ pound
   (150 g) each
1 tablespoon (15 ml) olive oil
2 teaspoons (10 ml) chopped fresh rosemary
freshly ground black pepper

Grapefruit and avocado salsa
1 ruby red or pink grapefruit
1 avocado
$\frac{1}{2}$ small red onion, finely chopped
2 tablespoons (30 ml) chopped fresh parsley

1   To make the salsa, cut the top and bottom from the grapefruit to make two flat ends. Use a small, sharp knife to cut downwards and remove the skin, taking off all the white pith. Hold the grapefruit in the palm of your hand and cut on either side of the membrane to remove the segments. Dice the segments.

2   Dice the avocado flesh the same size as the grapefruit. Gently toss the grapefruit and avocado in a bowl with the onion and parsley.

3   Brush the swordfish with the olive oil and sprinkle with the rosemary. Season well with freshly ground black pepper. Heat a large nonstick frying pan over high heat and cook the swordfish for 2 minutes on each side, until the flesh is just cooked through.

4   Transfer the swordfish to four serving plates and serve with the salsa.

Substitute salmon, tuna or trout fillets if the swordfish is not available.

EACH SERVING PROVIDES
368 calories, 32 g protein, 25 g fat (5 g saturated fat), 4 g carbohydrate (3 g sugars), 2 g fiber, 141 mg sodium

Citrus fruit such as *grapefruit* are high in brain-protective antioxidants. Red and pink grapefruit also contain lycopene, which is thought to help protect against cancer.

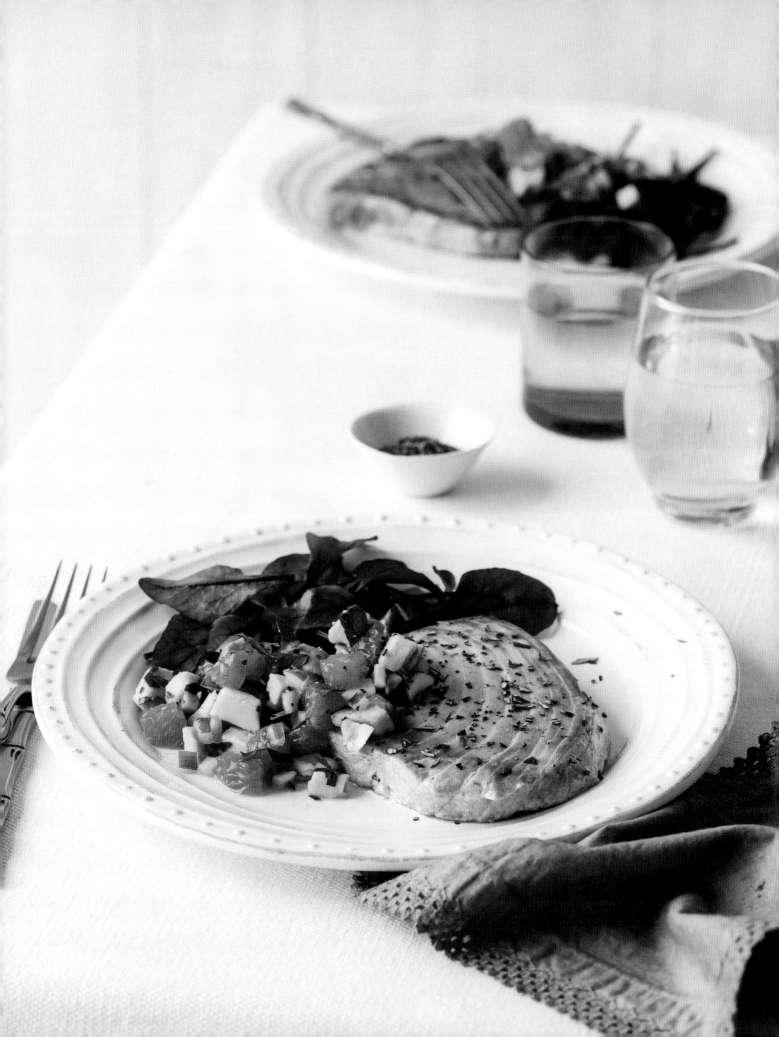

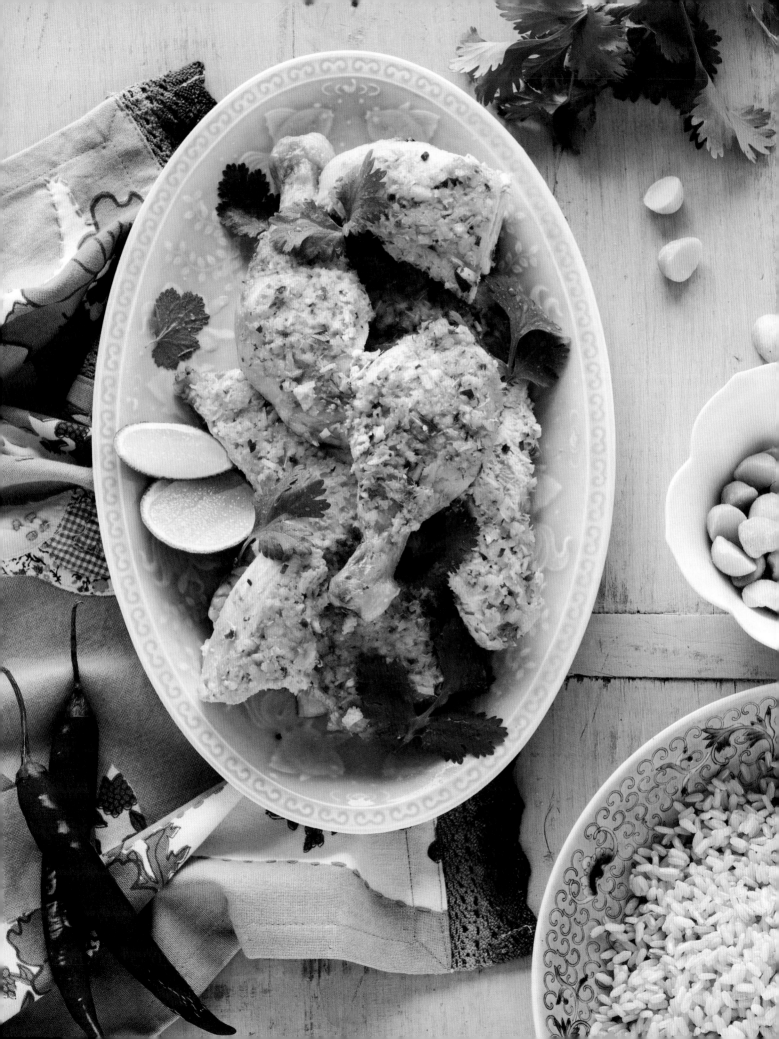

Roast chicken with lemongrass stuffing

Skinless chicken can be bland, but this Vietnamese-style roast chicken is full of flavor, using an antioxidant-rich paste of nuts, herbs, spices and lime. Serve the chicken with brown rice and your choice of steamed Asian greens.

PREPARATION **15 MINUTES, PLUS 2 HOURS MARINATING**
COOKING **1 HOUR**
SERVES **4**

1 whole 3 pound (1.5 kg) chicken
canola or olive oil spray
fresh cilantro leaves, to garnish

Lemongrass paste
3 lemongrass stems, white part only, thinly sliced
6 cloves garlic, diced
1/4 cup (20 g) fresh cilantro stems and roots, finely chopped
1 long red chile, seeded and thinly sliced
grated zest and juice of 1 lime
1/4 cup (50 g) unsalted toasted macadamia nuts or peanuts

1 To make the lemongrass paste, combine the lemongrass, garlic, cilantro, chile, lime zest and lime juice in a mortar or food processor, and grind the mixture into a paste. Add the nuts and grind until the paste is well combined but still slightly chunky.

2 Cut along the backbone of the chicken and flatten out the bird on a baking sheet. Remove and discard all of the skin.

3 Using a small, sharp knife, make a long, deep cut into the breast meat on either side of the center breastbone to form two long, deep pockets extending two-thirds of the way into the breast meat. Make similar cuts along the fleshy part of the thigh, drumstick and wing bottom on each side of the bird.

4 With your fingers, firmly press the lemongrass paste into the pockets, filling them completely. Spread any remaining paste over the chicken. Refrigerate for at least 1–2 hours.

5 Preheat the oven to 350°F (180°C). Brush or spray the top surfaces of the chicken with oil. Bake the chicken for 45–60 minutes, until the juices run clear from the side of the breast when pierced. Let the chicken stand in a warm place for 10 minutes.

6 Cut the chicken into eight pieces, garnish with cilantro leaves and serve immediately.

EACH SERVING PROVIDES
402 calories, 31 g protein, 29 g fat (8 g saturated fat), 5 g carbohydrate (1 g sugars), 2 g fiber, 123 mg sodium

Nuts are an energy-dense food but the fats they contain are beneficial to brain function. Here, macadamia nuts add their healthy fats to help moisten skinless chicken.

Chicken and mushrooms in red wine

This low-salt version of the classic French coq au vin omits the traditional bacon or pancetta but keeps its essential aromatic flavor with herbs, garlic and red wine. For best results, use a good-quality, full-flavored red wine.

PREPARATION **10 MINUTES**
COOKING **1 HOUR**
SERVES **4–6**

3 pounds (1.5 kg) whole chicken
1 tablespoon (15 ml) olive oil
8 baby onions, trimmed
1 clove garlic, crushed
1 cup (200 g) button mushrooms
2 cups (500 ml) low-sodium chicken stock
2 cups (500 ml) red wine
4 sprigs fresh flat-leaf parsley
4 sprigs fresh thyme
2 fresh bay leaves
6 black peppercorns
2 tablespoons (30 ml) chopped fresh
    flat-leaf parsley

1   Rinse the chicken and pat dry with paper towels. Cut the chicken into eight pieces.

2   Heat the oil in a large flameproof casserole dish. Cook the chicken in batches over medium heat for 5 minutes, until browned. Drain on paper towels.

3   Add the onions, garlic and mushrooms to the casserole dish. Cook, stirring, for a few minutes until the onions and mushrooms are browned.

4   Return the chicken to the dish, pour in the stock and red wine, and add the parsley sprigs, thyme sprigs, bay leaves and peppercorns. Bring to a boil, reduce the heat, cover and simmer for 40 minutes, until the chicken is tender.

5   Garnish the chicken with the chopped parsley and serve with green beans and steamed baby potatoes.

If you would like to thicken the sauce, blend 1 tablespoon (15 ml) cornstarch with a little of the hot liquid, return it to the pan and stir until the sauce boils and thickens.

EACH SERVING PROVIDES
486 calories, 32 g protein, 28 g fat (8 g saturated fat),
6 g carbohydrate (4 g sugars), 3 g fiber, 465 mg sodium

More than any other part of the body, the brain relies on *antioxidants* to protect it against damage. This dish combines antioxidant-rich ingredients such as red wine, garlic and mushrooms.

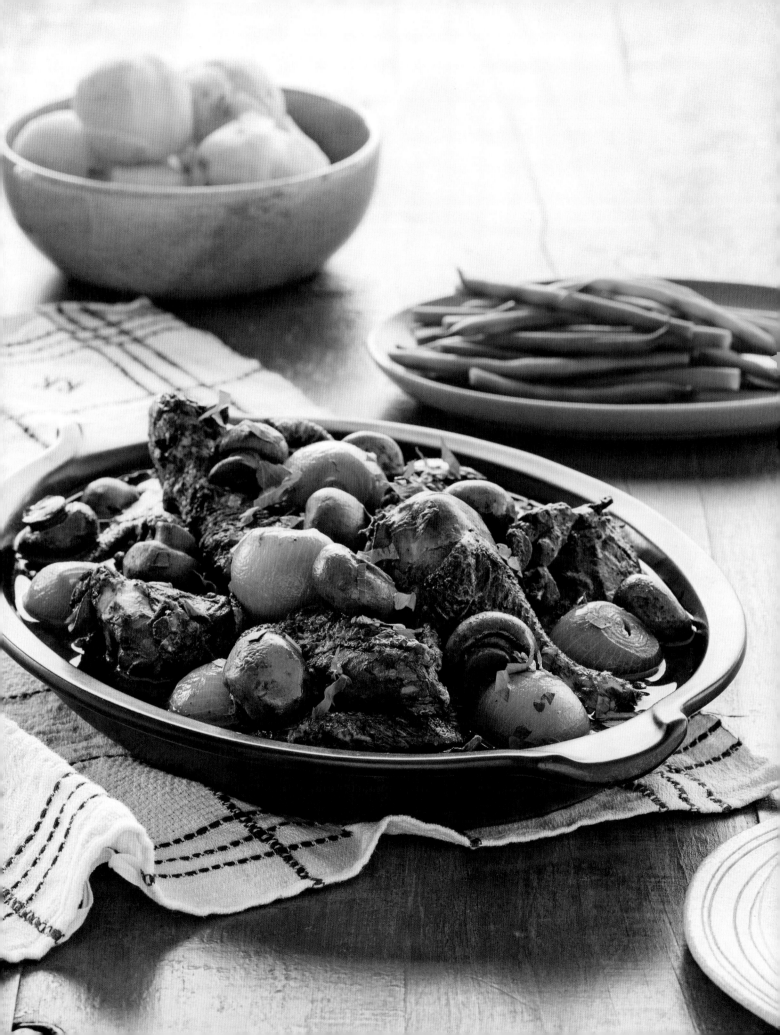

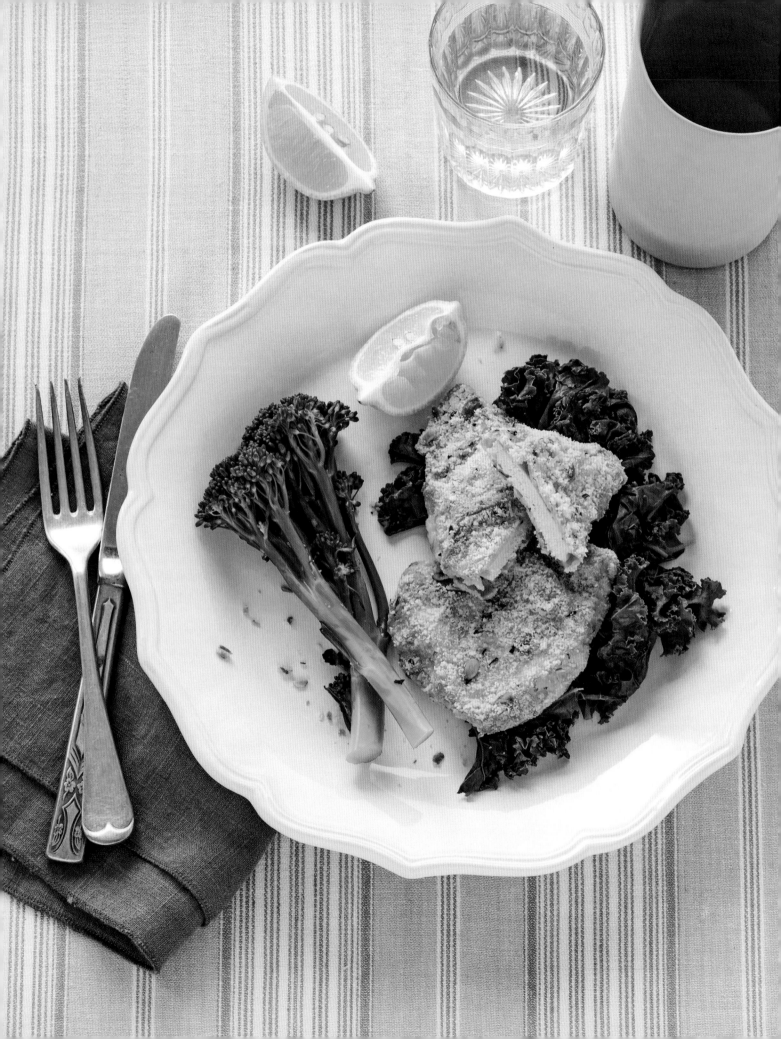

Almond-crumbed chicken schnitzels with steamed greens

To make the schnitzels into party bites, cut the chicken into strips, bread them with the crumbs and bake for 10 minutes, until golden brown and tender. Serve with a garlic yogurt dip.

PREPARATION **20 MINUTES**
COOKING **15 MINUTES**
SERVES **4**

2 boneless, skinless chicken breasts, about 1 pound (500 g) total
$1^{1}/_{2}$ cups (150 g) ground almonds
2 tablespoons (30 ml) pepitas (pumpkin seeds), roughly chopped
2 tablespoons (30 ml) finely grated parmesan
2 tablespoons (30 ml) fresh oregano
$^{1}/_{4}$ cup (30 g) cornstarch
2 eggs, lightly beaten
olive oil spray
$^{3}/_{4}$ pound (350 g) kale, stems removed, leaves roughly chopped
$^{1}/_{2}$ pound (250 g) broccolini, halved
lemon wedges, to serve

1   Preheat the oven to 400°F (200°C). Line a baking pan with parchment paper.

2   Cut the chicken breasts in half horizontally. Lay one chicken breast between two sheets of plastic wrap. Pound with a rolling pin until the chicken is about $^{1}/_{2}$ inch (1 cm) thick. Repeat with the remaining chicken.

3   Combine the ground almonds, pepitas, parmesan and oregano in a shallow bowl. Put the cornstarch and egg in separate shallow bowls.

4   Coat the chicken breasts in the cornstarch, shaking off any excess, then dip into the egg. Press into the almond mixture, making sure the chicken is evenly coated on both sides.

5   Place the chicken on the prepared pan, lightly spray with olive oil and bake for 15 minutes, until the chicken is golden and tender.

6   Meanwhile, combine the kale and broccolini in a metal colander over a saucepan of simmering water, making sure the base of the colander is not touching the water. Cover and steam for 5 minutes, until the vegetables are bright green and just tender.

7   Serve the chicken with the wilted kale, broccolini and a wedge of lemon.

EACH SERVING PROVIDES
583 calories, 46 g protein, 36 g fat (6 g saturated fat), 22 g carbohydrate (3 g sugars), 7 g fiber, 216 mg sodium

Pepitas (pumpkin seeds) are a good source of zinc, important to the body's immune system. Zinc deficiency is associated with impaired function, so it is important that you get enough of this beneficial nutrient.

Chicken and vegetable curry

This Indian-style aromatic curry is full of flavor and color. The coconut and tomato sauce is mildly spiced with turmeric, ginger, coriander and garam masala. Serve it with brown rice or whole-wheat naan bread.

PREPARATION **25 MINUTES**
COOKING **50 MINUTES**
SERVES **6**

1 tablespoon (15 ml) olive oil
1 large onion, chopped
1 red pepper, chopped
2 pounds (1 kg) boneless, skinless chicken thighs, trimmed of all fat, chopped
4 cloves garlic, crushed
1 tablespoon (15 ml) grated fresh ginger
3 teaspoons (15 ml) ground turmeric
2 teaspoons (10 ml) ground coriander
1 teaspoon (5 ml) garam masala
$\frac{1}{2}$ teaspoon (2 ml) cayenne pepper
1 cup (250 ml) low-sodium chicken stock
$14\frac{1}{2}$ ounce (400 ml) can diced tomatoes
$1\frac{1}{2}$ pounds (750 g) sweet potatoes, cut into chunks
$\frac{1}{2}$ pound (250 g) green beans, halved
$\frac{1}{2}$ cup (125 ml) light coconut milk
fresh cilantro leaves, to serve

1   Heat the oil in a large saucepan and cook the onion and pepper over medium heat for 5 minutes, until very soft. Add the chopped chicken and cook, stirring occasionally, for 5 minutes, until lightly browned. Stir in the garlic, ginger and spices, and cook, stirring, for 1 minute.

2   Stir in the stock, tomatoes and sweet potatoes. Cover and bring to a simmer, reduce the heat to low and cook for 30 minutes, until the sweet potatoes are tender.

3   Add the beans and return to a simmer. Increase the heat slightly and cook, uncovered, for 5 minutes, until the beans are just tender. Stir in the coconut milk and cook until the curry is heated through.

4   Serve the curry sprinkled with the cilantro leaves.

Prepare the garlic and ginger in advance and measure out the dry spices so you can add them all at once.

EACH SERVING PROVIDES
385 calories, 36 g protein, 15 g fat (5 g saturated fat), 27 g carbohydrate (12 g sugars), 6 g fiber, 272 mg sodium

Colorful *turmeric* has powerful antioxidant and anti-inflammatory properties that help to protect brain cells from damage. Its soothing effects have been used in traditional medicine for thousands of years.

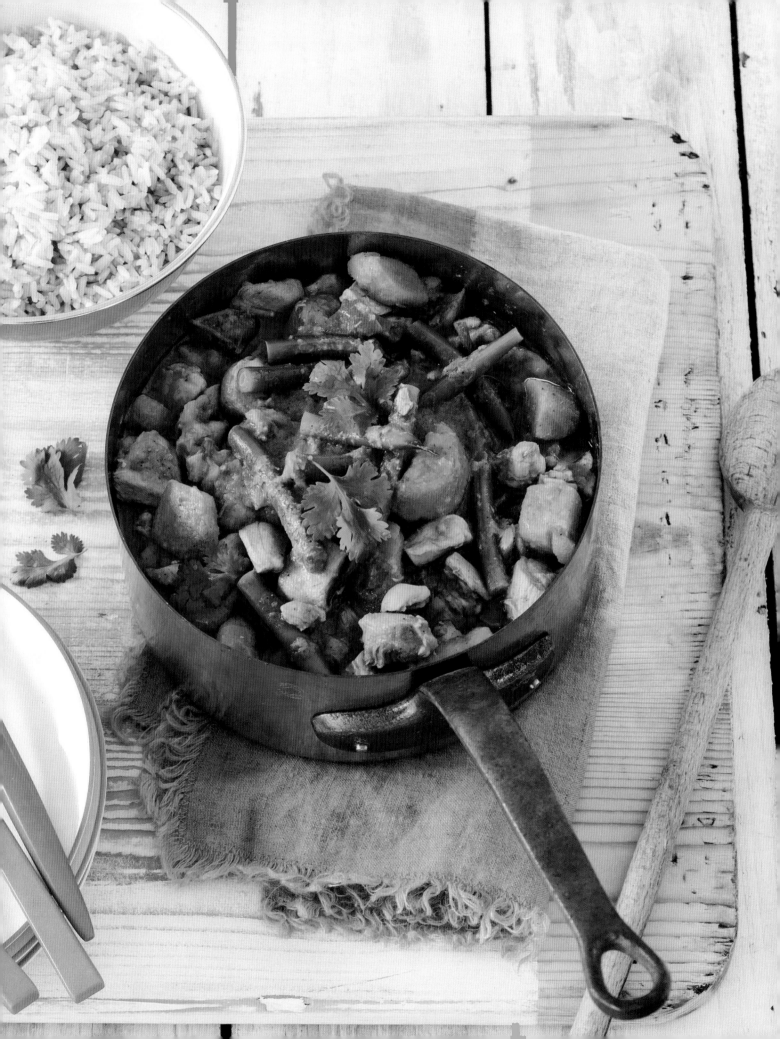

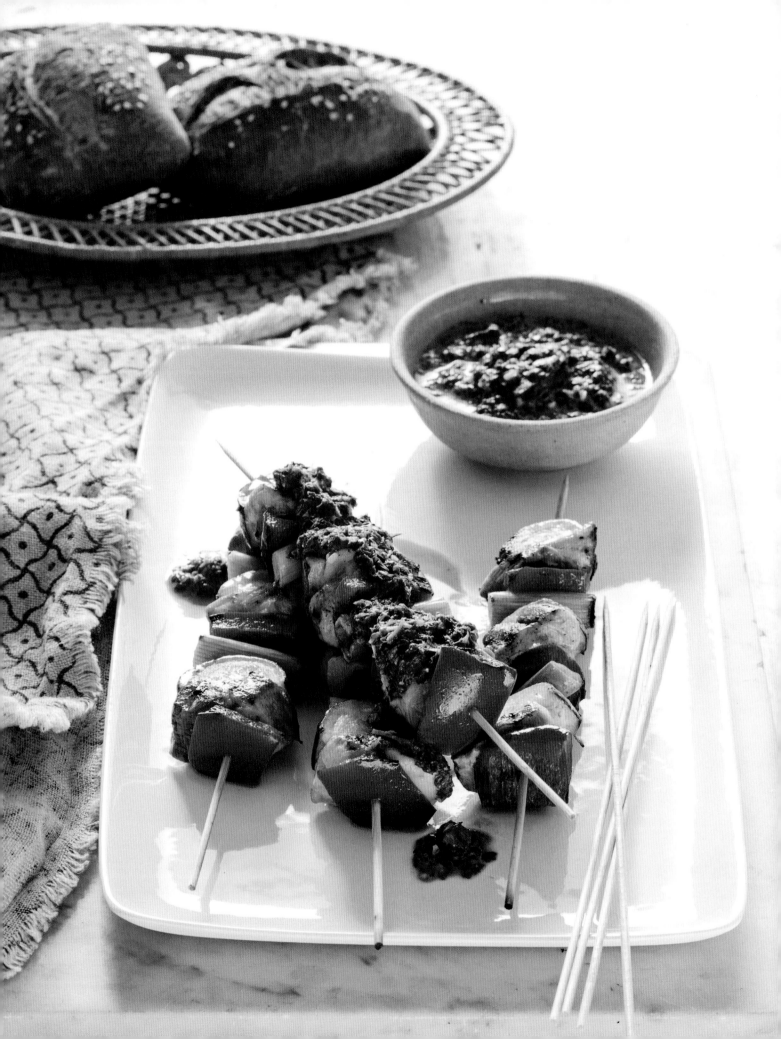

Chicken and pepper skewers with chimichurri sauce

Chimichurri is a versatile sauce that is very popular throughout South America. Prepare it just before serving so the herbs keep their bright color. Serve leftover sauce with grilled fish or tofu.

PREPARATION 20 MINUTES, PLUS 30 MINUTES SOAKING
COOKING 10 MINUTES
SERVES 4 (MAKES 8)

1 red pepper, cut into squares
4 boneless, skinless chicken thighs, trimmed and cut into large cubes
2 zucchini, halved and cut into thick slices
4 scallions, cut into short lengths
olive oil spray

Chimichurri sauce
½ cup (110 g) fresh cilantro, finely chopped
½ cup (120 g) fresh parsley, finely chopped
2 cloves garlic, finely chopped
1 large red chile, seeded and finely chopped
1 teaspoon (5 ml) ground cumin
½ teaspoon (2 ml) dried oregano
juice of 1 lemon
1 tablespoon (15 ml) red wine vinegar
¼ cup (50 ml) extra virgin olive oil

1   Soak eight bamboo skewers in water for 30 minutes.

2   To make the chimichurri sauce, combine the cilantro, parsley, garlic, chile, cumin and oregano in a bowl. Stir in the lemon juice, vinegar and olive oil. Set aside while you prepare the skewers.

3   Thread the pepper, chicken, zucchini and scallions onto the skewers. Lightly spray with olive oil.

4   Preheat a barbecue or grill pan. Cook the skewers over medium–high heat for 10 minutes, until the chicken is cooked through and the vegetables are tender, turning several times to be sure they cook evenly.

5   Drizzle the chicken skewers with the chimichurri sauce and serve the remainder on the side. Serve with a green salad and crusty whole-grain bread.

You can prepare the chimichurri sauce ahead and refrigerate it in an airtight container. Return the sauce to room temperature before serving.

EACH SERVING (2 SKEWERS) PROVIDES
233 calories, 13 g protein, 18 g fat (3 g saturated fat), 5 g carbohydrate (3 g sugars), 4 g fiber, 64 mg sodium

> *Leafy herbs* such as cilantro, parsley, basil and rosemary are very rich sources of a variety of antioxidants, as well as providing good amounts of vitamin C, folate and beta-carotene.

Roasted turkey breast stuffed with quinoa and herbs

This recipe uses turkey breast steaks, which are available in supermarkets all year round. The stuffing can also be used to fill a whole turkey breast. Use your choice of seeds and nuts.

PREPARATION **20 MINUTES**
COOKING **50 MINUTES**
SERVES **6**

¼ cup (50 g) red quinoa, rinsed
  and drained
1 tablespoon (15 ml) olive oil
1 leek, white part only, thinly sliced
2 tablespoons (30 ml) white wine
2 cloves garlic, chopped
2 tablespoons (30 ml) pine nuts
2 tablespoons (30 ml) sunflower seeds
1 tablespoon (15 ml) dried
  cranberries, chopped
1 tablespoon (15 ml) chopped fresh sage
2 tablespoons (30 ml) chopped fresh parsley
4 turkey breast steaks, skin removed
cranberry relish, to serve

1 Preheat the oven to 400°F (200°C). Line a baking pan with parchment paper.

2 Cook the quinoa in a large saucepan of boiling water for 20 minutes, until tender. Rinse under cold water and drain well.

3 Heat the oil in a large frying pan. Cook the leek over medium heat for 10 minutes, until soft and golden. Stir in the wine and cook until evaporated. Add the garlic, nuts, seeds and cranberries. Cook for 5 minutes, until the nuts have browned. Transfer to a bowl with the quinoa and herbs, and mix to combine.

4 Place one turkey breast steak between two sheets of plastic wrap and pound with a meat mallet or rolling pin to flatten it. Place 2 heaping tablespoons (35 ml) of the stuffing on one end of the turkey, then roll up and use a toothpick to secure the end. Repeat with the remaining turkey and stuffing.

5 Place the stuffed turkey on the prepared tray and bake for 15 minutes, until tender.

6 Serve the turkey with cranberry relish, sugar snap peas and roasted sweet potatoes.

If you are using a whole turkey breast, lay the turkey skin-side down, cut it three-quarters of the way through the center of the breast and open it out to lay flat. Spread the stuffing over the turkey breast, stopping about 1 inch (2.5 cm) from the edge. Roll up to enclose the filling and tie with several pieces of string. Rub the outside of the turkey with olive oil and place on a wire rack in a roasting pan. Pour 1 cup (250 ml) water into the dish. Bake for 10 minutes, reduce the oven to 350°F (180°C) and cook for 1 hour, until the turkey is tender. Cover and let stand for 10 minutes before slicing.

Skinless turkey is an excellent source of lean protein, as well as brain-boosting B-group vitamins including B_{12}, thought to help prevent cognitive decline by keeping homocysteine levels under control.

EACH SERVING PROVIDES
400 calories, 53 g protein, 18 g fat (4 g saturated fat), 8 g carbohydrate (1 g sugars), 3 g fiber, 5 mg sodium

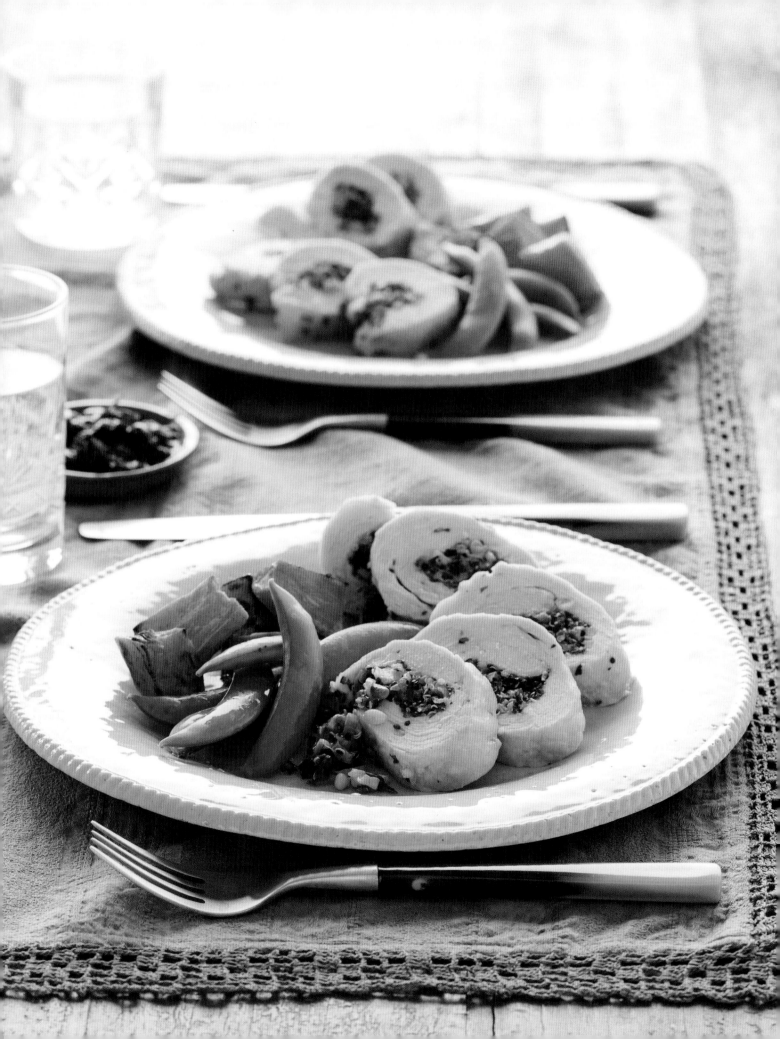

Nuts and seeds

Nuts and seeds are high in protein and beneficial fats. These fats help reduce cholesterol levels, and some nuts and seeds also contain plant sterols that block cholesterol absorption from other foods.

Different nuts and seeds offer a whole range of different nutritional benefits, so it's a good idea to eat a variety of them regularly. Cashew nuts, hazelnuts, macadamia nuts and almonds are high in monounsaturated fats, which lower cholesterol, while walnuts and flaxseeds are high in omega-3 fats with an anti-inflammatory effect. Brazil nuts are higher in saturated fat but contain particularly high levels of selenium, while pumpkin seeds are high in zinc. Both zinc and selenium are required in the body's antioxidant system. The brain has a high need for antioxidants as its metabolic activity generates a high load of oxidative stress. The brain also relies on a healthy cardiovascular system to supply all its needs, so it is very important to control cholesterol levels and blood pressure. Pistachios, pecans and hazelnuts are all high in cholesterol-lowering sterols, as are sunflower seeds and pine nuts. Sesame seeds are high in calcium, which aids in regulating blood pressure.

The protein in nuts and seeds includes the amino acid tryptophan, which is the precursor for the neurotransmitter serotonin, as well as the B-group vitamin niacin. To make these, adequate iron, riboflavin and vitamin B_6 need to be present. Riboflavin is also essential for obtaining energy for your cells, including brain cells, and this is thought to be the reason that riboflavin supplementation may help prevent migraines. Nuts and seeds are a good source of niacin and thiamine, which are important for good brain function. Niacin deficiency causes irritability and confusion, even dementia in extreme cases; thiamine deficiency can cause depression, irritability and impaired memory.

The US Physicians' Committee for Responsible Medicine has released dietary guidelines for preventing Alzheimer's disease and these include having a small handful of nuts or seeds each day, partly because of the importance of vitamin E in brain function. Vitamin E protects fats from being oxidized and helps to maintain the integrity of cell membranes. The high fat content of the brain means that it needs this protection more than other parts of the body. Vitamin E deficiency causes impairment of muscle function, vision, balance and sensory nerves.

Recent research indicates that depression risk may be reduced by improving the intake of monounsaturated fats and omega-3 fats. Traditional eating patterns that include nuts and seeds, such as Mediterranean diets, are good examples of this. Studies of people following a Mediterranean diet have shown a decreased risk of depression and heart disease, and improved cognition. This is attributed to a low intake of meat (associated with increased risk) and a high intake of plant foods as well as healthy fats from seafood, olive oil, nuts and seeds.

Because nuts and seeds are high in fat, they have a substantial calorie count, so it is important to limit serving sizes if you want to control your weight and use them to replace other less healthy foods rather than simply adding them to your daily intake. Use them in salads or as a replacement for some of the meat in a stir-fry; or eat just a small handful between meals as a nutritious and satisfying alternative to other snacks.

Clockwise from top left: almonds, sunflower seeds, hazelnuts, walnuts, pepitas (pumpkin seeds), cashew nuts, flaxseeds, sesame seeds, Brazil nuts

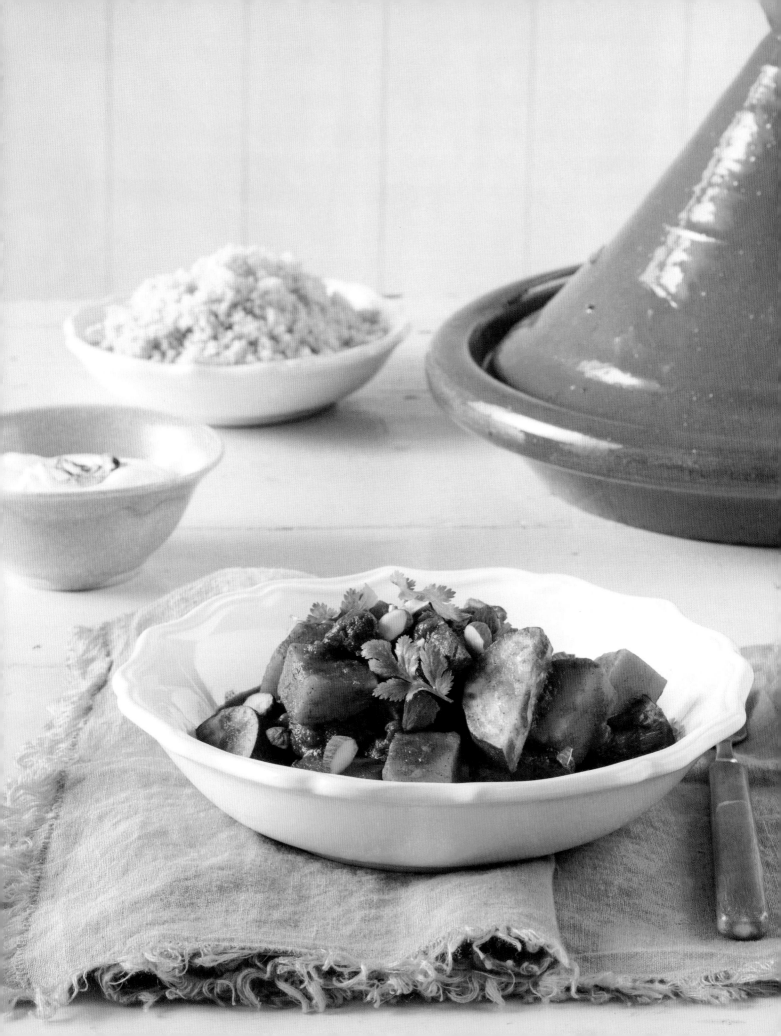

Beef and cranberry Moroccan-style tagine

The secret of a good tagine lies in the spices, so make sure your spices are very fresh. The longer you marinate the beef, the more intense the flavor will be.

PREPARATION **20 MINUTES, PLUS OVERNIGHT MARINATING**
COOKING **1 HOUR 30 MINUTES**
SERVES **4**

1 pound (500 g) beef chuck steak,
    cut into large cubes
1 teaspoon (5 ml) ground ginger
1 teaspoon (5 ml) ground allspice
1 teaspoon (5 ml) ground turmeric
2 tablespoons (30 ml) olive oil
pinch of saffron threads
1 red onion, chopped
1 cinnamon stick
$^1/_4$ cup (30 g) dried cranberries
$14^1/_2$ ounce (400 ml) can diced tomatoes
$^2/_3$ pound (300 g) sweet potatoes,
    cut into small chunks
1 zucchini, halved and thickly sliced
$1^1/_3$ cups (250 g) instant whole-wheat
    couscous
2 teaspoons (10 ml) harissa paste
$^3/_4$ cup (200 ml) low-fat Greek-style yogurt
2 tablespoons (30 ml) raw almonds,
    roughly chopped
fresh cilantro sprigs, to serve

1 Put the beef in a bowl, add the ginger, allspice, turmeric and 1 tablespoon (15 ml) of the olive oil. Toss to coat the beef, cover and refrigerate overnight, if time permits. Remove from the fridge about 30 minutes before cooking.

2 Put the saffron in a small bowl and soak in 2 tablespoons (30 ml) hot water for 10 minutes.

3 Meanwhile, heat the remaining oil in a large flameproof casserole dish over medium–high heat. Brown the beef in batches, then remove all of the beef from the pan.

4 Add the onion to the dish and cook over medium heat for 10 minutes, until golden. Return the beef to the pan. Add the saffron and soaking liquid, the cinnamon stick, cranberries, tomatoes and $1^1/_2$ cups (375 ml) water. Bring to a boil, reduce the heat, cover and simmer for 40 minutes.

5 Add the sweet potatoes and zucchini, and cook, uncovered, for 30 minutes, until the beef is tender and falling apart.

6 Put the couscous in a heatproof bowl, pour in $1^1/_2$ cups (375 ml) boiling water and let stand for 10 minutes, until the liquid has been absorbed. Use a fork to fluff up the grains.

7 Swirl the harissa through the yogurt. Serve the tagine sprinkled with the chopped almonds and cilantro, and accompanied by the yogurt and couscous.

Harissa is a fiery north African chile paste. You can omit it and leave the yogurt plain.

Spices provide a concentrated source of a variety of brain-protective antioxidants and beneficial minerals.

EACH SERVING PROVIDES
502 calories, 37 g protein, 20 g fat (5 g saturated fat),
44 g carbohydrate (15 g sugars), 7 g fiber, 242 mg sodium

Beef and vegetable stir-fry with almonds

A stir-fry is a good way to combine meat and vegetables in one dish. The trick with stir-fries is to have all the ingredients prepared and ready to go before you start cooking.

PREPARATION **15 MINUTES**
COOKING **15 MINUTES**
SERVES **4**

^{2}/$_3$ pound (300 g) lean round steak
2 cloves garlic, crushed
1 tablespoon (15 ml) finely grated
    fresh ginger
1^1/$_2$ tablespoons (22 ml) canola oil
^{3}/$_4$ pound (400 g) broccoli
1 red pepper, cut into thin strips
1 red onion, cut into thin wedges
1^1/$_2$ tablespoons (22 ml) kecap manis
    (sweet soy sauce)
1^1/$_2$ tablespoons (22 ml) lime juice
2 tablespoons (30 ml) toasted
    slivered almonds

1   Cut the beef across the grain into very thin strips. Place in a bowl with the garlic, ginger and half the oil. Mix well, and set aside.

2   Cut the broccoli into small florets, and cut the stem into thin slices.

3   Heat a wok or large frying pan over high heat. Stir-fry a third of the beef for 2 minutes, until well browned. Transfer to a plate and keep warm. Stir-fry the remaining beef in two batches, reheating the wok each time.

4   Heat the remaining oil in the wok. Add the vegetables and stir-fry over medium–high heat for 4–5 minutes, until just tender. Return the beef to the pan, add the kecap manis and lime juice, and stir until combined and heated through.

5   Sprinkle the beef and vegetables with the almonds and serve immediately with steamed brown rice.

You can use roasted, unsalted peanuts in place of the slivered almonds.

EACH SERVING PROVIDES
238 calories, 23 g protein, 13 g fat (2 g saturated fat),
9 g carbohydrate (7 g sugars), 5 g fiber, 395 mg sodium

This stir-fry is a good source of *iron* and *antioxidants* that protect the brain from free radical damage. Onion contains quercetin, one of the flavonoid group of antioxidants that have both antioxidant and anti-inflammatory powers. This means quercetin is beneficial in reducing the risk of stroke.

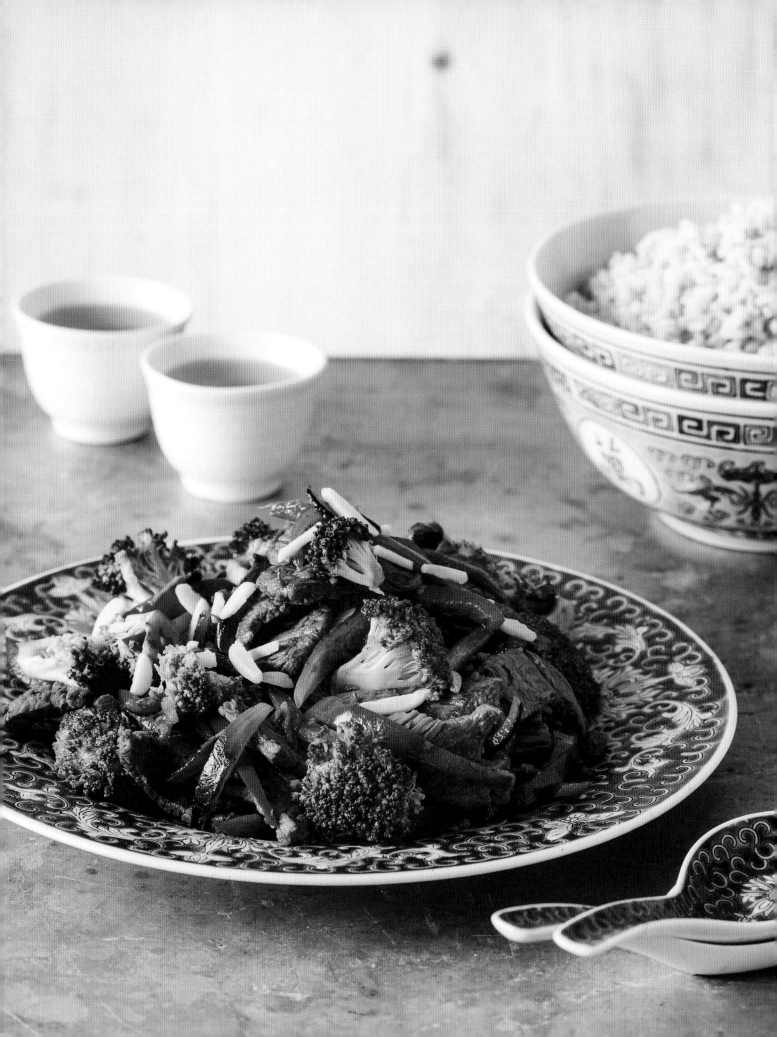

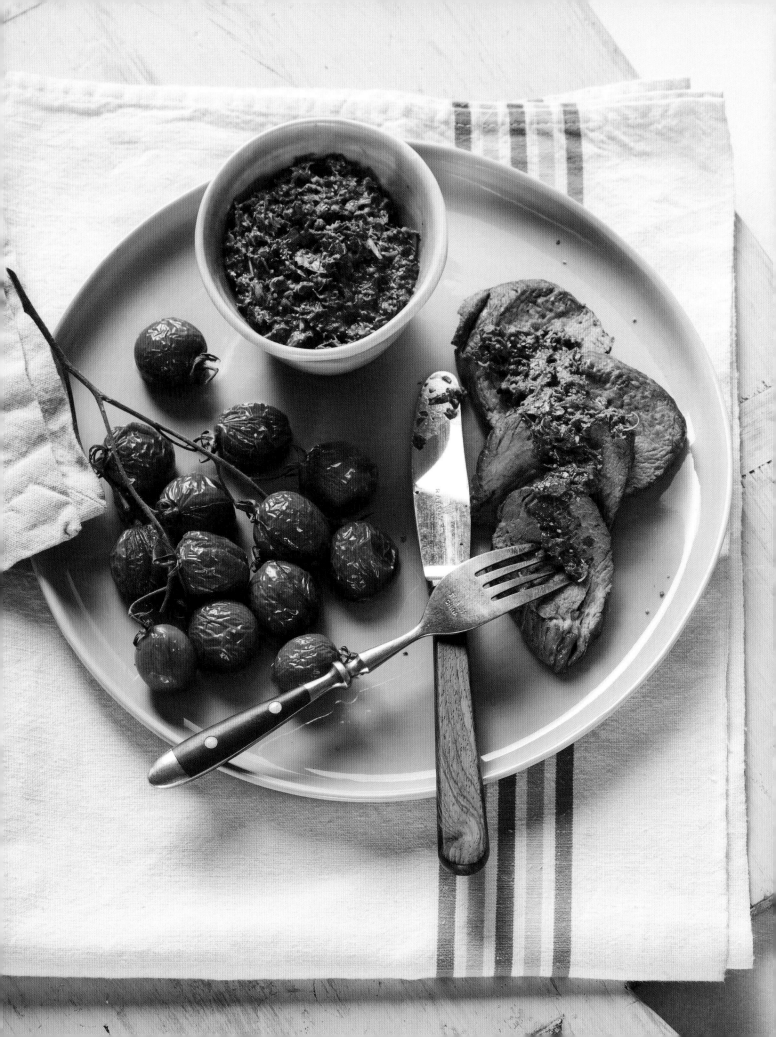

Roast beef with salsa verde

Lovely served hot or cold, this roast beef is a perfect match for a carbohydrate dish such as a rice pilaf or a quinoa salad. Refrigerate any leftover salsa verde and serve it with grilled meat or fish.

PREPARATION **20 MINUTES**
COOKING **35 MINUTES**
SERVES **6**

$1^{1}/_{2}$–$1^{2}/_{3}$ pound (750–800 g) beef fillet
1 tablespoon (15 ml) olive oil
freshly ground black pepper
1 pound (500 g) red cherry tomatoes
   on the vine

Salsa verde
3 anchovy fillets
milk, for soaking
2 cups (40 g) fresh flat-leaf parsley
$^{2}/_{3}$ cup (20 g) fresh basil
$^{1}/_{4}$ cup (5 g) fresh mint
2 teaspoons (10 ml) baby capers, rinsed
   and squeezed dry
1 clove garlic, chopped
2 tablespoons (30 ml) extra virgin olive oil
1 tablespoon (15 ml) red wine vinegar

1   Preheat the oven to 400°F (200°C).

2   Trim any visible fat and sinew from the beef fillet, and tie with kitchen string at 1 inch (2.5 cm) intervals so it holds its shape as it cooks.

3   Heat the olive oil in a large frying pan over medium–high heat. Cook the beef, turning often, for 5 minutes, until evenly browned. Transfer the beef to a roasting pan. Season with freshly ground black pepper.

4   Roast the beef for 30 minutes for medium, or until cooked to your liking. Add the cherry tomatoes for the last 20 minutes of cooking. Set the beef aside to rest, loosely covered with foil, for 10 minutes.

5   While the beef is cooking, make the salsa verde. Put the anchovies in a shallow bowl and cover with milk. Set aside to soak for 20 minutes. Drain the anchovies and pat dry with paper towels, then roughly chop. Combine the herbs, capers, garlic and anchovies in a food processor, and process until well chopped. Add the extra virgin olive oil and vinegar, and process until well combined.

6   Slice the roast beef and serve with the cherry tomatoes and salsa verde.

EACH SERVING PROVIDES
250 calories, 28 g protein, 14 g fat (4 g saturated fat), 2 g carbohydrate (2 g sugars), 2 g fiber, 203 mg sodium

Fresh herbs add nutritional benefits as well as distinctive flavor and aroma, providing a concentrated source of antioxidants important for protecting brain function.

Sweet potato and quinoa rosti with beef and basil dressing

A rosti is a Swiss dish traditionally made with potatoes. This version uses a sweet and nutty combination of quinoa and sweet potatoes that has a low glycemic index to keep you going longer.

PREPARATION **30 MINUTES**
COOKING **45 MINUTES**
SERVES **4**

¼ cup (50 g) red quinoa, rinsed and drained
1¼ cups (300 g) grated sweet potatoes
2 egg whites, lightly beaten
2 tablespoons (30 ml) all-purpose flour
¼ teaspoon (1 ml) ground cinnamon
2 tablespoons (30 ml) olive oil
4 porterhouse steaks, trimmed
olive oil spray
cracked black pepper
⅓ cup (100 g) watercress, trimmed

Basil dressing
½ cup (15 g) fresh basil, roughly chopped
1 tablespoon (15 ml) capers, rinsed and
    squeezed dry
1 tablespoon (15 ml) walnuts, roughly
    chopped
1 tablespoon (15 ml) white wine vinegar
2 tablespoons (30 ml) orange juice
1 clove garlic, crushed
1 tablespoon (15 ml) extra virgin olive oil

1 Cook the quinoa in a large saucepan of boiling water for 20 minutes, until tender. Drain well and transfer to a bowl. Add the sweet potatoes, egg whites, flour and cinnamon, and stir to combine.

2 Heat the oil in a nonstick frying pan over medium heat. Pour the sweet potato mixture into the pan, flatten and cook for 10 minutes. Invert the rosti onto a plate, slide back into the pan and cook for 10 minutes, until brown on both sides.

3 Spray the steaks on both sides with a little olive oil and season with cracked black pepper. Heat a large frying pan over medium–high heat. Cook the steaks for 3 minutes on each side, until done to your liking. Set aside to rest while you prepare the dressing.

4 To make the basil dressing, combine the basil, capers, walnuts, vinegar, orange juice, garlic and oil in a bowl.

5 Cut the rosti into wedges and arrange on plates with the steaks and basil dressing. Serve with watercress.

Prepare the basil dressing just before serving, to prevent the basil leaves from blackening if left to stand for too long.

EACH SERVING PROVIDES

405 calories, 26 g protein, 22 g fat (5 g saturated fat), 24 g carbohydrate (6 g sugars), 4 g fiber, 120 mg sodium

Vitamin B₆, essential for producing neurotransmitters, is found in good amounts in *sweet potatoes*, which also have a low glycemic index for long-lasting brain fuel.

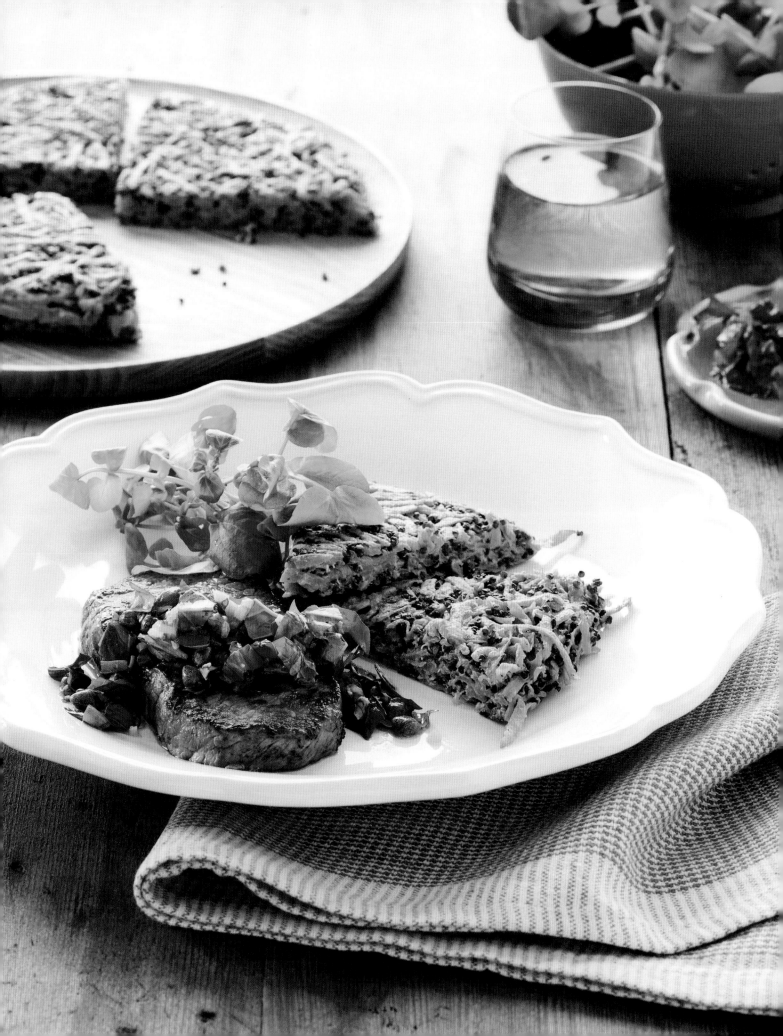

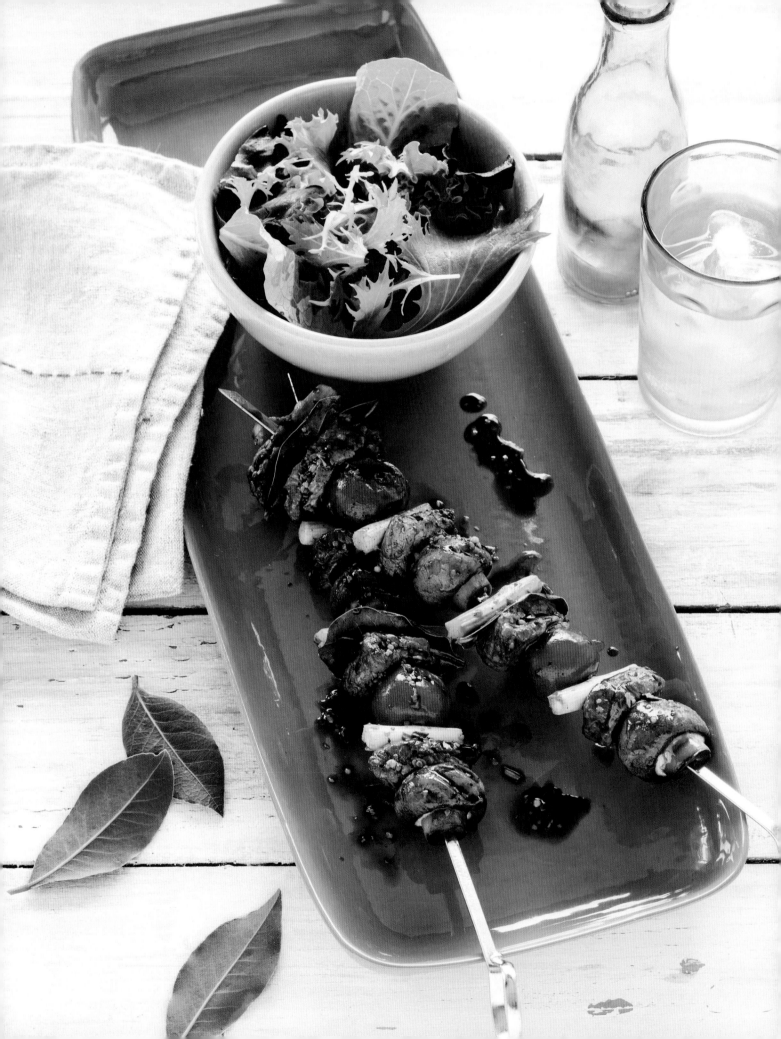

Beef and vegetable skewers

These skewers are wonderful for a summer barbecue—and equally good cooked indoors on a grill pan in the colder months. Cut the meat into pieces of a similar size so the skewers will lie flat.

PREPARATION **15 MINUTES**
COOKING **10 MINUTES**
SERVES **4 (MAKES 8)**

16 small cremini mushrooms
$^2/_3$ pound (300 g) round steak,
  cut into thin strips
4 scallions, cut into short lengths
16 red cherry tomatoes
16 fresh bay leaves
6 asparagus spears, cut into short lengths

Mustard dressing
1 tablespoon (15 ml) olive oil
1 tablespoon (15 ml) whole-grain mustard
1 tablespoon (15 ml) balsamic vinegar
1 teaspoon (5 ml) maple syrup
1 tablespoon (15 ml) chopped
  fresh rosemary

1 If using bamboo skewers, soak them in water for 30 minutes. Thread the mushrooms, steak, scallions, tomatoes, bay leaves and asparagus onto the skewers.

2 To make the mustard dressing, put the olive oil, mustard, vinegar, maple syrup, rosemary and 1 tablespoon (15 ml) water in a bowl, and whisk to combine.

3 Preheat a barbecue or grill pan. Brush the mustard dressing over the skewers and cook over medium–high heat for 10 minutes, until tender, turning several times to be sure they cook evenly.

4 Serve the hot skewers with a green salad and whole-wheat pita bread.

EACH SERVING PROVIDES
191 calories, 20 g protein, 10 g fat (3 g saturated fat),
13 g carbohydrate (4 g sugars), 4 g fiber, 49 mg sodium

Beef is an excellent source of protein, vitamins and minerals, which are all very important for brain function. Choose grass-fed meat, which is leaner and has a healthier blend of fats.

Beef and lentil shepherd's pie

Shepherd's pie is a classic comfort dish, and a great way to get extra vegetables into your diet. You can purée the vegetables to hide them if you are feeding children (or adults) who don't like vegetables.

PREPARATION **20 MINUTES**   COOKING **40 MINUTES**   SERVES **4**

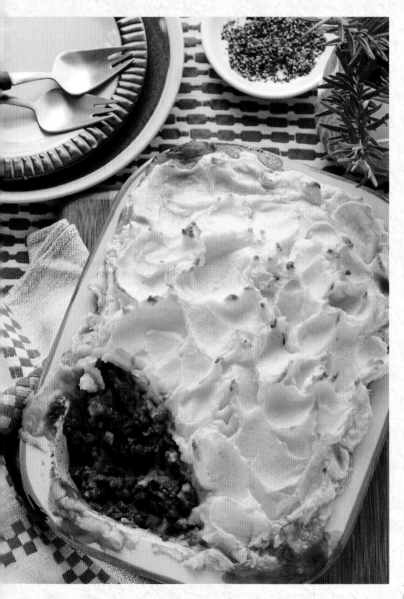

2 tablespoons (30 ml) olive or canola oil
1 small onion, finely chopped
2 cloves garlic, crushed
1 zucchini, cut into small cubes
1 small eggplant, cut into small cubes
3 potatoes, about 1 pound (500 g) total, chopped
½ cup (125 ml) low-fat milk
1 pound (500 g) 95 percent lean
  grass-fed ground beef or ground venison
15 ounce (425 ml) can brown lentils, rinsed
  and drained
½ cup (125 g) no-salt tomato paste
1 tablespoon (15 ml) chopped fresh herbs, such as
  parsley, oregano or rosemary, or 1 teaspoon
  (5 ml) dried herbs
freshly ground black pepper

1   Heat the oil in a large saucepan and cook the onion over low heat for 5 minutes, until translucent. Add the garlic and cook, stirring, for 2 minutes. Add the zucchini and eggplant cubes, and cook, stirring occasionally, for 15 minutes, until all the vegetables are soft and caramelized.

2   Meanwhile, cook the potatoes in boiling water until tender. Drain and mash with the milk.

3   Preheat the oven to 400°F (200°C).

4   Add the ground beef to the vegetables and cook, stirring, until well browned. Add the lentils, tomato paste and fresh herbs, season with freshly ground black pepper and stir until well combined.

5   Spread the beef and lentil mixture in a baking dish and spoon or pipe the mashed potatoes on top. Bake for 15 minutes, until the top is browned.

Replace the canned lentils with 2 cups (500 g) cooked lentils made from ⅔ cup (130 g) dried lentils.

Adding *lentils* increases the fiber content and allows you to use less meat.

EACH SERVING PROVIDES
367 calories, 36 g protein, 11 g fat (2 g saturated fat), 29 g carbohydrate (7 g sugars), 6 g fiber, 225 mg sodium

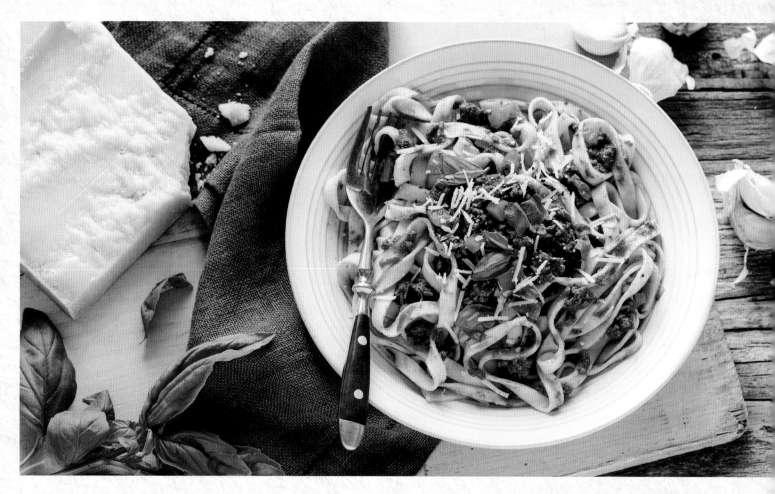

Beef bolognese with tagliatelle

Lean meat is a mineral-rich source of complete protein. For the lowest fat content (and more beneficial types of fat), look for grass-fed, wild or free-range types of meat and poultry.

PREPARATION **10 MINUTES** COOKING **4 HOURS 30 MINUTES** SERVES **4**

2 tablespoons (30 ml) olive oil
1 small onion, finely diced
2 cloves garlic, crushed
2 celery stalks, finely diced
2 small carrots, finely diced
1 pound (500 g) 95 percent lean grass-fed ground
  beef or ground venison
4 tomatoes, diced
$\frac{1}{2}$ cup (125 ml) red wine
$\frac{1}{2}$ cup (125 ml) low-fat milk
14 ounces (400 g) whole-wheat tagliatelle
12 fresh basil leaves, torn
grated parmesan, to serve

1 Heat the oil in a saucepan. Cook the onion for 10 minutes. Add the garlic and cook for 3 minutes. Add the celery and carrots. Cook, stirring until soft.

2 Add the ground beef and cook over medium heat, stirring, until browned. Add the tomatoes, red wine and milk. Bring to a boil, reduce the heat to low and very gently simmer for 2–4 hours.

3 Cook the tagliatelle in a large saucepan of boiling water according to the package directions, until al dente. Drain the pasta and add to the sauce, gently stirring to coat. Serve with the basil and parmesan.

EACH SERVING PROVIDES
595 calories, 44 g protein, 13 g fat (2 g saturated fat), 69 g carbohydrate (7 g sugars), 13 g fiber, 73 mg sodium

Smoked paprika lamb with whole-wheat couscous

Whole-wheat couscous is available from health food stores or specialty shops if you can't find it in your supermarket. Bulgur wheat is an alternative that works well.

PREPARATION **25 MINUTES**
COOKING **10 MINUTES**
SERVES **4**

³⁄₄ pound (400 g) loin lamb steak
1¹⁄₂ tablespoons (22 ml) olive oil
¹⁄₂ teaspoon (2 ml) smoked paprika
1 cup (250 ml) low-sodium vegetable stock
1 cup (185 g) whole-wheat couscous
1 teaspoon (5 ml) finely grated lemon zest
1 tablespoon (15 ml) lemon juice
¹⁄₂ cup (25 g) chopped fresh cilantro
2 tablespoons (30 ml) toasted pistachios,
  roughly chopped

Tahini yogurt dressing
¹⁄₃ cup (75 ml) low-fat Greek-style yogurt
1 tablespoon (15 ml) tahini
1 tablespoon (15 ml) lemon juice
1 small clove garlic, crushed

1   Brush the lamb all over with 3 teaspoons (15 ml) of the oil and sprinkle with the paprika. Heat a nonstick frying pan over medium–high heat. Cook the oiled lamb for 5 minutes on each side for a medium result, or until done to your liking. Transfer to a plate and let rest, loosely covered with foil, for 5 minutes.

2   Meanwhile, pour the stock into a saucepan, cover and bring to a boil. Remove from the heat and add the couscous, quickly replacing the lid. Briefly swirl the pan to mix the couscous and stock together, and set aside, tightly covered, for 5 minutes.

3   Add the lemon zest, lemon juice and remaining oil to the couscous. Use a fork to fluff up the grains. Transfer the couscous to a bowl and allow to cool slightly before mixing in the cilantro and pistachios.

4   To make the dressing, put the yogurt, tahini, lemon juice, and garlic in a small bowl. Add 1 tablespoon (15 ml) water and stir to combine.

5   Slice the lamb across the grain. Serve drizzled with the dressing, accompanied by the couscous and some lightly steamed mixed beans.

EACH SERVING PROVIDES

370 calories, 27 g protein, 22 g fat (6 g saturated fat), 16 g carbohydrate (3 g sugars), 2 g fiber, 368 mg sodium

Couscous is a miniature form of pasta. Like other pastas, it is available in whole-wheat varieties for a higher fiber, lower glycemic index, more satisfying meal.

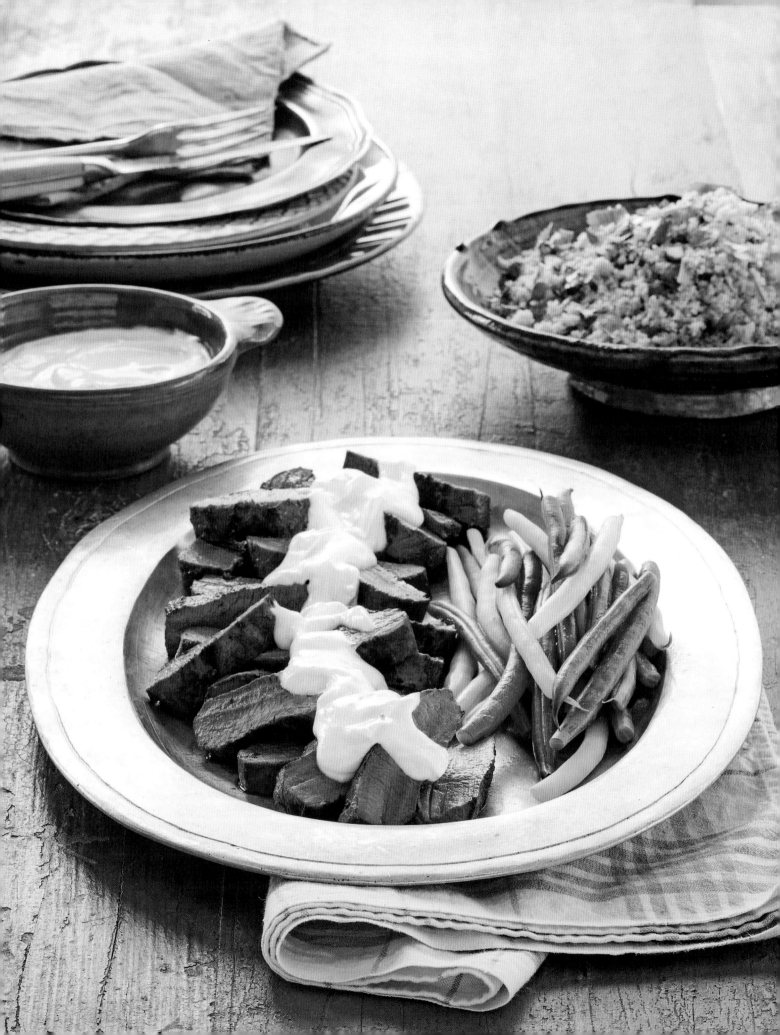

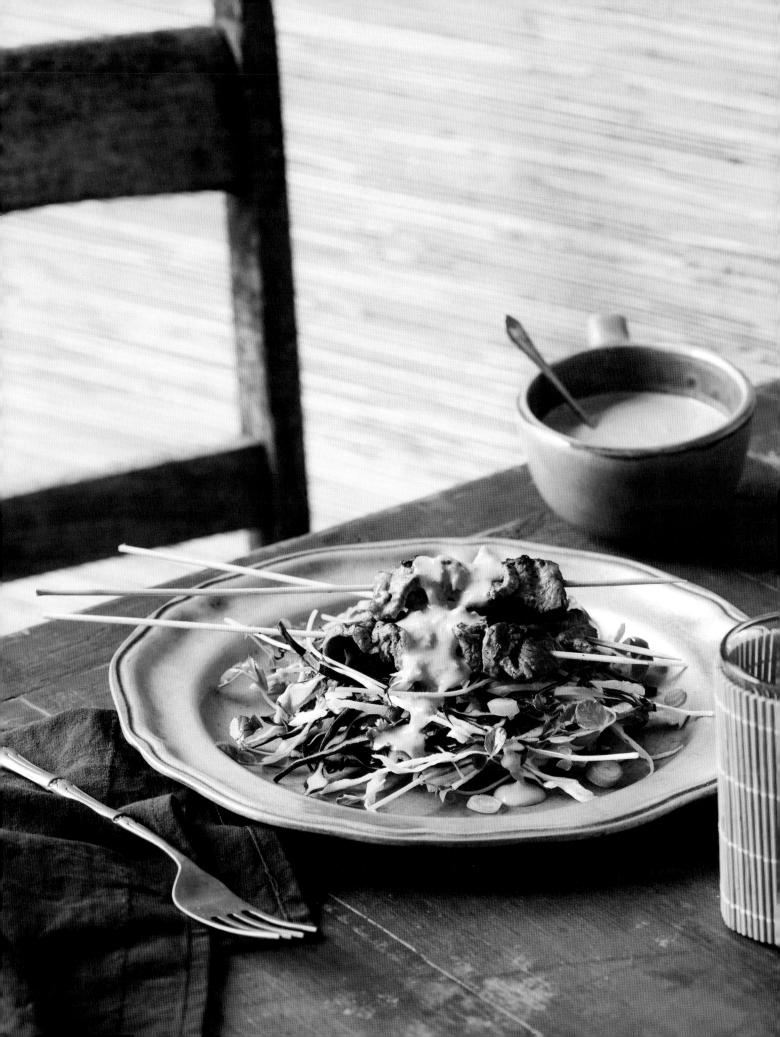

Lamb skewers with satay sauce and Asian-style slaw

Commercial satay sauces are usually higher in salt and unhealthy saturated fats. This version is quick, easy and healthy, and great served with brown rice or whole-wheat noodles.

PREPARATION **30 MINUTES, PLUS 30 MINUTES SOAKING AND MARINATING**
COOKING **10 MINUTES**
SERVES **4**

1 pound (500 g) loin lamb steaks
2 cloves garlic, crushed
3 teaspoons (15 ml) canola oil

Satay sauce
2 teaspoons (10 ml) canola oil
2 shallots, finely chopped
2 cloves garlic, crushed
1 teaspoon (5 ml) finely grated fresh ginger
½ teaspoon (2 ml) ground turmeric
⅔ cup (150 ml) light coconut milk
½ cup (125 g) creamy peanut butter
1 tablespoon (15 ml) low-sodium soy sauce
½ teaspoon (2 ml) brown sugar

Cabbage salad
½ cup (125 g) finely shredded red cabbage
½ cup (125 g) finely shredded white cabbage
¼ cup (50 g) snow pea sprouts
4 scallions, thinly sliced
¼ cup (10 g) fresh cilantro leaves, roughly
   chopped
2 tablespoons (30 ml) lime juice
2 teaspoons (10 ml) low-sodium soy sauce
1 teaspoon (5 ml) honey

1   Soak 12 bamboo skewers in water for 30 minutes.

2   Cut the lamb crosswise into thin slices. Toss with the garlic and oil, cover and refrigerate for 30 minutes.

3   To make the satay sauce, heat the oil in a small saucepan over medium–low heat. Cook the shallots, garlic and ginger, stirring, for 1 minute. Add the turmeric and cook for a few seconds. Stir in the coconut milk, peanut butter, soy sauce and sugar, and cook until smooth and heated through.

4   Thread the lamb onto the skewers. Heat a nonstick grill pan or barbecue grill. Cook the skewers for 3 minutes per side, until the lamb is tender and done to your liking. You may need to cook the skewers in batches, depending on the size of your pan or grill.

5   To make the salad, toss the cabbage, snow pea sprouts, scallions and cilantro in a large bowl. Combine the lime juice, soy sauce and honey. Just before serving, drizzle the dressing over the vegetables and toss to combine.

6   Serve the lamb skewers with the salad, drizzled with the satay sauce.

If the satay sauce is too thick, you can thin it with a little bit of water.

EACH SERVING PROVIDES
549 calories, 36 g protein, 38 g fat (13 g saturated fat),
14 g carbohydrate (8 g sugars), 4 g fiber, 588 mg sodium

Keep your brain healthy and well fueled by eating *cabbage*. Several large research studies have found an association between cruciferous vegetables and reduced inflammation, leading to a lower risk of heart disease.

Spiced lamb with roasted beets and herbed hummus

This dish of sliced lamb on hummus is a Lebanese-inspired recipe, and beets are a perfect match. Serve with some roasted baby carrots and cauliflower florets sprinkled with cumin seeds.

PREPARATION **20 MINUTES, PLUS OVERNIGHT MARINATING**
COOKING **50 MINUTES**
SERVES **4**

$^2/_3$ pound (300 g) loin lamb steaks
1 teaspoon (5 ml) ground allspice
1 teaspoon (5 ml) ground cinnamon
$^1/_2$ teaspoon (2 ml) freshly grated nutmeg
$^1/_2$ teaspoon (2 ml) ground black pepper
1 tablespoon (15 ml) olive oil
2 small beets, scrubbed
2 tablespoons (30 ml) red wine vinegar
1 tablespoon (15 ml) extra virgin olive oil
$^1/_2$ cup (60 g) chopped walnuts

Herbed hummus
15 ounce (425 ml) can chickpeas, rinsed
   and drained
1 tablespoon (15 ml) tahini
1 tablespoon (15 ml) lemon juice
1 clove garlic, roughly chopped
1 tablespoon (15 ml) chopped fresh cilantro
1 tablespoon (15 ml) chopped fresh dill
$^1/_3$ cup (75 ml) ice water

1   Trim any excess fat from the lamb and place in a shallow dish. Combine the allspice, cinnamon, nutmeg, pepper and olive oil, and rub all over the lamb. Cover and refrigerate overnight, if time permits.

2   Preheat the oven to 400°F (200°C). Put the beets on a large sheet of foil, fold in the sides to enclose and bake for 40 minutes, until tender. Cool slightly, then peel and dice the beets. Transfer to a bowl, add the vinegar and extra virgin olive oil, and gently toss to coat the beets.

3   To make the hummus, combine the chickpeas, tahini, lemon juice, garlic, cilantro and dill in a food processor, and process to a smooth paste. With the motor running, gradually add the ice water and process until smooth and creamy.

4   Heat a large frying pan over medium–high heat. Cook the lamb, turning once, for 5–10 minutes, or until cooked to your liking. Let stand for 5 minutes before slicing.

5   Spoon the hummus onto four serving plates and spread it into a large circle. Top with the lamb and beets, and sprinkle with the walnuts.

It is important that you use ice water to make the hummus, which will produce a smooth, creamy hummus, without adding any oil.

Replace the canned chickpeas with 1$^1/_2$ cups (375 g) cooked chickpeas made from $^1/_2$ cup (110 g) dried chickpeas.

EACH SERVING PROVIDES
409 calories, 23 g protein, 31 g fat (6 g saturated fat), 11 g carbohydrate (2 g sugars), 6 g fiber, 220 mg sodium

Chickpeas slowly release their energy to help keep you feeling full longer and help to maintain a steady supply of energy to the brain.

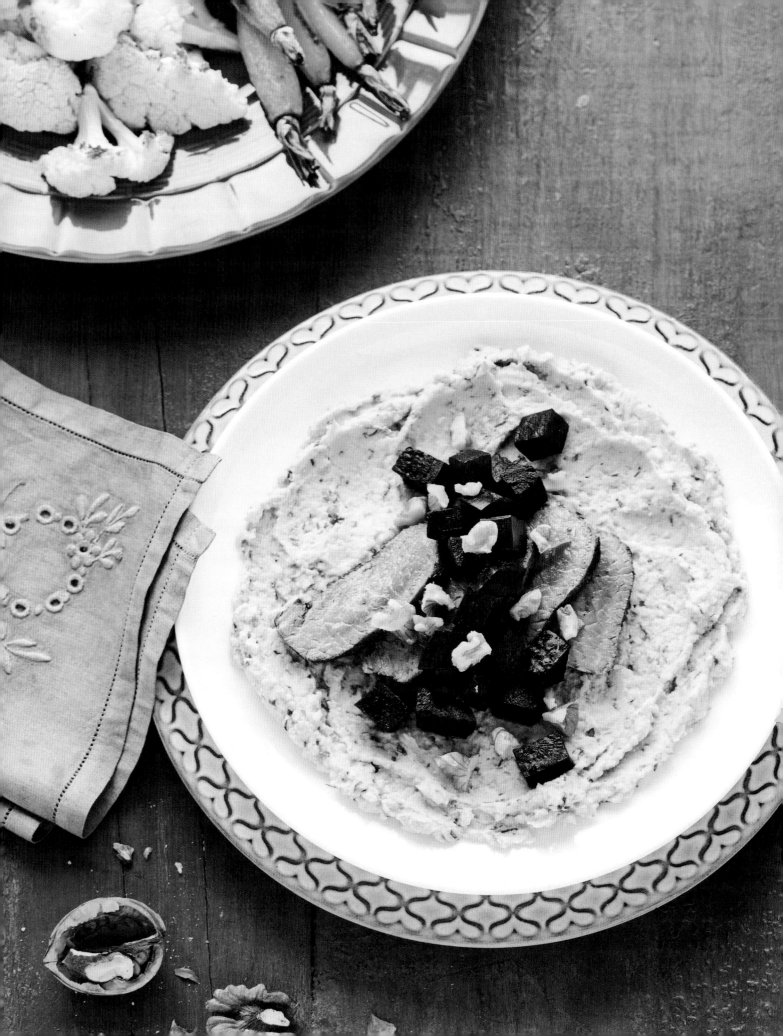

Brain-boosting treats and desserts

The nutrients in these treats make them brain-healthy and delicious.

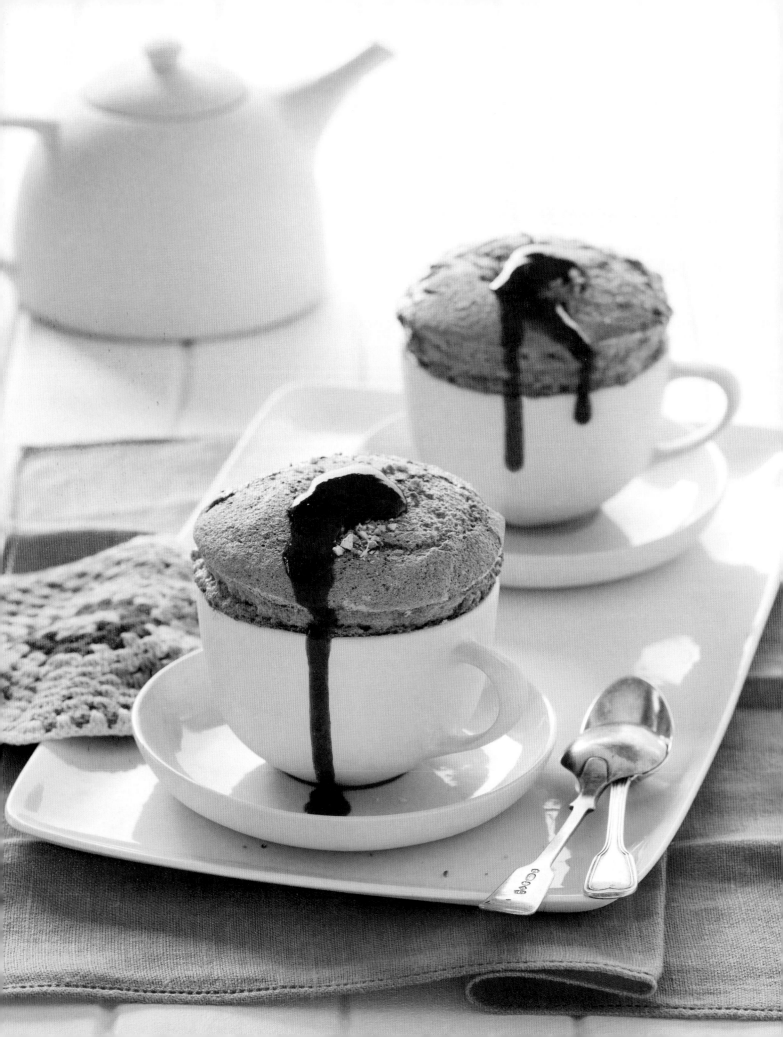

Hot raspberry soufflés

Don't be daunted by the thought of making soufflés—these pretty pink ones aren't difficult at all. Prepare the raspberry purée ahead, and measure all the ingredients so you can assemble and bake them right before serving.

PREPARATION **20 MINUTES**
COOKING **15 MINUTES**
SERVES **6**

$\frac{1}{2}$ cup (115 g) superfine sugar
1$\frac{2}{3}$ cups (400 g) raspberries
1 teaspoon (5 ml) vanilla extract
2 eggs, separated
2 egg whites, extra
1$\frac{1}{2}$ tablespoons (22 ml) finely
  chopped pistachios

1 Preheat the oven to 350°F (180°C). Lightly oil six 1 cup (250 ml) capacity ramekins. Sprinkle $\frac{1}{2}$ teaspoon (2 ml) of the sugar into each ramekin, turning to coat the sides.

2 Purée the raspberries in a blender or food processor, and press through a sieve to remove the seeds. Measure out a quarter of the purée and set it aside. Combine the remaining purée with the vanilla and egg yolks.

3 Using electric beaters, beat the 4 egg whites in a large, dry bowl until soft peaks form. Gradually add the rest of the sugar, beating after each addition until the sugar has dissolved and the mixture is thick and glossy.

4 Stir a large spoonful of the beaten egg whites into the raspberry and egg yolk mixture. Using a large metal spoon, gently fold in the remaining egg whites until the mixture is combined and there are no lumps of white. Be careful not to lose the volume in the mixture.

5 Spoon the mixture into the prepared ramekins and place on a baking pan. Bake for 15 minutes, until the soufflés are risen and lightly golden on top.

6 Serve the soufflés straight from the oven, topped with the pistachios and reserved raspberry purée.

You can use fresh or thawed frozen raspberries for this recipe. Use eggs at room temperature.

EACH SERVING PROVIDES
147 calories, 5 g protein, 3 g fat (<1 g saturated fat), 24 g carbohydrate (23 g sugars), 4 g fiber, 42 mg sodium

Make this recipe with a variety of different *berries*—all berries are a good source of fiber and antioxidants that are essential for good cardiovascular and brain health.

Pear, cranberry and ginger crisp

Full of fiber, antioxidants and potassium, versatile pears can be a healthy snack or a superb dessert—they become wonderfully fragrant when poached. In this crisp, they are combined with antioxidant-rich cranberries for a brain-boosting treat.

PREPARATION **25 MINUTES**
COOKING **40 MINUTES**
SERVES **6**

5 large pears, about 2 pounds (1 kg) total
2 teaspoons (10 ml) superfine sugar
$1/2$ cup (60 g) dried cranberries, halved
1 teaspoon (5 ml) vanilla extract

Topping
$1/3$ cup (55 g) whole-wheat all-purpose flour
$1/2$ teaspoon (2 ml) ground ginger
$1/4$ cup (60 g) olive oil spread
$1/2$ cup (50 g) rolled oats
2 tablespoons (30 ml) shredded coconut
2 tablespoons (30 ml) brown sugar
$1/3$ cup (40 g) chopped pecans

1   Preheat the oven to 375°F (190°C).

2   Peel, quarter and core the pears, roughly chop and place in a large saucepan. Sprinkle with the sugar, cover and bring to a boil. Reduce the heat to medium–low and cook for 5 minutes. Stir in the cranberries.

3   Using a slotted spoon, transfer the pears and cranberries to a 5 cup (1.25 L) capacity ovenproof dish, leaving behind most of the liquid. Stir in the vanilla.

4   To make the topping, sift the flour and ginger into a bowl. Add the olive oil spread and use your fingertips to rub it in until evenly combined. Mix in the oats, coconut, brown sugar and pecans.

5   Sprinkle the topping over the fruit in the dish and bake for 30 minutes, until golden brown.

6   Serve the crisp hot or warm, with a low-fat custard or low-fat ice cream.

Choose pears that are ripe but still firm so that they don't lose their shape when cooked.

EACH SERVING PROVIDES
307 calories, 4 g protein, 13 g fat (3 g saturated fat), 47 g carbohydrate (24 g sugars), 9 g fiber, 43 mg sodium

Cranberries are high in antioxidants. In some animal studies, cranberry extract has been shown to protect brain cells against the kind of damage seen in dementia and stroke. Dried cranberries have sugar added, but supermarkets often stock frozen cranberries which can be used in this recipe—just slice the berries in half.

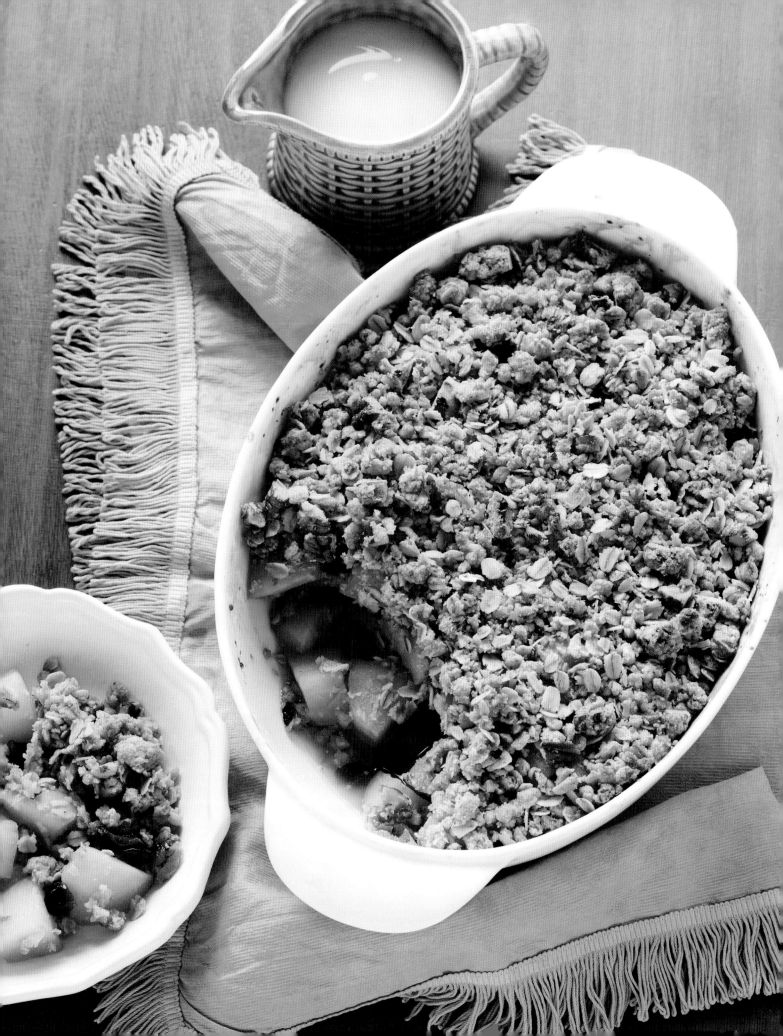

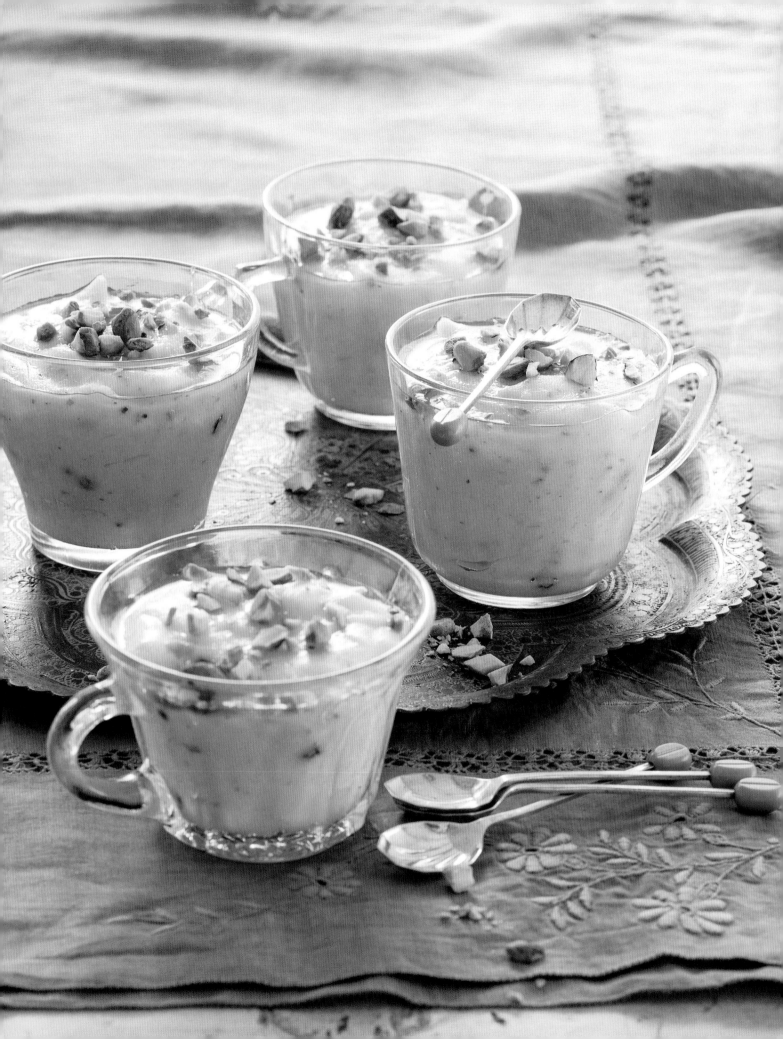

Saffron and pistachio puddings with cardamom and honey syrup

Creamy and mildly sweet, this Indian-style dessert makes a great finish to a spicy meal. It can also be used as an accompaniment to poached fruits such as pears, apples, quince or apricots.

PREPARATION **20 MINUTES, PLUS 1 HOUR SOAKING**
COOKING **15 MINUTES**
SERVES **4**

$^{1}/_{2}$ cup (75 g) raw pistachios
3 cups (750 ml) low-fat milk
$1^{1}/_{2}$ tablespoons (22 ml) currants
pinch of saffron threads
1 cinnamon stick
2 cardamom pods, crushed
2 tablespoons (30 ml) honey
$1^{1}/_{3}$ cups (185 g) fine semolina
1 teaspoon (5 ml) rosewater

Cardamom and honey syrup
$1^{1}/_{2}$ tablespoons (22 ml) honey
2 cardamom pods, crushed

1   Finely chop or process half the pistachios. Coarsely chop the remainder and set aside.

2   Combine the milk, currants, saffron threads, cinnamon stick and cardamom pods in a large saucepan. Allow the mixture to stand for 1 hour if time permits. Bring to a boil, remove the cinnamon stick and whisk in the honey and semolina.

3   Beat until the mixture is completely smooth, and stir in the finely chopped pistachios and the rosewater. Spoon or pour into four 1 cup (250 ml) serving glasses or dishes.

4   To make the syrup, combine the honey and cardamom pods in a small saucepan and bring to a boil.

5   Serve the puddings topped with the hot cardamom and honey syrup and the remaining pistachios.

EACH SERVING PROVIDES

432 calories, 18 g protein, 10 g fat (1 g saturated fat), 68 g carbohydrate (35 g sugars), 4 g fiber, 120 mg sodium

Saffron is believed to be a natural mood-enhancer, and may even protect against depression. Research studies are investigating how it might be used to treat mood disorders.

Raspberry chia pots with coconut yogurt

PREPARATION **10 MINUTES, PLUS 4 HOURS SETTING**
SERVES **4**

4 cups (500 g) fresh or frozen raspberries
1/2 cup (100 g) white chia seeds
1/2 cup (125 ml) low-fat Greek-style yogurt
2 tablespoons (30 ml) coconut cream (do not shake
 the can—use the thick cream from the top)
1 teaspoon (5 ml) maple syrup
2 tablespoons (30 ml) toasted slivered almonds
1/2 cup (60 g) fresh raspberries (optional),
 to serve

1　Use a fork to crush the raspberries until they are broken but not puréed. Stir in the chia seeds.

2　Divide the raspberry and chia mixture among four 1/2 cup (125 ml) glasses. Cover and chill for 4 hours, until set.

3　Just before serving, put the yogurt, coconut cream and maple syrup in a bowl, and mix until combined. Spoon over the chia pots and sprinkle with the almonds and fresh raspberries, if using.

Serve the chia pots sprinkled with your choice of nuts or seeds.

EACH SERVING PROVIDES
242 calories, 10 g protein, 14 g fat (4 g saturated fat), 23 g carbohydrate (11 g sugars), 16 g fiber, 52 mg sodium

This recipe is set using the fluid-absorbing power of *chia seeds*, which swell to increase in size and form a gel. They provide protein, fiber and healthy fats, including some brain-beneficial omega-3s.

Blueberry yogurt panna cotta

PREPARATION **15 MINUTES, PLUS 4 HOURS SETTING**
SERVES **4**

2 teaspoons (7 g) powdered clear gelatin
2 cups (500 ml) low-fat Greek-style yogurt
1 tablespoon (15 ml) honey
1/4 teaspoon (1 ml) ground ginger
1 teaspoon (5 ml) vanilla extract
1/2 cup (100 g) blueberries
shredded orange zest, to serve
pomegranate seeds, to serve (optional)
2 teaspoons (10 ml) honey

1　Pour 2 tablespoons (30 ml) of hot water into a bowl and sprinkle with the gelatin. Whisk until the gelatin has dissolved. Set aside to cool slightly.

2　In a small bowl, mix the yogurt with the honey, ginger and vanilla until combined.

3　Stir the cooled gelatin into the yogurt mixture. Spoon the mixture into four 1/2 cup (125 ml) molds and chill for 4 hours, until set.

4　Briefly dip the base of each mold in hot water and invert the panna cotta onto a serving plate. Top each panna cotta with blueberries, orange zest and pomegranate seeds, if using, and drizzle with honey.

EACH SERVING PROVIDES
195 calories, 11 g protein, 4 g fat (3 g saturated fat), 27 g carbohydrate (22 g sugars), <1 g fiber, 195 mg sodium

Yogurt is great as a low-fat, high-calcium ingredient for desserts that traditionally use cream or cream cheese. Calcium is not only important for strong bones but is also involved in nerve transmissions.

Flash-frozen berries are delicious and high in antioxidants, so you can enjoy them in desserts all year round.

Left: Raspberry chia pots with coconut yogurt
Right: Blueberry yogurt panna cotta

Low-fat dairy foods

Dairy foods are nutritious and highly versatile, with a wide variety of products and culinary uses. Many of these products are excellent sources of protein, calcium, phosphorus and vitamins, and most are available in a low-fat or reduced-fat form.

Clockwise from left: ricotta, evaporated milk, yogurt, low-fat milk, drained yogurt, skim milk, low-fat ice cream

The Internet is rife with recommendations to avoid dairy foods, but this advice is generally based on misconceptions. Dairy foods remain the best way for most people to obtain their calcium needs, as long as low-fat milk and yogurt are the main choices (low-fat cheeses are usually very high in salt). Low-fat varieties of dairy foods are higher in protein and calcium than full-fat varieties and it is simple to swap your milk, yogurt, cheese and ice cream to reduced-fat versions for more nutrition and less fat. Other great swaps using low-fat dairy foods include using drained low-fat yogurt as an alternative to cream cheese or sour cream in desserts; substituting skim evaporated milk for cream in soups and pasta sauces; and whipping low-fat ricotta to replace cream or cream cheese in dips and desserts. These all provide much less fat, and lots more protein, calcium, vitamins and minerals than their fatty alternatives.

Three to four servings per day of dairy foods can meet most people's calcium requirements. Everybody knows that calcium is important for healthy bones, but less well-known is the essential role it plays in neurotransmission. The body maintains strict control of calcium levels in the blood to enable proper nerve and muscle function. If you don't get enough calcium from your diet, it will be taken out of your bones to keep blood levels stable.

Dairy food is also a good source of vitamin B_{12}, essential for myelin and for processing inflammatory homocysteine to minimize its damage to brain cells. Magnesium, potassium, zinc and phosphorus are also important for brain function. These are all found in good amounts in low-fat dairy foods.

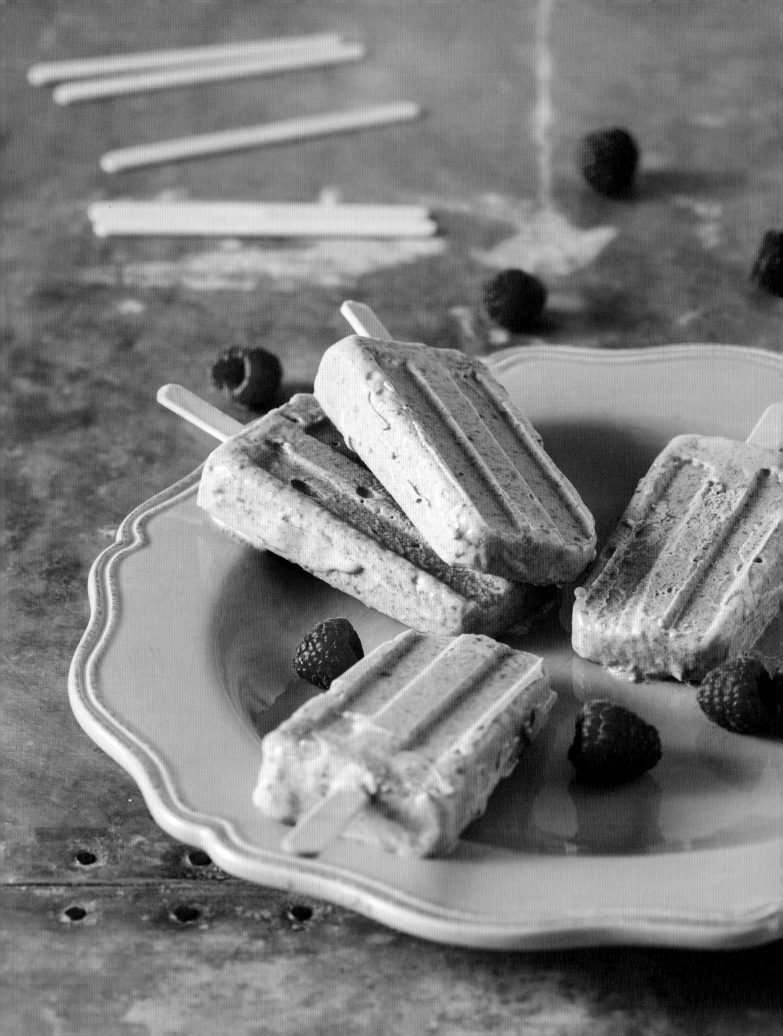

Banana and raspberry yogurt ice cream

Frozen berries are great for this recipe, so use your choice of berries or a mixture, instead of the raspberries. Yogurt is used here instead of cream for a healthier treat.

PREPARATION **20 MINUTES, PLUS FREEZING AND DRAINING**
SERVES **8**

3 large, ripe bananas, about 1 pound (500 g) total
1 cup (250 ml) low-fat Greek-style yogurt
1 cup (200 g) frozen raspberries
1 teaspoon (5 ml) vanilla extract

1   Cut the bananas into ³/₄-inch (2-cm) slices, and place in a ziplock plastic bag. Expel the excess air and tightly seal. Freeze for about 6 hours, until firm.

2   Meanwhile, line a sieve with cheesecloth and put it over a bowl, without the bottom of the sieve touching the bottom of the bowl. Spoon the yogurt into the cheesecloth, gather up the ends and twist to close. Place a saucer on the cheesecloth and weigh it down with a couple of heavy cans. Place the yogurt in the fridge to drain for 4 hours.

3   Combine the frozen banana slices, frozen raspberries, drained yogurt and vanilla in a food processor. Process until smooth and evenly combined, occasionally stopping to scrape down the sides with a rubber spatula.

4   Transfer the mixture to an airtight container and freeze for 6 hours, until firm. Remove from the freezer 10 minutes before serving, so it can soften. For individual servings, freeze the mixture in eight 1 cup (100 ml) popsicle molds.

EACH SERVING PROVIDES
238 calories, 14 g protein, 5 g fat (4 g saturated fat),
34 g carbohydrate (25 g sugars), 3 g fiber, 236 mg sodium

This method of *draining yogurt* is useful for many recipes that call for cream cheese, sour cream or thickened cream. Even if you substitute only half the cream for this yogurt cheese, you'll have four times the protein and calcium—and half the fat.

Buttermilk puddings with mixed berries

Bright berries add a dramatic contrast to these creamy, white puddings. Tangy, low-fat buttermilk lends a pleasing, slightly tart taste, making the puddings more refreshing than if they were made with sweet cream.

PREPARATION **15 MINUTES, PLUS 4 HOURS SETTING**
COOKING **10 MINUTES**
SERVES **4**

2 cups (500 ml) buttermilk
2 tablespoons (30 ml) superfine sugar
1 vanilla bean
$1/6$ ounce (5 g) gelatin sheets
2 cups (250 g) mixed frozen berries
1 tablespoon (15 ml) maple syrup

1 Combine the buttermilk and sugar in a small saucepan. Split the vanilla bean lengthwise, scrape the tiny seeds into the pan and add the vanilla bean. Gently heat the mixture until hot but not boiling. Turn off the heat and let stand for 10 minutes; remove the vanilla bean.

2 Soak the gelatin in a bowl of cold water for 5 minutes, to soften. Squeeze out the water, add the gelatin to the buttermilk mixture and stir until dissolved.

3 Lightly oil four $1/2$ cup (125 ml) molds. Pour in the buttermilk mixture and chill for 4 hours, until set.

4 Place the berries in a saucepan and gently heat until thawed and juicy. Stir in the maple syrup.

5 Just before serving, invert each mold onto a serving plate. Firmly hold the mold with your thumbs and the plate with your hands, and give a sharp shake to dislodge the pudding. Spoon the berries over the puddings.

To avoid using oil, simply pour the buttermilk mixture into the molds and, when set, briefly dip the base of each in hot water before inverting.

EACH SERVING PROVIDES
169 calories, 7 g protein, 3 g fat (2 g saturated fat), 26 g carbohydrate (23 g sugars), 3 g fiber, 82 mg sodium

Buttermilk is traditionally made by adding a yogurt culture to the fluid left over after butter is made. It is low in fat and high in calcium, great for cardiovascular health to help maintain a good blood supply to the brain.

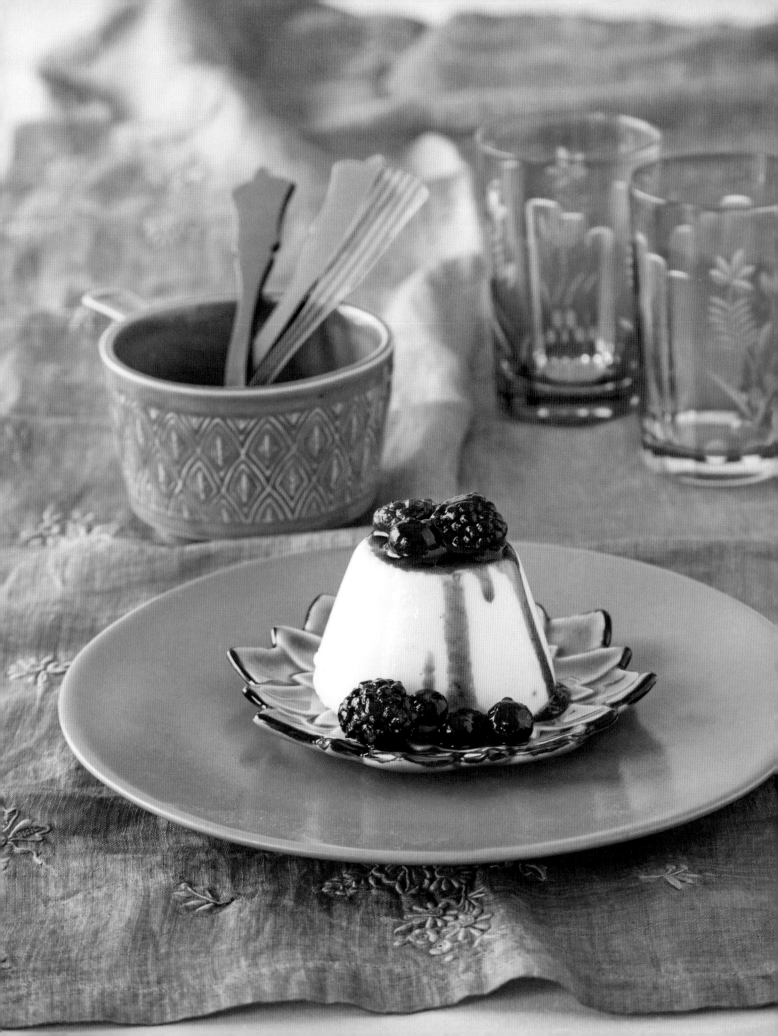

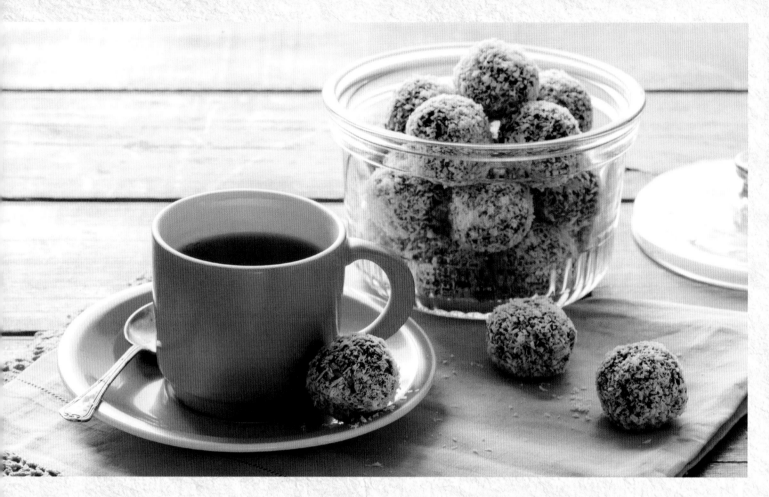

Coconut, mixed seed and almond-butter balls

These nutrient-dense balls are a great alternative to cakes and cookies.
Purchase the ingredients at the supermarket or health food store.

PREPARATION 20 MINUTES   MAKES 24 BALLS

³/₄ cup (125 g) dried figs, roughly chopped
2 teaspoons (10 ml) finely grated orange zest
¹/₄ cup (50 ml) orange juice
2 tablespoons (30 ml) chia seeds
¹/₄ cup (50 g) flaxseeds
¹/₃ cup (95 g) almond butter
¹/₄ cup (30 g) sunflower seeds
¹/₃ cup (30 g) shredded coconut

1 Combine the figs, orange zest, orange juice and
chia seeds in a bowl, and let stand for 10 minutes.

2 Coarsely grind the flaxseeds in a spice grinder,
coffee grinder or mortar and pestle. Put them in a
food processor with the almond butter, sunflower
seeds, half the coconut and fig mixture. Pulse in
short bursts until well combined.

3 Roll level tablespoons (15 ml) of the mixture into
balls. Toss the balls in the remaining coconut.

Refrigerate the balls in an airtight container for
up to 2 weeks.

If using a coffee or spice grinder, make sure it is very
clean to remove any trace of unwanted flavors. If you
don't have almond butter, you can use peanut butter.

EACH SERVING (2 BALLS) PROVIDES
120 calories, 3 g protein, 7 g fat (2 g saturated fat),
12 g carbohydrate (10 g sugars), 4 g fiber, 7 mg sodium

For a similar number of calories, two balls
provide twice the *protein* you would get
from a fun-size candy bar, as well as
beneficial fats and *fiber*.

Chewy nut bars

This chewy snack is packed with nutritious seeds, making them chock full of healthy fiber. You can use your own favorite combination of seeds or add chopped nuts to vary the flavor.

PREPARATION **10 MINUTES**   COOKING **20 MINUTES**   MAKES **24 BARS**

1⅓ cups (200 g) mixed seeds, such as sunflower
   seeds, pepitas (pumpkin seeds), sesame seeds
   and flaxseeds
1 cup (50 g) crushed whole-grain cereal flakes
⅔ cup (110 g) whole-wheat all-purpose flour
¼ cup (55 g) superfine sugar
½ cup (100 g) canola or olive oil spread
¼ cup (90 g) honey or molasses
1 teaspoon (5 ml) baking powder

1   Preheat the oven to 325°F (160°C). Line an
11 x 7 x ½ inch (28 x 18 x 1 cm) baking pan with
parchment paper.

2   Combine the seeds, crushed cereal, flour and
sugar in a bowl.

3   Put the canola or olive oil spread and honey or
molasses in a large saucepan. Cook over medium–
low heat until bubbling, about 3 minutes.

4   Add the baking powder and quickly stir—the
mixture will foam up. Working quickly, add the dry
ingredients and briefly stir until well combined.

5   Spread the mixture into the prepared pan and
smooth the surface. Bake for 15 minutes, until the
slice is puffed and golden all over. Allow to cool
completely before cutting into 24 bars.

EACH SERVING (1 BAR) PROVIDES
108 calories, 3 g protein, 7 g fat (<1 g saturated fat),
10 g carbohydrate (6 g sugars), 2 g fiber, 33 mg sodium

Nuts and seeds are true brain food,
containing beneficial fats essential
for brain function, as well as valuable
vitamins and minerals.

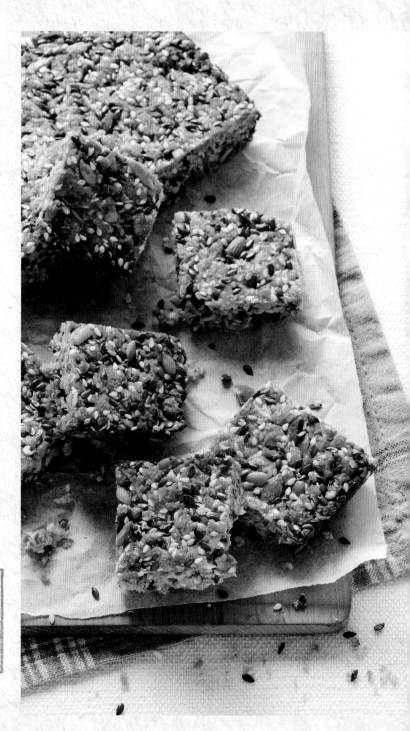

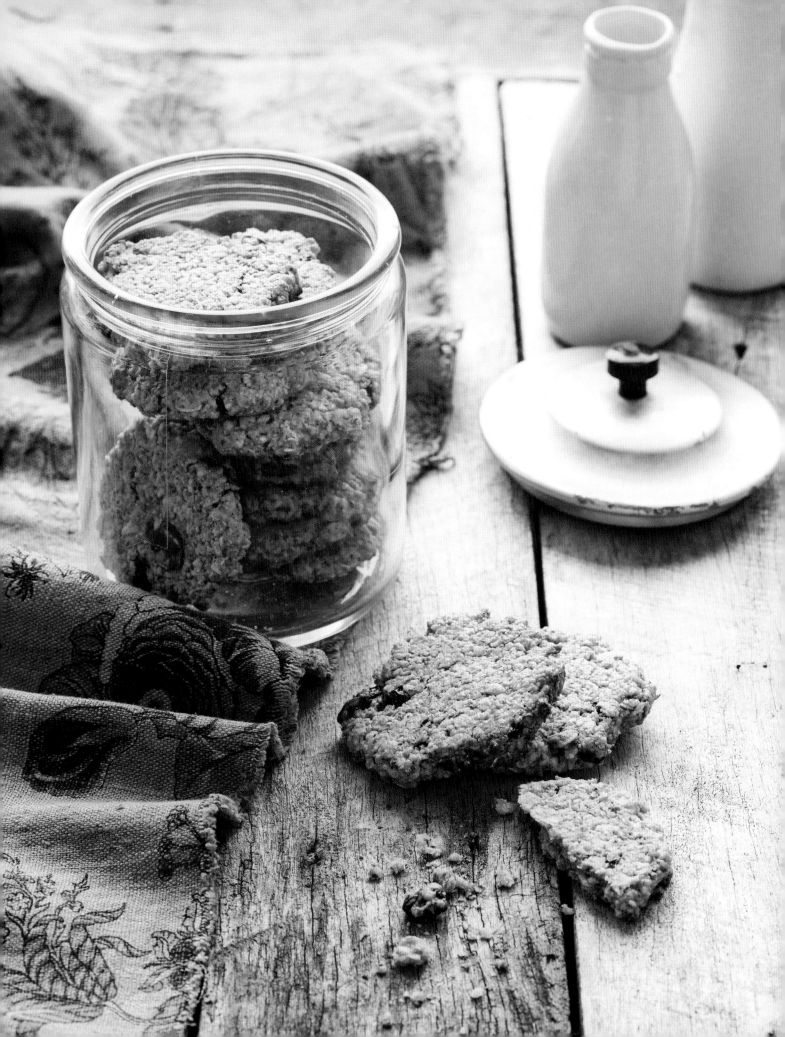

Almond, cranberry and quinoa cookies

These cookies are packed with fiber, beneficial fats and a good amount of protein from quinoa and almonds for a snack that will keep you satisfied longer.

PREPARATION **15 MINUTES**
COOKING **25 MINUTES**
MAKES **24**

2 tablespoons (30 ml) quinoa, rinsed and drained
1 cup (155 g) raw almonds
¼ cup (60 g) olive oil or canola spread
1 egg
¼ cup (90 g) molasses or honey
¼ cup (45 g) brown sugar
2 teaspoons (10 ml) vanilla extract
¾ cup (120 g) whole-wheat self-rising flour
½ cup (50 g) rolled oats
½ cup (65 g) dried cranberry halves

1   Cook the quinoa in a small saucepan of boiling water for about 10 minutes, until soft. Drain and set aside to cool.

2   Preheat the oven to 350°F (180°C). Line two cookie sheets with parchment paper.

3   Put the almonds in a blender or food processor and grind into a fine powder. Add the olive oil or canola spread, egg, molasses or honey, brown sugar and vanilla, and blend until well combined.

4   Combine the flour, oats and dried cranberries in a large bowl. Add the almond mixture and quinoa, and briefly stir to combine.

5   Using a slightly heaping tablespoon (20 ml) of the mixture for each cookie, spoon onto the prepared cookie sheets and press into flat circles.

6   Bake the cookies for 10–15 minutes, until dark golden.

These cookies soften quickly with storage, so bake only the amount you need. Freeze the remaining mixture, ready to bake another day. The cookies don't spread, so you can place them quite close together on the trays.

EACH SERVING (1 COOKIE) PROVIDES
105 calories, 3 g protein, 5 g fat (<1 g saturated fat),
12 g carbohydrate (5 g sugars), 2 g fiber, 46 mg sodium

Molasses is a good alternative to sugar, as its strong caramelized flavor means you use it in smaller amounts. It also contains extra nutrients that sugar doesn't have, such as uridine, iron, copper and magnesium.

Ginger and chocolate cannellini bean cookies

These cookies are full of surprises—no one will suspect that the main ingredient is beans, or that the fats contained in the cookies are healthy ones from almonds and olive oil.

PREPARATION **15 MINUTES**
COOKING **20 MINUTES**
MAKES **24**

14^1/$_2$ ounce (400 ml) can cannellini beans, rinsed and drained
1 egg
^{1}/$_2$ cup (95 g) brown sugar
^{1}/$_4$ cup (50 ml) olive oil
1 cup (100 g) rolled oats
^{1}/$_2$ cup (80 g) raw almonds, chopped
^{1}/$_4$ cup (60 g)) dark chocolate, at least 60% cocoa, chopped
^{1}/$_3$ cup (80 g) chopped crystallized or candied ginger
^{1}/$_2$ cup (80 g) whole-wheat, self-rising flour

1   Preheat the oven to 350°F (180°C). Lightly oil two cookie sheets.

2   Purée the beans in a blender or food processor. Add the egg, sugar and olive oil, and mix until well combined.

3   Combine the oats, almonds, chocolate and ginger in a large bowl. Add the bean mixture and stir well. Add the flour and briefly stir until combined.

4   Using two tablespoons (30 ml) of the mixture for each cookie, drop on the prepared sheets and flatten into circles.

5   Bake the cookies for 20 minutes, until evenly browned.

Replace the canned cannellini beans with 1^1/$_2$ cups (375 g) cooked beans made from ^{1}/$_2$ cup (100 g) dried beans. You can also use other beans, such as black beans.

The cookies won't spread, so you can place them quite close together on the cookie sheets.

EACH SERVING (1 COOKIE) PROVIDES
111 calories, 3 g protein, 6 g fat (1 g saturated fat),
12 g carbohydrate (7 g sugars), 2 g fiber, 55 mg sodium

The antioxidants contained in *dark chocolate*, including flavonoids and catechins, help to control blood pressure, improving blood flow to the brain.

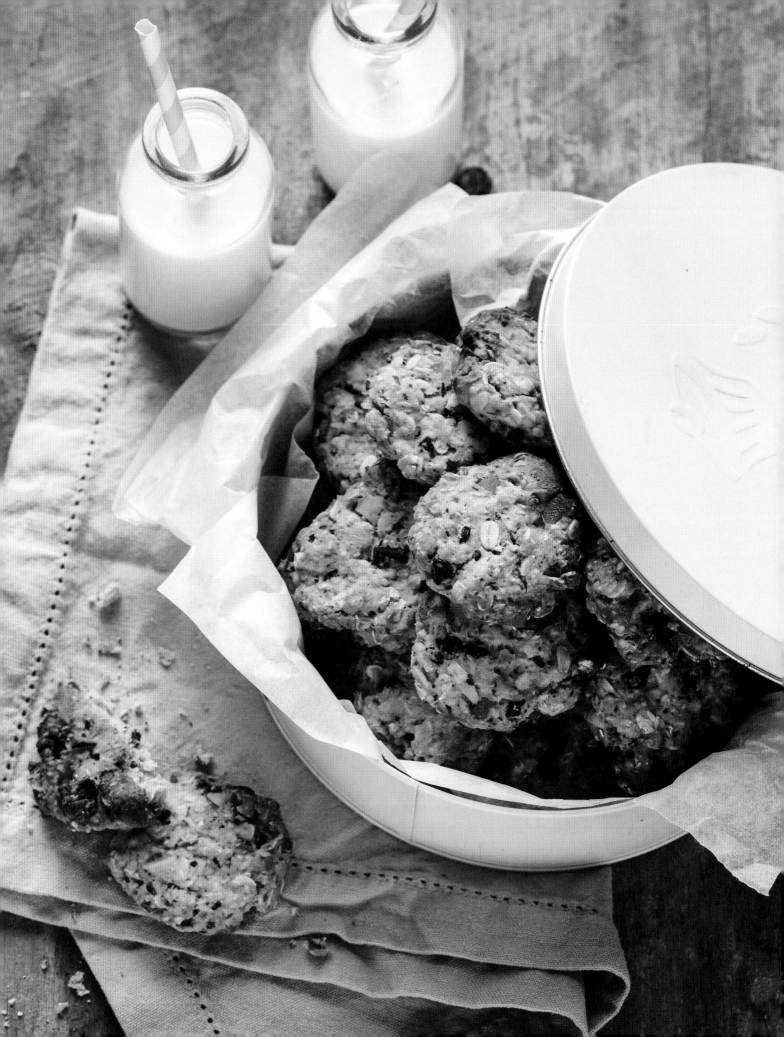

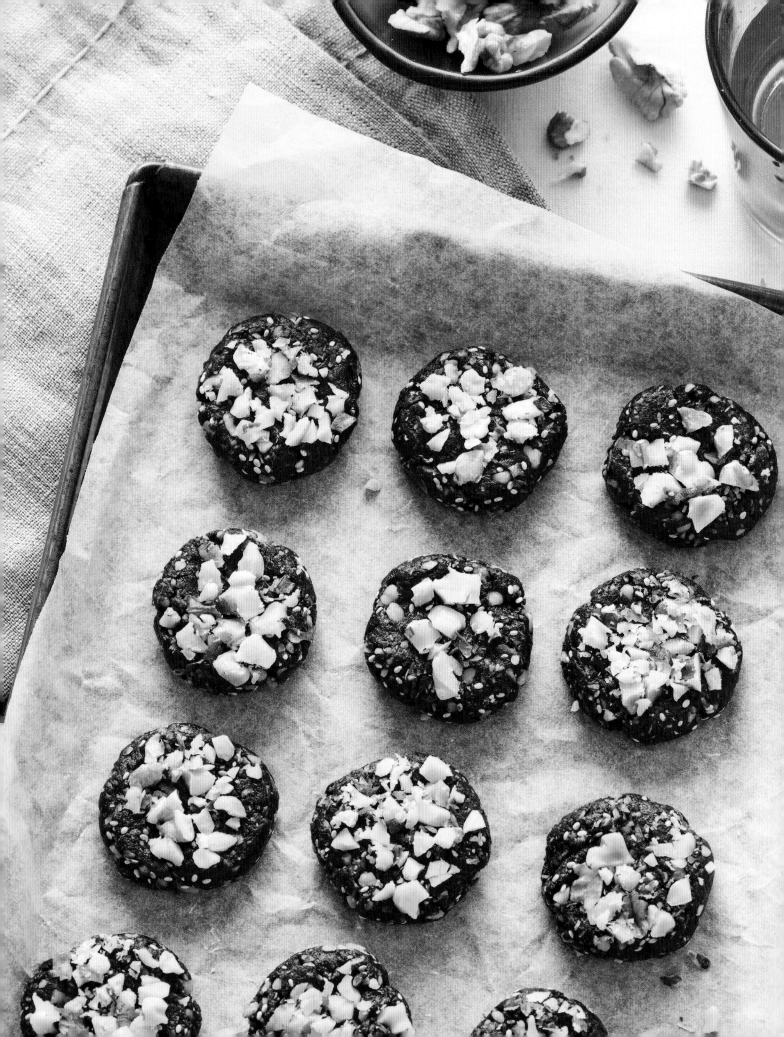

Chocolate, chia and coconut chilled cookies

These cookies are not baked, so they have a soft texture and are best kept in the fridge. While they contain many valuable nutrients, they are an energy-dense treat to enjoy in moderation.

PREPARATION **15 MINUTES**
COOKING **5 MINUTES**
MAKES **24**

½ cup (50 g) walnuts
1 cup (200 g) medjool dates, pitted
½ cup (45 g) shredded coconut
2 tablespoons (30 ml) dark (or Dutch-processed) cocoa powder or raw cacao powder
1 tablespoon (15 ml) chia seeds
1 teaspoon (5 ml) vanilla extract

1   Preheat the oven to 350°F (180°C). Spread the walnuts on a baking pan and bake for 4–5 minutes, until lightly toasted. Transfer the walnuts to a plate to cool, and roughly chop.

2   Put the dates in a food processor and add the coconut, cocoa powder, chia seeds, vanilla and ⅓ cup (40 g) of the walnuts. Process until well combined.

3   Put the remaining chopped walnuts in a bowl. Take a heaping teaspoon (7 ml) of the chocolate mixture and roll it into a ball. Slightly flatten it, and gently press the top into the walnuts. Repeat with the remaining mixture.

4   Put the cookies in a single layer in an airtight container, and chill until firm. The cookies can be refrigerated for up to 2 weeks.

Medjool dates, although dried, are still soft and moist. You will find them sold loose in the fruit and vegetable section of supermarkets, or packaged with the dried fruit. They are a deep amber color, are plump and slightly wrinkled. If you can't buy medjool dates, the recipe will also work well with regular dried dates. You can vary the cookies by using different nuts and other dried fruits.

Raw cacao powder is simply pulverized cacao beans. Regular or natural cocoa powder (the kind most commonly found in stores) is produced at higher temperatures. Dark or Dutch-processed cocoa powder is processed in an alkalized solution and has a richer taste.

EACH SERVING (1 COOKIE) PROVIDES
53 calories, <1 g protein, 3 g fat (1 g saturated fat),
6 g carbohydrate (6 g sugars), 1 g fiber, 3 mg sodium

Cacao powder and dark cocoa powder are both high in fiber and are good sources of minerals such as copper, iron and magnesium that the brain needs for optimal functioning.

Guilt-free chocolate brownies

Black beans boost the nutritional value of these brownies, adding fiber, minerals and low glycemic index carbohydrate to keep you feeling satisfied.

PREPARATION **15 MINUTES**
COOKING **25 MINUTES**
MAKES **16 PIECES**

15 ounce (425 ml) can black beans, rinsed and drained
2 eggs
2 tablespoons (30 ml) olive oil
1/2 cup (100 g) 85% cocoa dark chocolate, melted and cooled slightly
1/4 cup (30 g) dark cocoa powder
1 teaspoon (5 ml) baking powder
1/2 cup (100 g) brown sugar
2 teaspoons (10 ml) vanilla extract
pinch of salt
1 cup (100 g) pecans, chopped

1   Preheat the oven to 350°F (180°C). Lightly grease an 8-inch (20-cm) square cake pan, and line the bottom with parchment paper, extending over two opposite sides.

2   Combine all the ingredients except the pecans in a food processor. Process until smooth and well combined.

3   Spoon the mixture into the prepared pan and smooth the surface. Sprinkle the pecans over the top and gently press into the mixture.

4   Bake for 25 minutes, until the brownie is firm to a gentle touch in the center. Let cool in the pan for 5 minutes, lift out onto a wire rack and slide the paper off. Let cool completely, and cut into 16 squares.

Brownies will keep for up to a week in an airtight container. Make sure you wait until after people have tasted the brownies before revealing the secret ingredient.

Replace the canned black beans with 1 1/2 cups (375 g) cooked beans made from 1/2 cup (110 g) dried beans.

EACH SERVING (1 BROWNIE) PROVIDES
165 calories, 4 g protein, 12 g fat (3 g saturated fat),
13 g carbohydrate (7 g sugars), 3 g fiber, 68 mg sodium

> *Chocolate* tops most people's list of "naughty" foods, but recent research points to potential health benefits from a small regular intake of cocoa and cocoa products, such as dark chocolate. Chocolate that contains at least 65 percent cocoa solids appears to be protective against cardiovascular disease and good for keeping your brain healthy and functioning sharply.

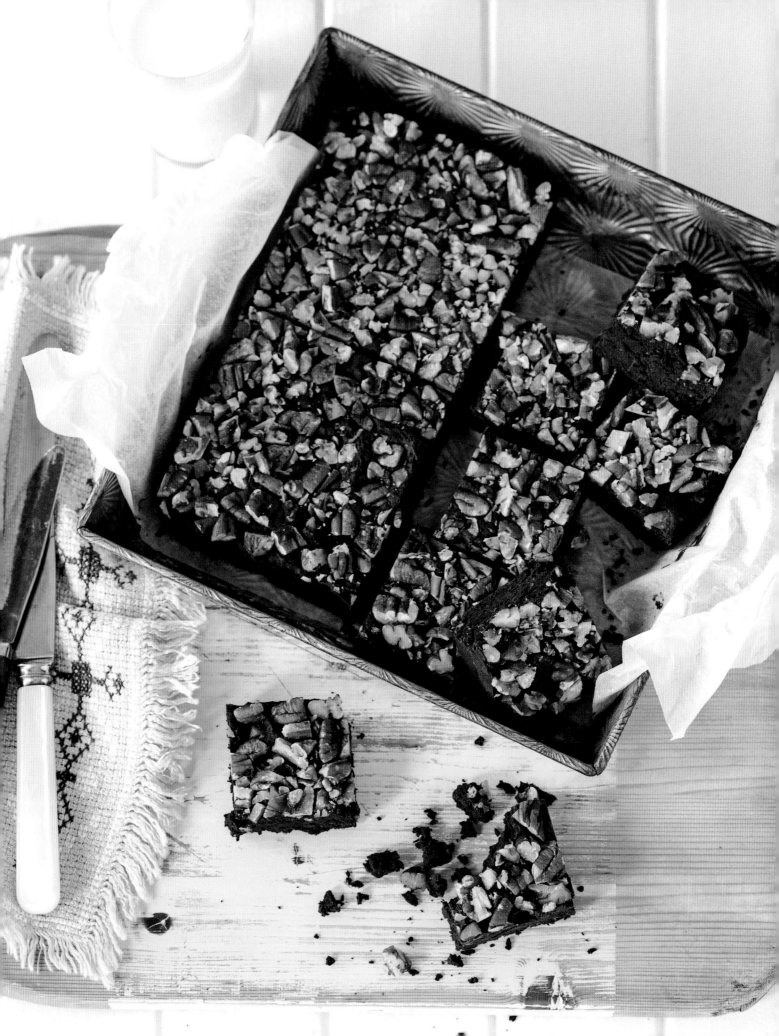

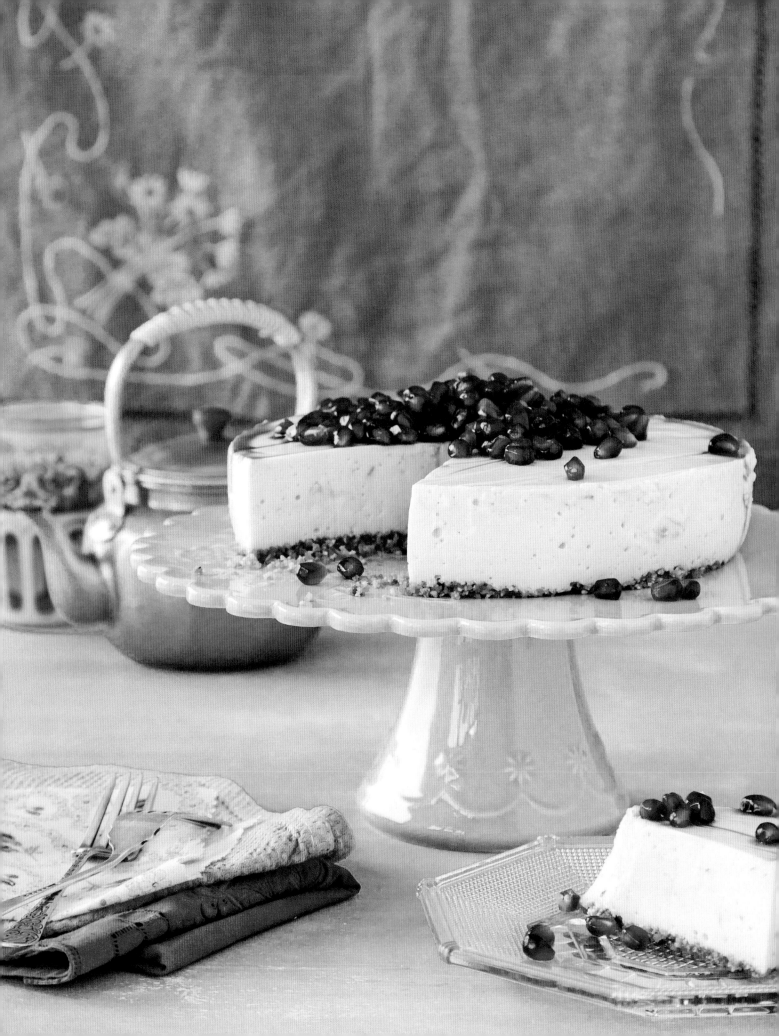

Chilled lime cheesecake

Silken tofu makes a light and creamy filling for this no-bake cheesecake, and the sweet–tart flavor of pomegranate complements it perfectly. If pomegranates aren't available, substitute blueberries or raspberries.

PREPARATION **30 MINUTES, PLUS 3 HOURS SETTING**
COOKING **5 MINUTES**
SERVES **8–10**

2 tablespoons (30 ml) canola oil
2 tablespoons (30 ml) brown sugar
$1/3$ cup (55 g) whole-wheat all-purpose flour
$1/3$ cup (35 g) ground almonds
20 ounces (600 g) silken tofu, drained
$2/3$ cup (150 ml) low-fat plain yogurt
$1/3$ cup (40 g) confectioners' sugar
1 teaspoon (5 ml) vanilla extract
1 tablespoon (15 ml) finely grated lime zest
2 tablespoons (30 ml) lime juice
1 tablespoon (14 g) powdered clear gelatin
1 pomegranate

1   Combine the oil, brown sugar, flour and almonds in a nonstick frying pan. Stir over medium heat for 5 minutes, until golden brown. Transfer the mixture to a plate and place in the fridge to cool.

2   Combine the tofu, yogurt, sugar, vanilla, lime zest and lime juice in a food processor, and process until smooth.

3   Pour $2^{1}/_{2}$ tablespoons (37 ml) cold water into a small heatproof bowl and sprinkle with the gelatin. Leave for 1 minute, until softened. Set the bowl in a larger bowl of boiling water, and whisk until the gelatin has dissolved. Stir a spoonful of the tofu mixture into the gelatin, add to the mixture in the food processor and process to combine.

4   Lay a large sheet of parchment paper on the bottom of an 7-inch (18-cm) springform pan, and clip the side into place, leaving the excess paper sticking out the side of the pan. Lightly oil the side of the pan. Pour in the tofu mixture, and evenly sprinkle the almond mixture over the top. Refrigerate for 3 hours, until set.

5   Remove the seeds from half the pomegranate, and press the other half using a citrus squeezer to extract the juice.

6   Run a nonserrated knife around the pan to loosen the cheesecake. Invert onto a serving plate, remove the side of the pan and peel off the paper. Spoon the pomegranate seeds over the cheesecake and drizzle with the pomegranate juice. Cut into wedges and serve immediately.

Turn the cheesecake out just before serving.

To extract the pomegranate seeds, cut the pomegranate in half crosswise. Holding the pomegranate under water, break apart and pry out all of the seeds, discarding the white membrane.

> *Almonds* are an excellent source of vitamin E, part of the body's antioxidant system that protects the brain and cardiovascular system from damage. Use a food processor or blender to grind raw almonds for this recipe.

EACH SERVING PROVIDES
194 calories, 8 g protein, 9 g fat (<1 g saturated fat), 20 g carbohydrate (14 g sugars), 1 g fiber, 25 mg sodium

Blueberry yogurt tart with ginger crust

Draining the yogurt overnight removes a large amount of moisture, leaving a thick yogurt cream that is a healthy alternative to cream cheese and makes this perfect tart filling. The longer you leave it draining, the thicker it will become.

PREPARATION **20 MINUTES, PLUS OVERNIGHT DRAINING**
SERVES **8**

2 cups (500 ml) low-fat Greek-style yogurt
2 teaspoons (10 ml) maple syrup
2 teaspoons (10 ml) rosewater
1 tablespoon (15 ml) white chia seeds (optional)
1 tablespoon (15 ml) 100% blueberry fruit spread (optional)
1½ cups (185 g) blueberries
⅓ cup (50 g) pistachios, roughly chopped

Ginger crust
1 cup (250 g) dried pitted dates, roughly chopped
¼ cup (60 g) almonds, roughly chopped
1 tablespoon (15 ml) tahini
1 teaspoon (5 ml) ground ginger
1 tablespoon (15 ml) white chia seeds (optional)

1   Combine the yogurt, maple syrup, rosewater and chia seeds, if using, in a bowl.

2   Line a sieve with cheesecloth and put it over a bowl, with the bottom of the sieve clear of the bottom of the bowl. Spoon the yogurt into the cheesecloth, gather up the ends and twist to close. Place a saucer on the cheesecloth and weigh it down with two heavy cans. Place in the fridge to drain overnight.

3   To make the ginger crust, put the dates and almonds in a food processor, and chop until the mixture resembles fine breadcrumbs. Add the tahini, ginger and chia seeds, if using, and process until the mixture just comes together.

4   Grease an 8-inch (20-cm) springform pan and line with parchment paper. Firmly press the crust mixture into the bottom of the pan.

5   Spread the blueberry fruit spread, if using, over the crust, and sprinkle with ¼ cup (30 g) of the blueberries. Spread the yogurt mixture over the top and scatter with the remaining blueberries and chopped pistachios. Serve immediately.

Remember to start preparation the day before as the yogurt has to be drained. The ginger crust and yogurt can also be served in individual dishes or bowls.

EACH SERVING PROVIDES
267 calories, 9 g protein, 11 g fat (2 g saturated fat), 34 g carbohydrate (30 g sugars), 5 g fiber, 101 mg sodium

Long valued for their intense sweetness, *dates* are high in fiber, antioxidants and valuable minerals that are important for brain function.

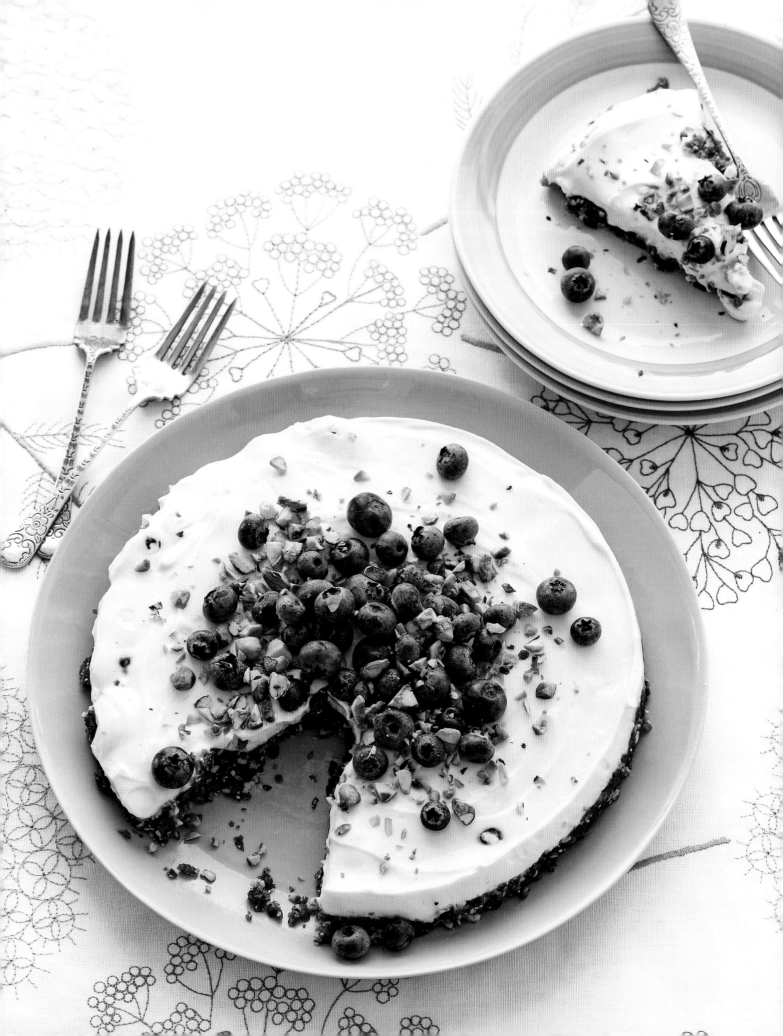

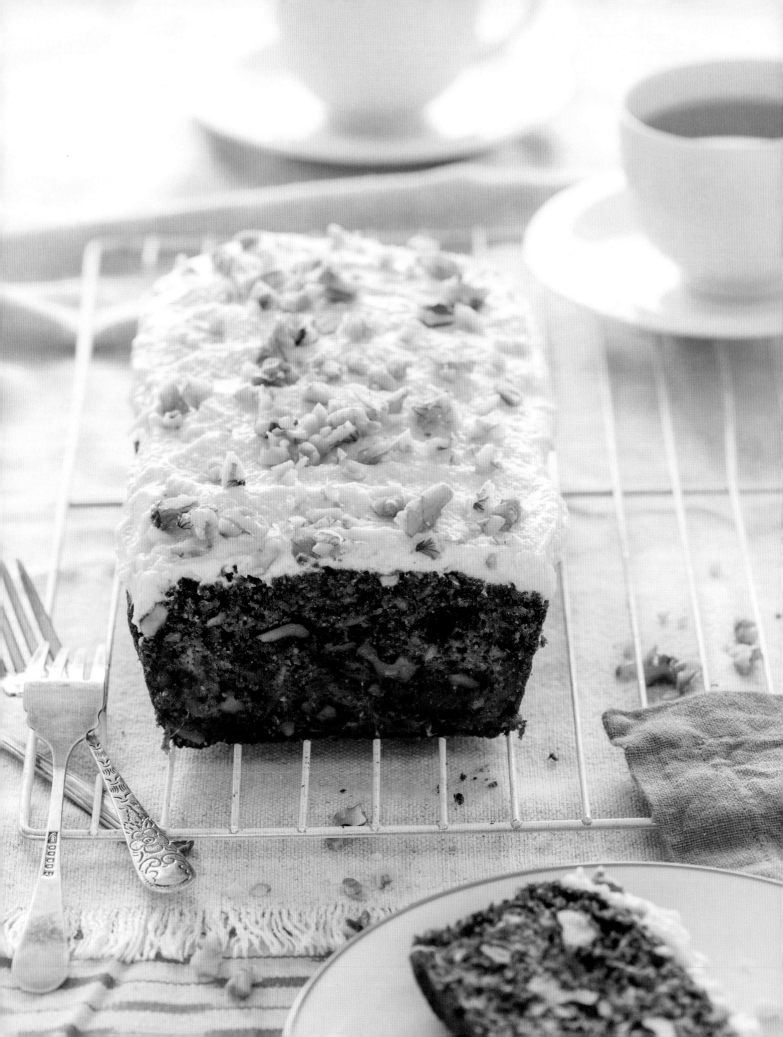

Carrot and walnut cake with tofu frosting

The frosting on this dense cake is made using tofu as a low-fat, high-protein alternative to cream cheese. It crowns a cake that features beneficial fats from almonds, walnuts and olive oil.

PREPARATION **20 MINUTES, PLUS OVERNIGHT DRAINING**
COOKING **40 MINUTES**
MAKES **16 SLICES**

1/4 cup (40 g) raw almonds
1 tablespoon (15 ml) ground nutmeg
1 tablespoon (15 ml) ground cinnamon
1/2 cup (95 g) brown sugar
2 large carrots, grated
1/4 cup (55 g) chopped crystallized or
    candied ginger (optional), plus extra
    to garnish
1 cup (100 g) walnut halves, chopped,
    plus extra to garnish
1/2 cup (125 ml) extra virgin olive oil
2 eggs
1 teaspoon (5 ml) vanilla extract
1/4 cup (40 g) whole-wheat all-purpose flour
1/4 cup (35 g) self-rising flour
1 teaspoon (5 ml) baking soda
1 teaspoon (5 ml) baking powder

Tofu icing
10 ounces (300 g) silken firm tofu
1/2 cup (60 g) confectioners' sugar
2 tablespoons (30 ml) olive oil spread
1 teaspoon (5 ml) vanilla extract
finely grated zest of 1 lemon

1 To prepare the tofu for the icing, line a sieve with cheesecloth and put it over a bowl, without the bottom of the sieve touching the bottom of the bowl. Spoon the tofu into the sieve and refrigerate overnight to drain and thicken.

2 Preheat the oven to 340°F (175°C). Line a 7 1/2 x 3 1/2 inch (19 x 9 cm) loaf pan with parchment paper.

3 Using a blender or food processor, grind the almonds into a coarse powder. Transfer to a large bowl with the nutmeg, cinnamon, brown sugar, carrots, ginger and walnuts. Stir until well combined.

4 Add the olive oil, eggs and vanilla, and beat well. Add the flours, baking soda and baking powder, and briefly stir to combine.

5 Spread the batter into the prepared pan and bake for 40 minutes, until the top springs back when touched. Cool slightly, then turn out onto a wire rack to cool completely.

6 To make the frosting, beat the drained tofu with the sugar, olive oil spread, vanilla and lemon zest until smooth and creamy.

7 Spread the icing over the cooled cake and sprinkle with the extra ginger and walnuts.

You can use 3 tablespoons (45 g) ground almonds instead of grinding the almonds yourself.

EACH SERVING (1 SLICE) PROVIDES
213 calories, 4 g protein, 16 g fat (2 g saturated fat),
15 g carbohydrate (11 g sugars), 2 g fiber, 91 mg sodium

Instead of the traditional butter and cream cheese, this carrot cake features healthy fats from *tofu, nuts* and *olive oil*, which are beneficial for the heart and brain.

Olive, rosemary and walnut bread

Homemade bread is best eaten the day it is made, but can be toasted and kept for a few days or frozen. This savory bread makes a fine base for bruschetta, topped with tomatoes and basil.

PREPARATION **30 MINUTES, PLUS 1 HOUR 35 MINUTES PROOFING**
COOKING **35 MINUTES**
SERVES **12**

2 teaspoons (7 g) dry yeast
2 cups (500 g) whole-wheat all-purpose
  flour, plus extra for kneading
$\frac{1}{4}$ cup (40 g) pitted kalamata olives, halved
$\frac{1}{3}$ cup (40 g) roughly chopped walnuts
1 tablespoon (30 ml) chopped fresh
  rosemary

1 Measure $1\frac{1}{2}$ cups (375 ml) lukewarm water into a bowl, stir in the yeast and a sprinkle of the flour. Let stand for 10 minutes, until frothy.

2 Place the flour in a large bowl and make a well in the center. Pour in the yeast mixture and mix, with a wooden spoon at first and then your hands, until well combined. Turn the dough out onto a lightly floured surface. Knead for 10 minutes, until smooth and elastic.

3 Place the dough in a large, lightly oiled bowl, cover with plastic wrap and let stand in a draft-free place for 45 minutes, until doubled in size.

4 Punch down the dough to expel the air, then briefly knead. Press the dough out flat and sprinkle the olives, walnuts and rosemary over it. Fold the dough over these ingredients, and knead again, folding and turning to incorporate them. Roll the dough into a smooth ball and place on a lightly oiled baking pan.

5 Press the dough into a long oval shape. Cover with a clean dish towel and let rise in a warm place for 30 minutes, until it has doubled in size. Meanwhile, preheat the oven to 400°F (200°C).

6 Brush the top of the bread with water and use a small, sharp knife to cut six slashes across the top of the loaf. Bake for 35 minutes, until the bread is golden brown and sounds hollow when tapped on the bottom.

EACH SERVING (1 SLICE) PROVIDES
179 calories, 6 g protein, 4 g fat (<1 g saturated fat),
29 g carbohydrate (<1 g sugars), 6 g fiber, 40 mg sodium

Rosemary has powerful antioxidant and anti-inflammatory properties that are thought to enhance and stimulate brain function and sharpen mental clarity. This bread also contains beneficial fats from the *olives* and *walnuts*.

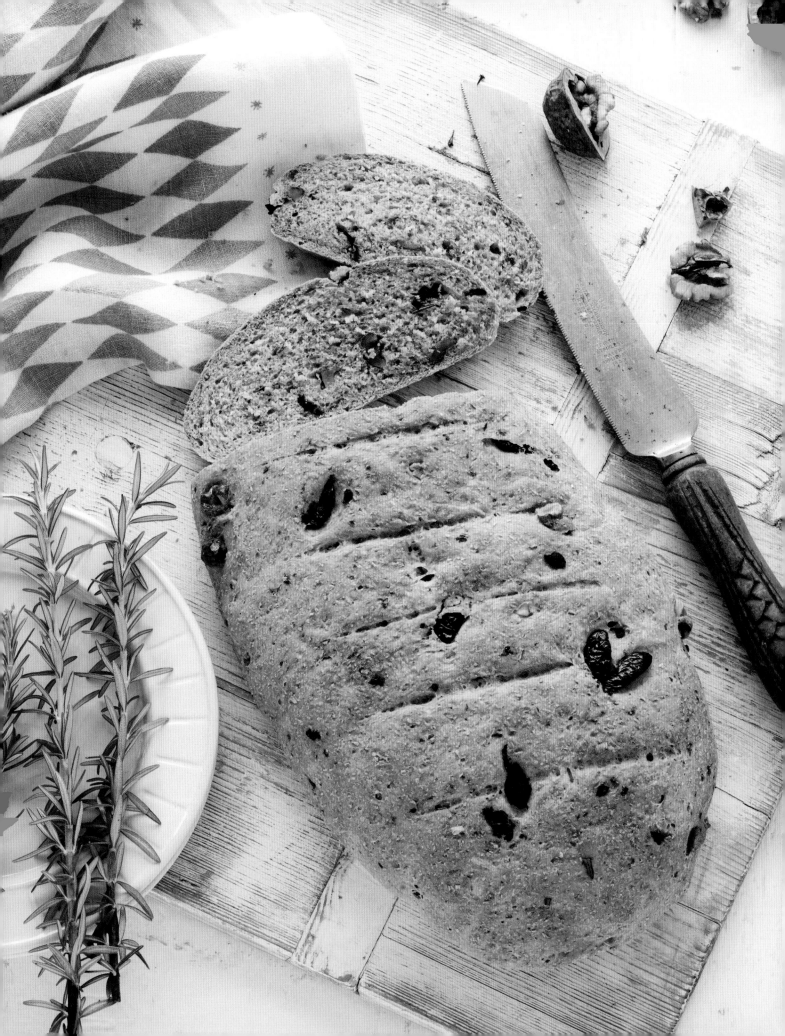

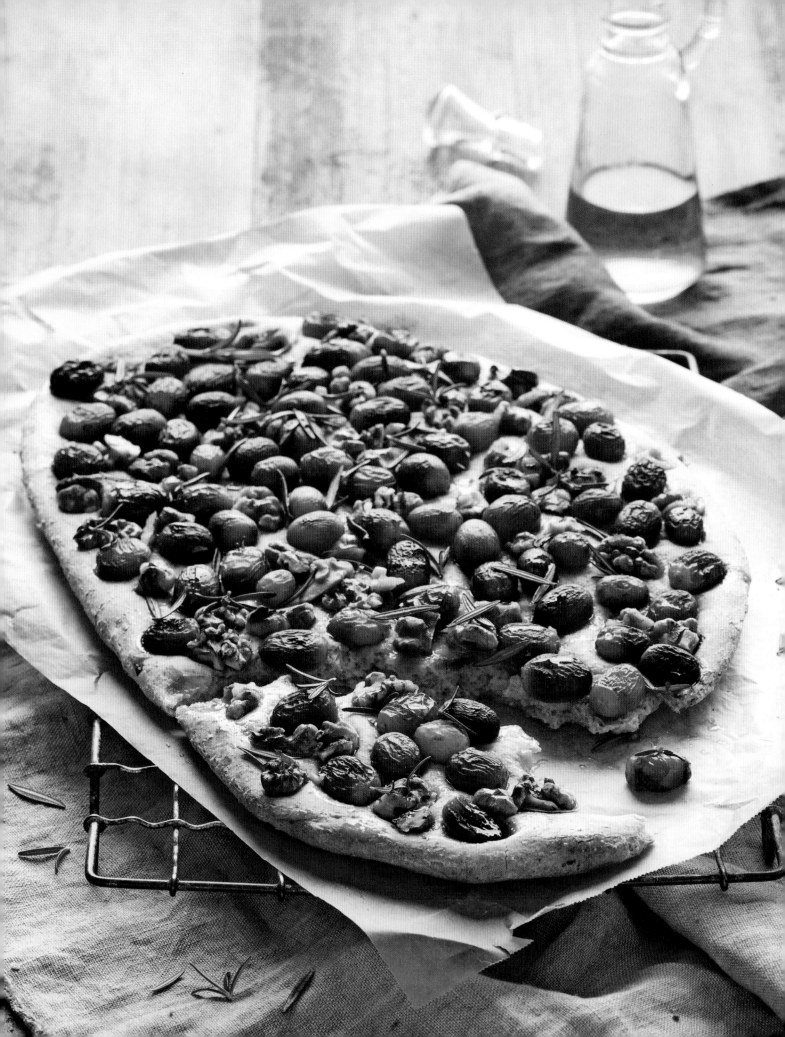

Whole-wheat walnut and grape focaccia

Red grapes, walnuts and rosemary combine beautifully in this elegant and wholesome Italian-style bread that is high in antioxidants and rich in traditional flavors.

PREPARATION **25 MINUTES, PLUS 55 MINUTES PROOFING**
COOKING **25 MINUTES**
SERVES **8**

2 teaspoons (7 g) dry yeast
2 cups (320 g) whole-wheat all-purpose
 flour, plus extra for kneading
2 tablespoons (30 ml) seedless grapes
1 cup (100 g) walnuts
2 tablespoons (30 ml) extra virgin olive oil
1 tablespoon (15 ml) fresh rosemary

1 Measure $\frac{3}{4}$ cup (175 ml) lukewarm water into a bowl, stir in the yeast and a sprinkle of the flour. Let stand for 5 minutes, until frothy.

2 Place the flour in a large bowl and make a well in the center. Pour in the yeast mixture and olive oil, and stir with a wooden spoon until almost combined. Gather the dough together with your hands.

3 Turn the dough out onto a lightly floured surface and knead for 5 minutes, until smooth and elastic.

4 Place the dough in a lightly oiled bowl, cover with plastic wrap and let stand in a warm place for 45 minutes, until doubled in size.

5 Preheat the oven to 400°F (200°C). Lightly oil a large baking sheet. Punch down the dough to expel the air, and knead again for a couple of minutes. Roll out the dough to a 13 x 9 inch (33 x 23 cm) oval or rectangle. Place on the prepared baking sheet.

6 Scatter the grapes and walnuts over the surface and firmly press them into the dough. Bake for 25 minutes, until golden brown. Cool slightly, then drizzle with the extra virgin olive oil and sprinkle with the rosemary.

EACH SERVING PROVIDES
338 calories, 8 g protein, 19 g fat (2 g saturated fat), 34 g carbohydrate (5 g sugars), 7 g fiber, 7 mg sodium

Recent animal studies indicate that age-related changes in the brain may be inhibited by high-antioxidant foods such as *walnuts* and *grapes*. The polyphenols in these foods appear to reduce the effects of oxidative stress on the brain and also improve neural communication, enhancing cognitive performance.

Flaxseed and sesame whole-wheat rolls

Making your own bread is a very satisfying project. Homemade bread doesn't keep as well as store-bought bread, so eat it the day it is made. Leftover rolls can be frozen in a ziplock bag for up to a month. Thaw at room temperature and reheat.

PREPARATION 30 MINUTES, PLUS 1 HOUR 10 MINUTES PROOFING
COOKING 20 MINUTES
MAKES 8

1 tablespoon (14 g) dry yeast
²/₃ cup (135 g) flaxseeds, plus 2 tablespoons (30 ml) extra for sprinkling
4 cups (640 g) whole-wheat all-purpose flour, plus extra for kneading
¼ cup (40 g) sesame seeds, plus 1 tablespoon (15 ml) extra for sprinkling

High *salt* intake can harm the brain. Most of the salt we eat comes from processed foods, added by the manufacturer and some, such as breads and breakfast cereals, don't even taste salty. If you make your own bread, you can significantly reduce the amount of salt or leave it out completely, as in this recipe.

1   Measure 1³/₄ cups (425 ml) lukewarm water into a bowl, stir in the yeast and a sprinkle of the flour. Let stand for 10 minutes, until frothy.

2   Meanwhile, use a clean spice grinder, coffee grinder or mortar and pestle to grind the flaxseeds.

3   Combine the flaxseeds with the flour and sesame seeds in a large bowl, and make a well in the center. Pour in the yeast mixture and mix, with a wooden spoon at first and then your hands, until well combined. Turn the dough out onto a lightly floured surface. Knead for 10 minutes, until smooth and elastic.

4   Place the dough in a large, lightly oiled bowl, cover with plastic wrap and stand in a draft-free place for 45 minutes, until doubled in size.

5   Preheat the oven to 480°F (250°C). Lightly oil a large baking pan. Punch down the dough to expel the air, and briefly knead. Divide into eight portions, and make 5-inch (13 cm) long rolls. Brush the tops with water, then sprinkle with the extra flaxseeds and sesame seeds. Place on the pan, loosely cover with plastic wrap and let stand for 15 minutes.

6   Bake the rolls for 20 minutes, until they are risen, crusty and golden brown.

EACH SERVING (1 ROLL) PROVIDES
416 calories, 16 g protein, 12 g fat (1 g saturated fat), 60 g carbohydrate (2 g sugars), 16 g fiber, 16 mg sodium

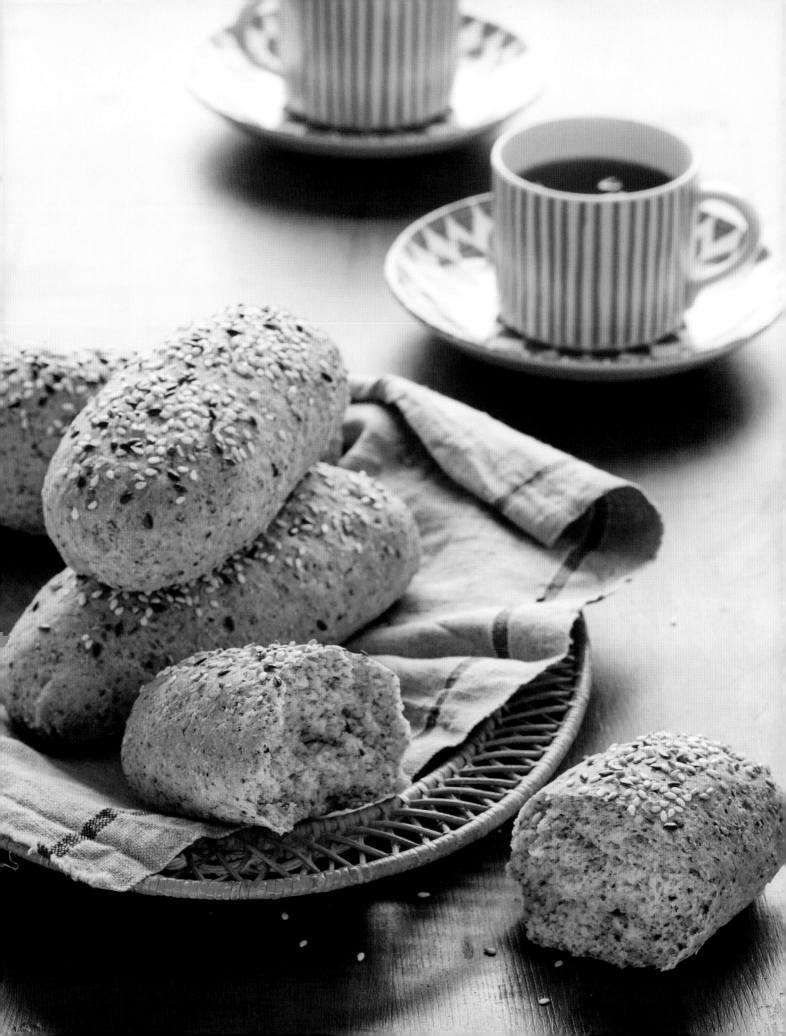

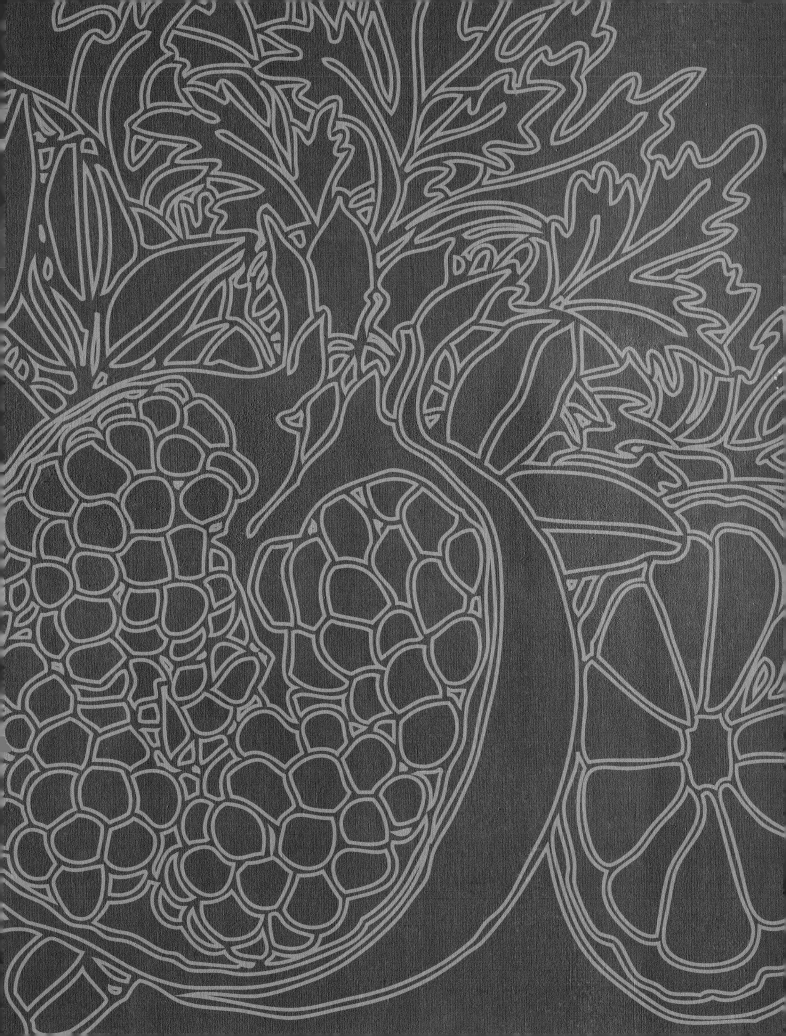

Recipes and puzzles to boost your brainpower

Give yourself the edge with dishes for specific situations and exercises to sharpen your brain.

Kick-start your day

You're much less likely to stick to healthy choices later in the day if you start out being hungry. Doughnuts and pastries will be too tempting when your stomach is grumbling mid-morning. Numerous studies of memory, alertness and cognitive function have found significant disadvantages to skipping breakfast—it really is the most important meal of the day. A good breakfast should include low glycemic index carbohydrates to provide long-lasting fuel for the brain, in combination with satisfying protein, fiber and plenty of brain-boosting micronutrients.

Apple and cinnamon oatmeal

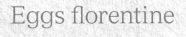

PREPARATION 5 MINUTES COOKING 15 MINUTES

½ cup (50 g) rolled oats
1 green apple
1 teaspoon (5 ml) ground cinnamon
½ cup (125 ml) low-fat milk
pure maple syrup or honey, to serve

1   Combine the rolled oats and 1 cup (250 ml) water in a heavy-bottom saucepan, and bring to a boil.
2   Meanwhile, grate the apple, leaving the skin on if you like, and add it to the boiling oats along with the cinnamon. Stir until well combined.
3   Simmer the oatmeal for about 3–5 minutes, until thick and sticky, pour in the milk and stir well.
4   Simmer over low heat for another 5 minutes, until smooth and thick, and the oats are completely cooked. Serve with a little maple syrup or honey. **SERVES 2**

Eggs florentine

PREPARATION 5 MINUTES COOKING 5 MINUTES

4 very fresh eggs
1 bunch spinach, about ⅔ pound (300 g), stems trimmed
4 slices whole-grain bread
freshly ground black pepper

1   Break each egg into a small cup. Bring a large saucepan of water to a boil.
2   Meanwhile, put the spinach in a large heatproof bowl and cover with boiling water. Set aside until the spinach is completely wilted.

3   Turn the heat down under the pan so the water is just simmering. Gently slip each egg into the water, avoiding splashing or spreading the egg white. Cook for 3–5 minutes, until set.
4   While the eggs are cooking, toast the bread and place a slice on each of four warmed plates.
5   Drain the wilted spinach and when cool enough to handle, firmly squeeze to release as much liquid as possible. Chop the spinach into four portions, and arrange one portion on each slice of toast to make a nest for the poached egg.
6   Remove the eggs from the water with a slotted spoon and place on top of the spinach. Grind fresh black pepper on top and serve. **SERVES 4**

Whole-grain avocado and prosciutto toasts

PREPARATION 10 MINUTES COOKING 5 MINUTES

1 tablespoon (15 ml) olive oil
½ small red onion, finely chopped
¼ cup (50 g) finely diced prosciutto, pancetta or lean bacon
4 slices whole-grain bread
1 large avocado
1 tomato, thickly sliced
4 sprigs fresh parsley or basil, finely chopped

1   Heat the oil in a small nonstick frying pan and cook the onion over medium heat for 1–2 minutes, until translucent. Add the prosciutto, pancetta or bacon and cook, stirring, for 1 minute, until the fat has melted.
2   Meanwhile, toast the bread and place a slice on each of four warmed plates.
3   Mash the avocado well and stir in the onion mixture. Spread the avocado on the toasts and top with the tomato slices and chopped parsley or basil. Serve immediately. **SERVES 4**

Parmesan and herb scrambled eggs

PREPARATION **10 MINUTES** COOKING **5 MINUTES**

6 eggs
$^1\!/_2$ cup (125 ml) low-fat milk
1 tablespoon (15 ml) olive oil
$^3\!/_4$ cup (75 g) finely grated parmesan
4 sprigs fresh basil, finely chopped
4 sprigs fresh thyme, finely chopped
4 sprigs fresh chervil, finely chopped
4 sprigs fresh parsley, finely chopped

1 Crack the eggs into a bowl, pour in the milk and use a fork to break the yolks and very gently stir a few times, keeping the egg texture chunky.
2 Heat the oil in a large nonstick saucepan and add the egg mixture. Cook for 1 minute, and use a wooden spoon or spatula to move the cooked egg to the side and allow the runny egg to move to the center. Add the parmesan and herbs, and repeat. Repeat again if needed.
3 When only a small amount of runny egg is still visible, give the eggs one more stroke of the spoon, and turn them out onto warmed plates (the egg will continue to cook slightly after serving). Serve with whole-grain toast. **SERVES 4**

Yogurt and oatmeal smoothie

PREPARATION **5 MINUTES, PLUS OVERNIGHT SOAKING IF DESIRED**

$^1\!/_2$ cup (50 g) rolled oats
$^3\!/_4$ cup (175 ml) low-fat plain yogurt
2 tablespoons (30 ml) honey or pure maple syrup, to taste
vanilla extract, to taste
1 cup (250 g) fruit: try berries, bananas, pineapple or a mix of fruit
low-fat milk (optional)

1 Grind the rolled oats in a blender until finely ground. For a softer, smoother drink, combine the oats with the yogurt and soak overnight to soften.
2 Combine all the ingredients and process until smooth using a food processor or stick blender. Add some milk if needed to achieve the desired consistency. **SERVES 2**

Fruity barley breakfast loaf

PREPARATION **10 MINUTES** COOKING **1 HOUR**

$^1\!/_2$ cup (90 g) dried apricots, chopped
$^1\!/_2$ cup (65 g) dried cranberries
$^1\!/_2$ cup (60 g) rolled barley or other whole grain
$^1\!/_2$ cup (50 g) walnut halves
1 teaspoon (5 ml) ground allspice
1 teaspoon (5 ml) ground ginger
$^1\!/_4$ cup (90 g) molasses
1 cup (250 ml) buttermilk or $^3\!/_4$ cup (175 ml) low-fat plain yogurt
2 cups (320 g) whole-wheat self-rising flour

1 Combine the apricots, cranberries and barley in a large mug. Pour in enough boiling water to cover the mixture. Set aside to soak for 10 minutes.
2 Preheat the oven to 300°F (150°C). Line a 12 x 4 inch (30 x 10 cm) loaf pan with parchment paper.
3 Combine the walnuts, spices, molasses and buttermilk or yogurt in a large bowl. Pour in the soaked barley mixture and stir well.
4 Gently stir in the flour until the mixture is just combined. Spread the mixture in the prepared pan and bake for 1 hour, until a knife inserted in the center comes out clean. **MAKES 12 THICK SLICES**

Nut and cranberry muesli

PREPARATION **5 MINUTES**

$1^1\!/_2$ cups (150 g) rolled whole grains of your choice, such as oats, rye, barley, quinoa or rice
$^1\!/_4$ cup (40 g) Brazil nuts, sliced
$^1\!/_4$ cup (35 g) hazelnuts, roughly chopped
$^1\!/_2$ cup (35 g) dried apple, chopped
1 cup (120 g) dried cranberries
$^1\!/_2$ cup (60 g) golden raisins
low-fat milk or low-fat plain yogurt, to serve

1 Combine all the ingredients except the milk or yogurt in a large bowl.
2 Store the muesli in an airtight container, ready for use. Serve with milk or yogurt.
MAKES 4 CUPS

Boost your performance

When you have to deal with a stressful situation, such as an exam, job interview, driving test or an important business meeting, you should consider extra ways you can boost your performance. The last thing you need is a greasy snack that leaves you feeling queasy from indigestion or too much sugar and caffeine that first make you jumpy and then sluggish afterwards. These food ideas are designed to optimize brain function by providing a nutritious blend of protein and healthy fats, with a low glycemic load for long-lasting energy. To improve your memory and concentration, always eat breakfast, keep lunch light and high in protein, include carbohydrates and healthy fats in your daytime snacks, and have some protein such as meat or tofu for dinner.

Mixed-grain muesli with cranberries and nuts

PREPARATION **5 MINUTES, PLUS 20 MINUTES COOLING** COOKING **10 MINUTES**

1 cup (100 g) rolled whole grains of your choice, such as oats, rye and quinoa
1/2 cup (70 g) mixture of pepitas (pumpkin seeds), sunflower seeds, flaxseeds, unhulled sesame seeds or chia seeds
1/2 cup (80 g) Brazil nuts and hazelnuts, roughly chopped
1 tablespoon (15 ml) ground cinnamon
1 teaspoon (5 ml) pumpkin pie spice
1 tablespoon (15 ml) pure maple syrup, honey or agave syrup
1 tablespoon (15 ml) canola or light olive oil
1/2 cup (35 g) dried apple, chopped
1 cup (130 g) dried cranberries
1/2 cup (60 g) golden raisins
low-fat milk or low-fat plain yogurt, to serve

1   Preheat the oven to 400°F (200°C).
2   Combine the grains and seeds in a large bowl. Add the nuts and spices, and toss to mix well. Drizzle with the maple syrup, honey or agave syrup, and mix thoroughly. Add the oil and mix again.
3   Spread the mixture on a baking sheet and bake for 10 minutes, until it starts to turn light golden brown. Stir every 3–4 minutes with a spatula or spoon so the mixture toasts evenly. Set aside to cool on the pan, about 20 minutes.
4   Turn the grain mixture into a large bowl. Add the dried fruit and mix well. Divide the muesli among four bowls and serve with milk or yogurt.
SERVES 4

Oatcakes with berry ricotta

PREPARATION **20 MINUTES, PLUS 15 MINUTES STANDING** COOKING **20 MINUTES**

3/4 cup (110 g) all-purpose flour
1/3 cup (40 g) rolled oats
3 eggs
3/4 cup (175 ml) low-fat milk
1 tablespoon (15 ml) canola or olive oil, plus extra for brushing
1 cup (250 g) low-fat ricotta
1 tablespoon (15 ml) honey
vanilla extract, to taste
2 cups (250 g) fresh berries or thawed frozen berries

1   Process the flour and oats in a blender or food processor until finely ground. Turn into a large bowl.
2   Beat the eggs, milk and oil until well combined. Whisk in the flour and oat mixture until smooth. Let the batter stand for 15 minutes.
3   Meanwhile, process the ricotta with the honey and vanilla in a blender or food processor until smooth. Gently fold in the berries.
4   Brush an 8 inch (20 cm) nonstick frying pan with oil and place over medium heat. Pour 1/4 cup (50 ml) of the batter into the pan, quickly tilting the pan in a circular motion to coat with a thin circle of batter. Cook the oatcake for 1–2 minutes each side, until golden brown. Repeat with the remaining batter to make eight oatcakes total.
5   Divide the berry and ricotta mixture among the oatcakes, roll up and serve. Alternatively, serve with savory fillings such as cheese or egg, or simply spread with jam. **SERVES 4 (MAKES 8)**

Creamy almond oatmeal

PREPARATION **5 MINUTES** COOKING **20 MINUTES**

$\frac{1}{2}$ cup (80 g) raw almonds or $\frac{1}{2}$ cup (55 g)
  ground almonds
$1\frac{1}{2}$ cups (150 g) rolled grains, such as oats,
  barley and rye
1 teaspoon (5 ml) ground cinnamon
1 teaspoon (5 ml) freshly grated nutmeg
low-fat milk or soy milk, to serve
honey, to serve (optional)

1 If using whole almonds, process in a food
processor or blender to your preferred coarseness.
2 Combine the chopped or ground almonds, rolled
grains, cinnamon, nutmeg and 4 cups (1 L) water
in a large, heavy-bottom saucepan. Bring to a boil,
stirring occasionally, reduce the heat and simmer for
15 minutes, until soft and creamy.
3 Serve the oatmeal with milk or soy milk, and a
little honey, if desired. **SERVES 4**

Scrambled tofu with rye toast

PREPARATION **15 MINUTES** COOKING **10 MINUTES**

2 teaspoons (10 ml) light olive oil
1 teaspoon (5 ml) sesame oil
$\frac{1}{2}$ green pepper, finely diced
$\frac{1}{2}$ large green chile, seeded and finely chopped
1 teaspoon (5 ml) grated fresh ginger
3 scallions, finely chopped
10 ounces (300 g) silken tofu, drained
2 teaspoons (10 ml) salt-reduced soy sauce
1 tablespoon (15 ml) snipped fresh chives
2 slices rye bread, toasted

1 Heat the olive oil and sesame oil in a small frying
pan over medium–high heat. Add the pepper, chile
and ginger. Cook, stirring frequently, for 3 minutes,
until softened. Add the scallions and cook, stirring,
for 2 minutes, until softened.
2 Reduce the heat to medium and add the tofu and
soy sauce. Using a wooden spoon, break the tofu into
small pieces and cook, gently stirring to combine the
tofu with the pepper mixture, for 2 minutes, until
heated through. Gently stir in the chives. Don't
overcook the tofu, otherwise it will release too
much liquid.
3 Spoon the scrambled tofu onto the toasted rye
bread and serve hot. **SERVES 2**

Mushroom and corn omelet

PREPARATION **10 MINUTES** COOKING **20 MINUTES**

1 corn on the cob, husk removed
1 tablespoon (15 ml) canola or olive oil
1 small red onion, finely chopped
3–4 mushrooms, diced
2 tablespoons (30 ml) chopped fresh parsley
freshly ground black pepper
1 tablespoon (15 ml) olive oil spread
6 eggs, lightly beaten

1 Boil the corn until tender. When cool enough to
handle, cut the corn kernels off the cob.
2 Meanwhile, heat the oil in a frying pan over low
heat. Cook the onion for 5 minutes, until starting to
color. Add the mushrooms and cook, stirring, for
5 minutes, until soft. Put the mixture into a bowl and
add the corn kernels, chopped parsley and some
freshly ground black pepper.
3 Place the cleaned pan over medium heat. Add the
olive oil spread and allow to melt. Pour in one-quarter
of the beaten eggs. As the egg heats, use a spatula to
push the cooked egg to the middle of the pan and tilt
to allow the uncooked egg to run to the edges. When
most of the egg is cooked, spoon one-quarter of the
mushroom and corn mixture on top of the eggs and
cook for 1 minute.
4 Slide the omelet onto a plate and fold over to
enclose the filling. Repeat with the remaining eggs
and filling to make four omelets total.
SERVES 4

Mexican muffins

PREPARATION **5 MINUTES** COOKING **2 MINUTES**

1 whole-grain English muffin, split in half
2 tablespoons (30 ml) tomato paste
1 small tomato, thinly sliced
$\frac{1}{2}$ small avocado, sliced
$\frac{1}{2}$ cup (125 g) low-sodium baked beans
chili sauce, to taste (optional)
2 slices low-fat cheddar cheese

1 Preheat the broiler to high.
2 Spread the muffin halves with the tomato paste
and top with the tomato and avocado. Spoon the
baked beans on top, sprinkle with the chili sauce,
if using, and top with the cheese.
3 Broil for 2 minutes until the cheese has melted.
SERVES 1

Avoid the afternoon slump

Slow-release carbohydrates are featured in these lunchbox ideas in combination with protein-rich foods to prevent excess serotonin release, which induces sleepiness. These foods will also keep your blood glucose levels steady for sustained energy.

Chicken and avocado rolls

PREPARATION **10 MINUTES**

1 large avocado
juice of $\frac{1}{2}$ lime or lemon
freshly ground black pepper
$\frac{1}{2}$ cup (50 g) pecan or walnut halves,
   finely chopped
1 celery stalk, finely chopped
1 scallion, thinly sliced
2 sprigs fresh parsley, finely chopped
4 whole-grain sandwich rolls
$\frac{2}{3}$ cup (100 g) cooked chicken, trimmed
   of skin and fat
1 cup (45 g) arugula

1   Mash the avocado with the lime or lemon juice and some freshly ground black pepper until smooth. Add the nuts, celery, scallion and parsley, and stir until well combined.
2   Cut open the rolls and spread each side with the avocado mixture. Divide the chicken and arugula among the rolls and serve. **SERVES 4**

Satay beef rye wraps

PREPARATION **10 MINUTES** COOKING **10 MINUTES**

1 tablespoon (15 ml) olive or canola oil
$\frac{1}{2}$ pound (250 g) sirloin steak, trimmed of fat
1 small clove garlic, crushed
$\frac{1}{3}$ cup (90 g) creamy unprocessed peanut butter
2 tablespoons (30 ml) fish sauce
2 teaspoons (10 ml) chili sauce
4 rye lavash or flatbreads
$\frac{1}{2}$ carrot, grated
$\frac{1}{2}$ cup (50 g) white mung bean sprouts
8 snow peas, sliced
1 cup (45 g) baby spinach leaves
8 sprigs fresh cilantro

1   Heat the oil in a nonstick frying pan over high heat and cook the steak for about 3 minutes on each side. Transfer to a warm dish and cover until needed.
2   Add the garlic to the pan and cook, stirring, for 1 minute, add the peanut butter, fish sauce and chili sauce, and stir until well combined.
3   Thinly slice the beef and add it to the satay sauce in the pan. Stir to coat with the sauce, and set aside to cool.
4   Lay out the flatbreads and pile with the carrot, sprouts, snow peas, baby spinach and cilantro. Divide the beef slices among the breads, firmly roll up and serve. **SERVES 4**

Whole-grain lentil salad wraps

PREPARATION **10 MINUTES**

1 cup (170 g) cooked lentils
$\frac{1}{4}$ cup (35 g) currants
$\frac{1}{4}$ cup (30 g) pepitas (pumpkin seeds)
$\frac{1}{2}$ carrot, finely diced
$\frac{1}{2}$ small red onion, finely diced
$\frac{1}{4}$ red pepper, finely diced
$\frac{1}{2}$ tomato, finely diced
$\frac{1}{4}$ cup (35 g) sun-dried tomatoes, finely chopped
4 sprigs fresh parsley
4 sprigs fresh cilantro
2 sprigs fresh mint leaves (about 16 leaves)
1 tablespoon (15 ml) finely grated lemon
   or lime zest
$\frac{1}{2}$ teaspoon (2 ml) ground cumin
$\frac{1}{2}$ teaspoon (2 ml) paprika
freshly ground black pepper
4 whole-grain lavash or other flatbreads

1   Combine all the ingredients except the flatbreads in a large bowl.
2   Arrange the flatbreads on a flat surface, divide the salad among them and firmly roll up. Cut on the diagonal to serve.
SERVES 4

Cannellini bean and tuna salad

PREPARATION **10 MINUTES**

2 tablespoons (30 ml) extra virgin olive oil
juice of $1/2$ lemon
$1/4$ preserved lemon, flesh discarded, skin rinsed
   and finely diced
$1/2$ small red onion, finely chopped
1 tomato, finely chopped
15 ounce (425 ml) can cannellini beans, rinsed and
   drained, or 2 cups (500 g) cooked cannellini beans
   made from $2/3$ cup (135 g) dried beans
2 cups (90 g) baby spinach leaves, arugula or lettuce
5 ounce (150 g) can low-sodium tuna in water,
   drained

1 Combine the oil, lemon juice, preserved lemon,
onion and tomato in a bowl. Add the beans, stirring
well to coat. (If preparing the salad for a lunchbox,
put this mixture in a separate container to marinate,
and combine with the remaining ingredients when
ready to serve.)
2 Arrange the salad leaves in a large bowl and add
the bean mixture, gently tossing to coat the leaves
with the dressing.
3 Spoon the tuna on top of the salad and gently fold
into the leaves, keeping the chunks intact. **SERVES 4**

Egg and bacon tarts

PREPARATION **15 MINUTES** COOKING **35 MINUTES**

1 tablespoon (15 ml) olive oil
1 small red onion, halved and thickly sliced
$1/4$ cup (50 g) finely diced prosciutto, pancetta
   or lean bacon
olive oil, for spraying or brushing
8 sheets phyllo pastry, about 16 x 12 inches
   (40 x 30 cm) each
2 cups (90 g) baby spinach leaves or
   shredded spinach
8 eggs
freshly ground black pepper

1 Heat the oil in a small saucepan and cook the
onion over low heat for 15 minutes, until soft and
caramelized. Add the prosciutto and cook, stirring,
for 2–3 minutes.
2 Meanwhile, preheat the oven to 400°F (200°C).
Grease 8 cups of a 12-cup standard muffin pan.

3 Stack the phyllo sheets on a clean surface.
Working with one sheet at a time, spray or brush the
entire surface of the phyllo with oil. Fold in half
lengthwise and use your hands to press out all the
air. Spray or brush the top surface of the folded sheet
with oil and then fold again into three, pressing out
the air to make a 6 inch (15 cm) square.
4 Fold back the corners of the square so they don't
stick out and burn. Fit the square into a muffin cup
and press all around the inside with your fingers to
make room for the filling. Repeat with the remaining
phyllo sheets.
5 Divide the onion and prosciutto mixture among
the muffin cups, add the spinach and crack an egg
into each one, keeping the yolk intact. Season with
freshly ground black pepper. Bake the tarts for
15 minutes, until the egg whites are set.
SERVES 4 (MAKES 8)

Quinoa and apple pudding

PREPARATION **10 MINUTES** COOKING **30 MINUTES**

1 cup (200 g) white quinoa
$3^{1}/2$ cups (800 ml) low-fat milk
1 teaspoon (5 ml) ground cinnamon
1 teaspoon (5 ml) freshly grated nutmeg
3 apples, about 1 pound (500 g) total, peeled,
   cored and cut into small cubes
$1/2$ cup (100 g) dried cherries or dried cranberries
$1/4$ cup (50 ml) pure maple syrup or honey

1 Put the quinoa in a fine sieve and rinse under cold
water; drain. Transfer the quinoa to a saucepan and
stir in the milk. Bring to a boil, reduce the heat and
simmer, stirring occasionally, for 15 minutes.
2 Stir in the cinnamon, nutmeg, apples and cherries,
and cook for 15 minutes, until the quinoa is tender.
3 Add a little more milk if the pudding is too thick.
Stir in the maple syrup or honey, to taste. Serve the
pudding hot or divide it into individual containers
and serve cold as an afternoon snack. **SERVES 4**

Keep calm under stress

Life is full of stressful moments—from the first day in a new job to a dreaded dentist's appointment. In such situations, you need to eat foods that will calm your nerves and avoid anything that will increase your edginess. These recipes include foods that produce soothing substances in the body like serotonin and dopamine—the relaxing pleasure chemical that forms the basis of some addictions. Some foods, such as dairy foods, help to produce extra dopamine, making them ideal comfort foods in stressful situations or to relax you before bedtime.

Chinese-style chinese and rice

Chinese-style chicken and rice

PREPARATION **15 MINUTES** COOKING **1 HOUR**

1 cup (200 g) brown rice
2–3 pound (1–1.5 kg) whole chicken, cut into four
    pieces, skin and fat removed
4 cloves garlic, peeled and bruised
2 inch (5 cm) piece fresh ginger, peeled and sliced
4 star anise
8 scallions, white parts cut into short lengths and
    green parts finely chopped
4 baby bok choy or other Asian greens, trimmed
2 tablespoons (30 ml) soy sauce
1 tablespoon (15 ml) sesame oil
1 tablespoon (15 ml) chili sauce
1 kirby or other short cucumber, diagonally sliced
8 sprigs fresh cilantro

1 Rinse the rice, then combine with 2 cups
(500 ml) water in a 12 cup (3 L) saucepan. Bring to
a boil, reduce the heat to low, cover and simmer
for 10 minutes.
2 Arrange the chicken on top of the rice so that the
pieces neatly fit together. Tuck the garlic, ginger, star
anise and white parts of the scallions into the gaps
between the chicken. Cover, bring to a boil, reduce
the heat and gently simmer for 40 minutes.
3 Transfer the chicken to a warmed dish and pour
off as much of the stock as possible into a bowl. Put
the bok choy on top of the rice in the pan, cover and
cook over low heat for 5–10 minutes, until the rice is
fully cooked and there is no liquid remaining.
4 Combine the green parts of the scallions, soy
sauce, sesame oil and chili sauce to make a sauce.
5 Slice the chicken and serve with the rice, greens
and sauce, topped with the cucumber and cilantro
sprigs, with the stock on the side. Alternatively, serve
as a soup by dividing all the ingredients among four
large serving bowls. **SERVES 4**

Beef and lemongrass rice paper rolls

PREPARATION **20 MINUTES, PLUS 1 HOUR MARINATING**
COOKING **5 MINUTES**

1 lemongrass stem
2 cloves garlic, crushed
$^1/_2$ pound (250 g) lean beef, cut into thin strips
    across the grain
2 tablespoons (30 ml) canola or olive oil
8 large rice paper wrappers
16 fresh mint leaves
16 fresh Vietnamese mint leaves
16 small sprigs fresh cilantro
8 fresh basil leaves
1 scallion, cut into short lengths
    and then finely shredded
$^1/_2$ red pepper, cut into thin strips
1 kirby or other short cucumber, cut into
    thin strips
2 cups (90 g) baby spinach leaves

1 Thinly slice the white part of the lemongrass,
pounding any solid parts with a kitchen mallet or
knife handle before finely chopping. Combine the
lemongrass with the garlic and toss with the beef
until completely coated. If time permits, marinate
the beef in the refrigerator for at least 1 hour.
2 Heat a wok until very hot and add the oil. Stir-fry
the beef strips for 5 minutes, until browned all over.
3 Fill a large shallow dish with hot water. Working
with one rice paper wrapper at a time, dip a wrapper
into the water for 1 second, drain off the excess and
place on a board.
4 Put two mint leaves, two Vietnamese mint leaves,
two cilantro sprigs and a basil leaf in the center
of the wrapper. Top with some scallion, pepper,
cucumber, spinach leaves and a few beef strips. Roll
up to enclose the filling, folding in the sides. Repeat
to make eight rolls in total. **SERVES 4**

Cheesy potato and spinach bake

PREPARATION **5 MINUTES**
COOKING **1 HOUR 20 MINUTES**

2 tablespoons (30 ml) olive or canola oil
1 onion, finely chopped
4 cloves garlic, crushed
1$^{1}/_{2}$ cups (375 ml) skim evaporated milk
1 pound (500 g) potatoes, skin on, sliced
4 ounces (100 g) low-fat cheddar, sliced
1 bunch spinach, about $^{2}/_{3}$ pound (300 g),
   very finely chopped

1 Preheat the oven to 350°F (180°C).
2 Heat the oil in a small frying pan over low heat
and cook the onion for 5 minutes, until starting to
color. Add the garlic and cook for 3 minutes. Pour in
the evaporated milk to deglaze the pan. Set aside.
3 Spread half the potato slices in an 8 cup (2 L)
ovenproof dish and top with half the cheese slices.
Spread the spinach over the top, then pour the milk
and onion mixture on top.
4 Arrange the remaining cheese slices in the dish,
and top with the remaining potato slices. Cover
with foil and bake for 30 minutes. Uncover and bake
for another 30–40 minutes, until the potato is soft
and there is no liquid remaining around the edges
of the dish. **SERVES 4**

Hot caramel eggnog

PREPARATION **5 MINUTES** COOKING **10 MINUTES**

2 eggs, beaten
vanilla extract
2 tablespoons (30 ml) superfine sugar
1$^{1}/_{4}$ cups (300 ml) low-fat milk

1 Beat the eggs with the vanilla in a heatproof bowl.
2 Combine the sugar and 1 tablespoon (15 ml)
water in a small saucepan. Cook, stirring, over
medium heat until the sugar has dissolved.
3 Bring to a boil without stirring any further, then
cook for 4 minutes, until the caramel turns golden
brown. Quickly pour in the milk, being careful as it
will splatter at first. Cook, stirring, until the caramel
has dissolved in the milk.
4 Bring the mixture to a boil, and pour into the
eggs, beating constantly. Pour back into the pan and
gently heat until the mixture starts to thicken, about
2 minutes. Divide the eggnog between two warmed
mugs to serve. **SERVES 2**

Brazil nut cookies

PREPARATION **20 MINUTES, PLUS COOLING**
COOKING **20 MINUTES**

$^{1}/_{3}$ cup (75 g) light olive oil spread
$^{1}/_{4}$ cup (55 g) firmly packed soft brown sugar
2 tablespoons (30 ml) honey
1$^{1}/_{4}$ cups (185 g) all-purpose flour
2 teaspoons (10 ml) ground ginger
$^{1}/_{2}$ teaspoon (2 ml) ground cinnamon
$^{1}/_{2}$ teaspoon (2 ml) baking soda
$^{1}/_{4}$ cup (35 g) chopped Brazil nuts, plus
   16 small Brazil nuts, for decorating
1 tablespoon (15 ml) chopped candied ginger

1 Preheat the oven to 350°F (180°C). Line two
cookie sheets with parchment paper.
2 Combine the olive oil spread, sugar and honey
in a saucepan. Stir over low heat until melted and
smooth. Remove the pan from the heat.
3 Sift together the flour, ground ginger, cinnamon
and baking soda. Stir into the melted mixture. Stir
in the chopped Brazil nuts and ginger until well
combined. Set aside to cool for 10 minutes.
4 Roll into 16 equal balls of the mixture. Place
on the prepared cookie sheets, about 1$^{1}/_{4}$ inches
(3 cm) apart. Using your fingers, slightly flatten the
balls, and press a Brazil nut into each one. Bake for
12–15 minutes, until golden. Set aside to cool on the
cookie sheets. **MAKES 16**

Think fast

If you are attending a quiz night, bridge game or trivia contest, give your team the edge by providing some brain-buzzing food beforehand. Have snacks that keep your brains fueled and fired up—spicy nuts, roasted soybeans and wasabi peas are great choices. Avoid overloading on carbohydrate-rich foods like chips or sugary treats, which may give you a brief high but leave you feeling sleepy and depleted before you reach the final round. These recipes emphasize good sources of antioxidants, thiamine and protein and tyrosine, an amino acid that helps to produce adrenaline for alertness and quick thinking.

Chile pork tortillas

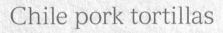

PREPARATION **15 MINUTES**
COOKING **2 HOURS 10 MINUTES**

1 pound (500 g) boneless pork, trimmed
1 onion, cut into thin wedges
1 long green chile, seeded and thinly sliced
1 tablespoon (15 ml) fennel seeds
1 tablespoon (15 ml) smoked paprika
1 tablespoon (15 ml) ground cumin
1 cup (250 ml) balsamic vinegar
8 large tortillas
shredded lettuce, grated carrot, grated cheese,
    diced tomato and diced avocado, to serve
hot chili sauce, to taste

1   Preheat the oven to 400°F (200°C).
2   Combine the pork, onion, chile, spices and balsamic vinegar in a large ovenproof dish. Cover and bake for 2 hours, until the pork is tender and falling apart. Remove the lid and bake for another 10 minutes if needed to thicken the liquid.
3   Divide the pork mixture among the tortillas, top with the remaining ingredients and roll up. **SERVES 4**

Nutty beef stir-fry

PREPARATION **10 MINUTES** COOKING **10 MINUTES**

2 tablespoons (30 ml) canola or olive oil
3/4 pound (375 g) lean beef, cut into strips
1 onion, cut into thin wedges
4 cloves garlic, crushed
3/4 inch (2 cm) piece fresh ginger, grated
1 carrot, halved lengthwise and thinly sliced
    on the diagonal

1/2 red pepper, cut into thin strips
1/4 cup (50 g) snow peas, trimmed
1 cup (60 g) broccoli florets
3 baby bok choy, thickly sliced on the diagonal
1/2 cup (80 g) raw cashew nuts
1/2 cup (50 g) raw walnut halves
2 tablespoons (30 ml) low-sodium soy sauce
1 tablespoon (15 ml) honey

1   Heat half the oil in a wok until smoking, then stir-fry the beef for 5 minutes, until brown on all sides. Remove and set aside.
2   Clean the wok and heat the remaining oil until smoking. Stir-fry the onion for 1 minute. Add the garlic and ginger, and stir-fry for 1 minute.
3   Add the carrot and pepper, and stir-fry for 2 minutes. Add the snow peas, broccoli, bok choy and nuts, and stir-fry until all the vegetables are just tender.
4   Return the beef to the wok and stir in the soy sauce and honey. Cook for 1 minute, until heated through. Serve with brown rice. **SERVES 4**

Chicken salad with ruby red grapefruit

PREPARATION **15 MINUTES** COOKING **10 MINUTES**

1 clove garlic, crushed
juice of 1/2 lime
1 tablespoon (15 ml) fish sauce
1 tablespoon (15 ml) dark brown sugar
6 boneless, skinless chicken thighs, about
    11/2 pounds (750 g) total, trimmed of all fat
1 long red chile, seeded and thinly sliced on
    the diagonal
1 tablespoon (15 ml) chopped scallions
11/2 tablespoons (22 ml) chopped fresh cilantro
11/2 tablespoons (22 ml) chopped fresh mint

2 cups (90 g) baby spinach leaves
1 ruby red grapefruit, cut into segments
¼ cup (40 g) unsalted peanuts, chopped

1 Combine the garlic, lime juice, fish sauce and sugar in a large bowl.
2 Heat a grill pan or barbecue grill to very hot and cook the chicken thighs for 5 minutes on each side, until golden and cooked through. Transfer to the bowl with the dressing and turn to coat.
3 When the chicken is cool enough to handle, shred it into bite-sized pieces. Add the chile, scallions and herbs, and stir to combine.
4 Add the spinach leaves and gently toss. Top with the grapefruit segments and serve scattered with the peanuts. **SERVES 4**

Crepes with coffee cream

PREPARATION **10 MINUTES** COOKING **30 MINUTES**

⅓ cup (25 g) ground or instant coffee
½ cup (50 g) walnut halves, chopped
½ cup (125 ml) pure maple syrup or molasses
1 cup (250 g) ricotta or soft silken tofu
1 egg
2 tablespoons (30 ml) superfine sugar
1½ cups (375 ml) low-fat milk
½ cup (75 g) all-purpose flour
½ cup (80 g) whole-wheat all-purpose flour
oil, for brushing

1 Put the coffee in a mug, pour in ¼ cup (50 ml) boiling water and let stand.
2 Meanwhile, stir the walnuts in a dry frying pan over medium heat for 2 minutes, until fragrant and starting to color. Transfer to a plate to cool.
3 Strain the coffee into a small bowl and stir in the maple syrup. Beat the ricotta or tofu in a blender or food processor until smooth. Stir in ½ cup (125 ml) of the coffee syrup, and fold in the walnuts.
4 Beat the egg, sugar and 1 cup (250 ml) of the milk in a bowl. Whisk in the flour to make a smooth, thin batter, adding more milk if needed.
5 Brush an 8 inch (20 cm) nonstick frying pan with oil and place over medium heat. Pour ¼ cup (50 ml) of the batter into the pan, quickly tilting the pan in a circular motion to coat with a thin circle of batter. Cook for 1–2 minutes on each side, just until set and starting to color. Repeat with the remaining batter to make eight crepes in total.
6 Divide the coffee cream among the crepes and fold or roll up. Serve warm or chilled, drizzled with the remaining coffee syrup.
SERVES 4 (MAKES 8)

Chocolate and raspberry cake

PREPARATION **10 MINUTES** COOKING **1 HOUR**

2 eggs
½ cup (95 g) brown sugar
½ cup (115 g) superfine sugar
1 cup (125 g) raw cacao or cocoa powder
¾ cup (175 ml) olive oil, plus 1 tablespoon (15 ml)
    extra for topping
½ cup (125 ml) buttermilk or low-fat plain yogurt
¾ cup (110 g) self-rising flour
2 cups (250 g) fresh or frozen raspberries
4 ounces (100 g) dark chocolate, at least 65% cocoa

1 Preheat the oven to 300°F (150°C). Grease an 8 inch (20 cm) round cake pan and line with parchment paper.
2 Beat the eggs and sugars until the sugars have dissolved. Stir in the cacao or cocoa powder, oil and buttermilk or yogurt. Gently fold in the flour until combined, then gently fold in the raspberries.
3 Spread the batter in the pan and bake for 1 hour, until a knife inserted in the center comes out clean.
4 Melt the chocolate and stir in the extra oil. Spread over the cooled cake to serve. **MAKES 12–16 SLICES**

Frozen yogurt with mixed berry compote

PREPARATION **10 MINUTES, PLUS FREEZING**

2 cups (500 ml) low-fat plain yogurt
2 tablespoons (30 ml) honey
vanilla extract, to taste
2 cups (250 g) mixed fresh berries or thawed
    frozen berries
2 tablespoons (30 ml) confectioners' sugar

1 Put the yogurt in a bowl and beat in the honey and vanilla until well combined. Spread the mixture into a shallow tray lined with plastic wrap and freeze until firm, about 1–1½ hours.
2 Meanwhile, put the berries and sugar in a small saucepan. Gently stir over low heat for 3–5 minutes, until the sugar has dissolved and the berries have collapsed. Set aside to cool.
3 Break the frozen yogurt into pieces. Whip until smooth in a blender or food processor. Layer the frozen yogurt with the berry coulis in four chilled glasses, and serve immediately. **SERVES 4**

Sleep well

Getting ready for sleep means inducing a relaxed, comfortable state, reducing stimulants such as loud noise, bright lights, caffeine and spicy food. Although alcohol makes you drowsy, it interferes with deep, refreshing sleep and should be avoided before bed. These recipes are designed to be relatively low in fat—high-fat foods prevent the emptying of your stomach, leaving you with an uncomfortable feeling of fullness or causing gastric reflux. The foods here are also rich in tryptophan, an amino acid that the body uses to make serotonin, which induces drowsiness. For best absorption of the tryptophan, have some carbohydrate just before bed. Low glycemic index carbohydrate helps prevent an overnight drop in blood glucose levels, which can also disturb your sleep.

Butternut squash and currant frittata

PREPARATION **10 MINUTES** COOKING **35 MINUTES**

$^{1}/_{2}$ butternut squash, about 2 pounds (1 kg), seeded, peeled and cut into small chunks
$^{1}/_{4}$ cup (50 ml) olive oil
1 onion, sliced
$^{1}/_{4}$ cup (35 g) currants
4 eggs, beaten

1   Preheat the oven to 480°F (250°C).
2   Toss the butternut squash with 2 tablespoons (30 ml) of the olive oil and spread out on a baking pan. Bake for 20 minutes, until golden and starting to caramelize.
3   Preheat the broiler to high.
4   While the butternut squash is cooking, heat the remaining olive oil in a nonstick frying pan with an ovenproof handle. Cook the onion over low heat for 5 minutes, until starting to color. Add the squash chunks and press into place to fill the pan. Scatter the currants over the top and carefully pour in the eggs, gently shaking the pan to evenly distribute them.
5   Cook the frittata for 10 minutes, until set around the edges. Place the pan under the broiler and cook for 5 minutes, until the top is set. Alternatively, cover the pan with a large plate, turn it over to release the frittata, and gently slide the frittata back into the pan and cook the other side, about 5 minutes.
6   Cut the frittata into wedges and serve with mixed salad greens and whole-grain bread. **SERVES 4**

Turkey rye pilaf

PREPARATION **15 MINUTES** COOKING **2 HOURS**

1 tablespoon (15 ml) olive or canola oil
1 onion, finely chopped
4 cloves garlic, crushed
1 small carrot, finely diced
$^{1}/_{2}$ red pepper, finely diced
2 large mushrooms, finely diced
$^{1}/_{2}$ pound (250 g) boneless, skinless turkey, chopped
1 tablespoon (15 ml) paprika
1 tablespoon (15 ml) ground cumin
1 teaspoon (5 ml) ground ginger
1 cup (200 g) whole rye grain or other whole grain, such as wheatberries or pearl barley
$^{3}/_{4}$ pound (400 g) fresh cherry tomatoes
2$^{1}/_{2}$ cups (625 ml) low-sodium chicken stock or water
4 sprigs fresh parsley, finely chopped

1   Preheat the oven to 350°F (180°C).
2   Heat the oil in a large flameproof casserole dish over low heat. Cook the onion for 5 minutes, until translucent, add the garlic and cook, stirring occasionally, for 3 minutes.
3   Add the carrot, pepper and mushrooms. Cook, stirring, for 10 minutes, until caramelized. Add the turkey and spices, and cook, stirring, for 5 minutes, until the turkey starts to brown.
4   Stir in the rye to coat with the spices, add half the tomatoes and the stock or water. Cover and transfer to the oven to cook for 1 hour 20 minutes, until the rye grains are tender and all the liquid has been absorbed.
5   Stir in the remaining tomatoes and the chopped parsley. Bake, uncovered, for another 10 minutes. **SERVES 4**

Lentil and spinach bake

PREPARATION **15 MINUTES** COOKING **25 MINUTES**

1 bunch spinach, about $^2/_3$ pound (300 g), trimmed
2 tablespoons (30 ml) olive or canola oil
1 leek, white part only, thinly sliced
14$^1/_2$ ounce (400 ml) can or fresh tomatoes, diced
15 ounce (425 ml) can lentils, rinsed and drained,
   or 2 cups (500 g) cooked lentils made from $^2/_3$ cup
   (125 g) dried lentils
2 eggs, beaten
$^1/_3$ cup (35 g) finely grated parmesan

1   Preheat the oven to 400°F (200°C).
2   Put the spinach in a large heatproof bowl and
cover with boiling water. Set aside until completely
wilted. Drain the spinach and, when cool enough to
handle, firmly squeeze to release as much liquid as
possible. Finely chop the spinach.
3   Heat the oil in a large frying pan. Cook the leek
over low heat for 5 minutes, until soft and starting
to color. Add the tomatoes and stir well. Add the
lentils and eggs, and stir until well combined.
4   Spread the lentil and spinach mixture in a 4 cup
(1 L) ovenproof dish, and top with the parmesan.
Bake for 20 minutes, until the middle is completely
set and the top is deep golden. **SERVES 4**

Cheesy baked potoatoes

PREPARATION **10 MINUTES** COOKING **55 MINUTES**

4 potatoes, about $^1/_2$ pound (250 g) each
1 cup (250 g) low-fat ricotta
$^1/_2$ cup (50 g) finely grated parmesan
5 sprigs fresh parsley, finely chopped
freshly ground black pepper

1   Preheat the oven to 400°F (200°C).
2   Place the potatoes directly on the oven rack and
bake for 30–45 minutes, until soft when squeezed.
3   When the potatoes are cool enough to handle, cut
off the tops and scoop out the insides with a spoon,
reserving the skins. Mash the potato flesh with the
ricotta, half the parmesan and the parsley. Season
with freshly ground black pepper.
4   Spoon the potato mixture back into the skins and
sprinkle with the remaining parmesan. Return to the
oven for 10 minutes, until the parmesan has melted.
Serve as a light meal with salad greens. **SERVES 4**

Duck breast with orange sauce

PREPARATION **10 MINUTES** COOKING **20 MINUTES**

olive oil, for brushing
4 shallots, finely chopped
4 boneless, skinless duck breasts, about
   $^1/_2$ pound (250 g) each
1 tablespoon (15 ml) all-purpose flour
finely grated zest and juice of 2 oranges
freshly ground black pepper

1   Brush a large nonstick frying pan with oil and
cook the shallots over low heat for 3–5 minutes, until
translucent. Increase the heat to medium and add the
duck breasts. Cook for 5 minutes on each side, until
browned and just pink in the middle. Transfer the
duck breasts to a warm covered dish to rest.
2   Add the flour to the pan. Gently cook, stirring, until
just starting to color, and gradually add the orange
juice, stirring to deglaze the pan and scraping up any
browned bits. Add the orange zest, reserving a little
for garnishing, and some freshly ground black pepper.
3   Slice the duck breasts on the diagonal and pour
any juices into the pan. Dilute the sauce with a little
water, if needed, until it reaches a nice consistency.
4   Arrange each sliced duck breast on a plate topped
with a stripe of orange sauce and garnished with the
reserved orange zest. Serve with a grain such as
quinoa or brown rice, and a green salad. **SERVES 4**

Saffron rice pudding

PREPARATION **5 MINUTES** COOKING **1 HOUR**

1 cup (200 g) brown rice
2 pinches saffron threads
1 teaspoon (5 ml) freshly grated nutmeg
1$^1/_2$ cups (350 ml) low-fat milk
2 tablespoons (30 ml) pure maple syrup
$^1/_4$ cup (30 g) golden raisins

1   Combine the rice, saffron threads, nutmeg and
1 cup (250 ml) water in a saucepan. Bring to a boil,
reduce the heat, cover and simmer the rice for
30 minutes, until all the water has been absorbed.
2   Preheat the oven to 350°F (180°C).
3   Stir the milk and maple syrup into the rice and
saffron mixture. Stir in the raisins, then pour into an
8 cup (2 L) ovenproof dish. Cover with foil and bake
for 30 minutes, stirring after 10 minutes to be sure it
cooks evenly. **SERVES 4**

Words and language

Puzzles that require you to recognize and understand words—no matter how well hidden or disguised—sharpen your verbal skills, expand your vocabulary and improve your powers of reasoning and observation.

1 Healthy pairs

Combine these 16 words to form 8 brain-friendly compound words. Use each word only once.

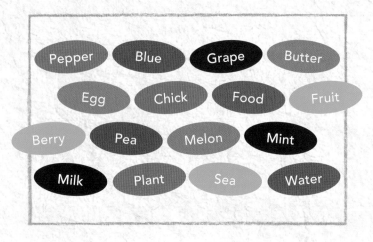

3 Spell out

Starting with W, spell out a 10-letter word, moving through each circle only once. *Hint* unprocessed crop.

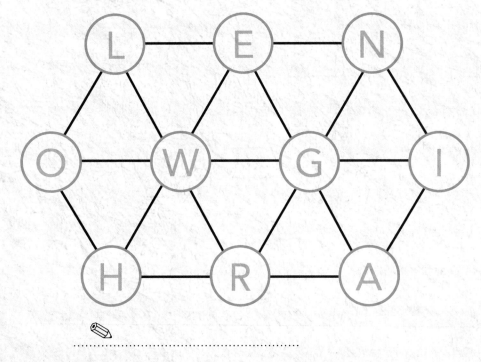

2 Word ladder

In a word ladder puzzle, you change one word into another by changing just one letter at each rung. Each of the four rungs on the word ladder must be a valid word.

Turn **corn** into **rice**

Clues:
1. center
2. concern
3. quite unusual
4. rush

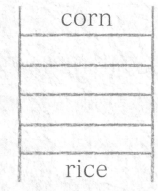

Turn **meat** into **ball**

This time, we have taken out the clues to make it a little more difficult.

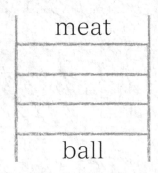

4 Word search

Can you spot the following herbs hidden in the grid? They may be found across, up, down or diagonally in any direction and may overlap.

BASIL
CAMOMILE
CHERVIL
CHIVES
CORIANDER
DILL
FENNEL
LOVAGE
MARJORAM
MINT
OREGANO
PARSLEY
ROSEMARY
RUE
SAGE
SORREL
TARRAGON
THYME

A	N	I	M	A	L	M	A	G	I	C	F	R	Y
C	O	R	I	A	N	D	E	R	H	O	R	S	E
A	G	R	A	R	I	A	N	F	E	N	N	E	L
M	A	E	M	Y	H	T	C	H	A	M	O	I	S
O	R	I	O	N	N	A	I	L	E	A	V	E	R
M	R	I	M	I	N	I	X	Y	L	R	E	Q	A
I	A	R	M	A	D	A	L	L	E	I	X	U	P
L	T	R	O	S	E	V	I	H	C	O	D	O	E
E	E	D	J	O	P	S	C	A	L	A	L	R	Y
E	G	G	R	O	O	B	A	R	R	I	D	E	K
F	A	I	R	R	R	U	G	U	N	S	G	I
O	V	E	R	H	I	A	C	R	E	A	M	A	W
D	O	E	A	G	L	E	M	I	N	A	H	N	B
A	L	L	I	G	R	Y	R	A	M	E	S	O	R

5 Scrambled words

Unscramble the letters in each berry to produce two words that are important for good brain function.

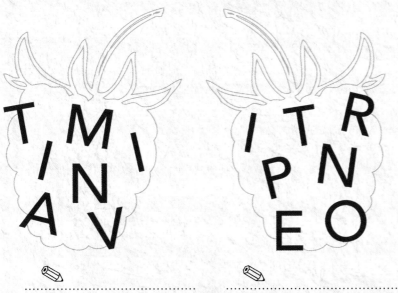

6 Hidden foods

Find the food words hiding in the following anagrams.

a. RUSTIC ....

b. STEAD ....

c. LUMP..........................

d. STUPORS ....

e. AGES..........................

f. LEAK ....

g. REPLAYS ....

h. PAGERS.......................

i. SANDIER......................

j. ARROGANT ....

k. AUNT ....

l. VEINED ....

Numbers and logic

Solving these puzzles will involve logic, common sense and strategy as well
as memory, as you will need to recall and make use of skills learned in school.
So ditch the calculator and exercise your brain instead.

1 Balancing act
How many forks are needed to balance scale C?

....

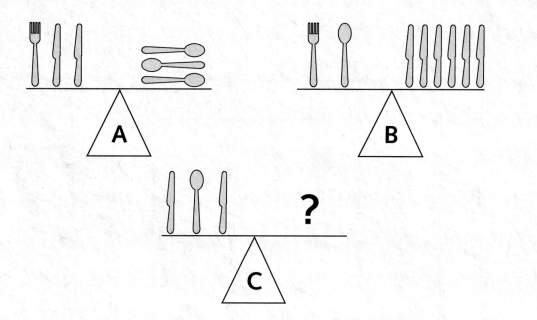

2 Magic square
In a magic square, all the rows, columns and
main diagonal lines must add up to the same
number. In this magic square, all the empty
squares contain an odd number. Can you work
out what they all are?

	10	6
4		16
14		2
	8	12

3 Problem pyramid
Each of the numbered blocks in this pyramid
carries the total of the two blocks on which it
rests. From the figures given, can you find all
the missing numbers?

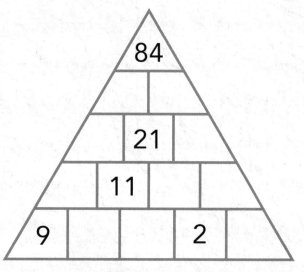

4 Hexagonal place mats

Dinner is almost ready. Which number should replace the x on the fourth place mat (D)? The key is to uncover the logic of the sequence.

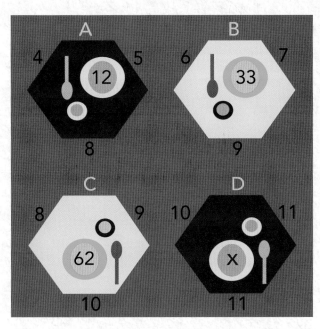

5 Orange segments

One slice is missing a number. Which number should replace the x?

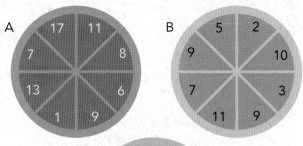

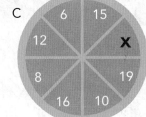

6 Fruit corner

If 6 apples + 3 bananas cost $8.70 and 5 apples + 7 bananas cost $12.20, what is the value of a single apple and a single banana?

7 If... then

Clear, careful thinking will help you to solve the logic problems here.

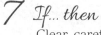
If... then

A. A certain café's lunch menu has three choices for sandwiches: tuna for $3, chicken salad for $4, and beef for $4.50. Three friends come into the café for lunch, and each one orders a sandwich. If the total cost of the three sandwiches ordered is $10, do we know how many of each sandwich were ordered?

....

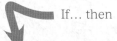
If... then

B. If in a yearly calendar of events National Egg Month comes before National Peanut Butter Month, National Strawberry Month comes after National Potato Month, and National Potato Month comes after National Egg Month, is National Egg Month before or after National Strawberry Month, or do we not have enough information to tell?

....

Answers on page 288

Spatial and visual

These puzzles challenge your ability to visualize objects from various angles and interpret them accurately. Mazes help improve your spatial reasoning skills and, as you may need to change direction several times, promote mental flexibility.

1 Draw a line

Can you divide this picture by drawing two straight lines to produce three sections, each containing two apples, two lemons, two pears, a banana and an orange?

2 Double trouble

Can you solve this doubly complicated maze, starting at the arrow in the top left and escaping by the exit marked with an X?

3 Fitting it together

Which four of these five pieces fit together to form the complete plate? You will need to mentally rotate and reposition the pieces of broken plate to eliminate the piece that does not belong and then fit the remaining four pieces together.

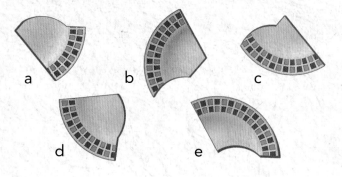

a   b   c

d   e

4 Reach your reward

Can you find your way through to the middle of
this square maze to get to the brain-friendly snack?

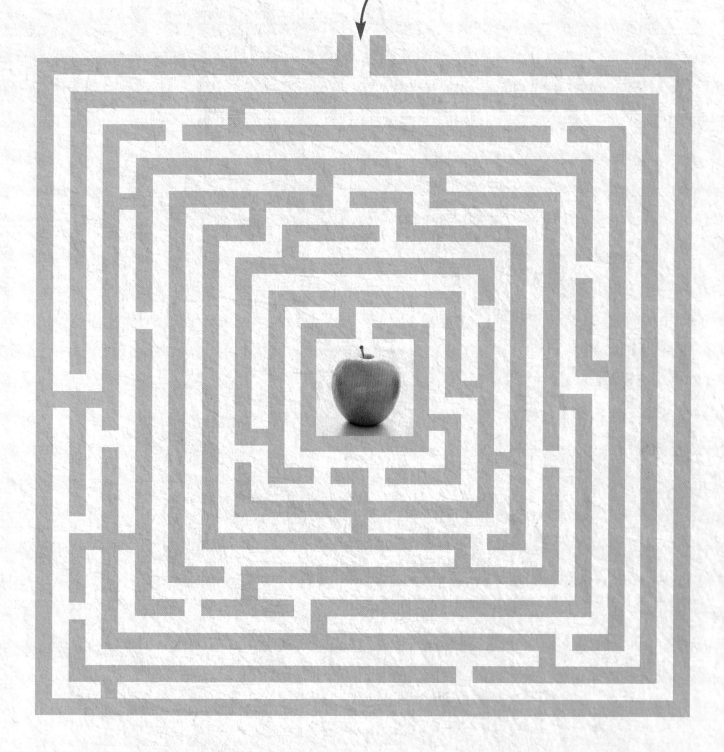

Answers on page 289

Memory
and concentration

Puzzles of this type train your visual memory, improve your powers of observation and attention to detail, increase your concentration skills, and expand your ability to retain information in your short-term memory. Puzzles to be completed in a given time also test your reaction speed.

1 Spot the differences

Can you spot the eight differences between Picture 1 and Picture 2?

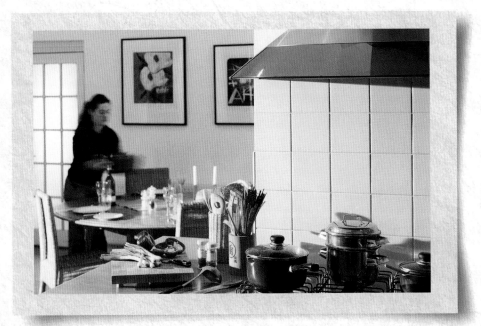

Picture 1

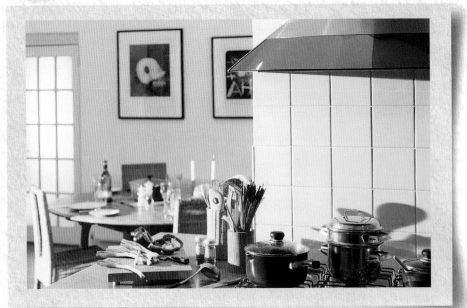

Picture 2

2 Time to eat

Look at these ten objects for one minute then cover the picture. List as many as you can remember. You will find it helps if you mentally link as many like objects as possible (e.g., two pieces of fruit, two containers, or four things).

red wine

whole-grain bread

pear

cup and saucer

parsley

napkins

pepper

saucepan

apples

pitcher of water

1. ....
2. ....
3. ....
4. ....
5. ....
6. ....
7. ....
8. ....
9. ....
10. ....

3 True or false? The brain and food

How good is your knowledge about the effect of food on the brain and its operation?

True False

1. Serotonin, the "feel-good" hormone, makes you feel alert and full of energy..................... ☐ ☐
2. Dopamine "switches off" melatonin to wake you up when the sun rises......................... ☐ ☐
3. The brain is fueled mainly by fiber and fat........ ☐ ☐
4. Because the brain works during the night, you should eat a substantial meal in the evening..... ☐ ☐
5. Chicken is the principal animal source of omega-3. .... ☐ ☐
6. Eating mainly high GI foods helps brain function. ☐ ☐
7. Too much vitamin B_{12} can make you irritable and confused. .... ☐ ☐
8. Skipping breakfast keeps you hungry, making you more alert.............................. ☐ ☐

True False

9. The colorful pigments in fruits and vegetables can help protect brain cells from damage........ ☐ ☐
10. A high-fat, high-sugar diet can impair memory function. .... ☐ ☐
11. Rich, fatty foods have a low glycemic index (GI)................................... ☐ ☐
12. A deficiency of the trace element zinc is common in people with depression.............. ☐ ☐
13. Dairy foods and poultry are high in the amino acid tryptophan, used to produce serotonin. .... ☐ ☐
14. Caffeine, which delays sleep, peaks in your bloodstream about an hour after consumption. ... ☐ ☐
15. A very low carbohydrate diet makes the brain work better. .... ☐ ☐

4 Odd one out

Look closely at these jugs. Which one is different from all the others?

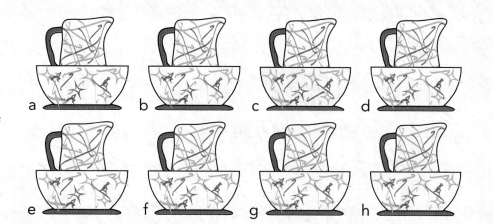

a   b   c   d

e   f   g   h

Answers to puzzles

Words and language

1 Healthy pairs
blueberry; buttermilk; chickpea; eggplant;
grapefruit; peppermint; seafood; watermelon

2 Word ladder
Turn corn into rice
corn, core, care, rare, race, rice

Turn meat into ball
meat, beat, belt, bell, ball

3 Spell out
whole-grain

4 Word search

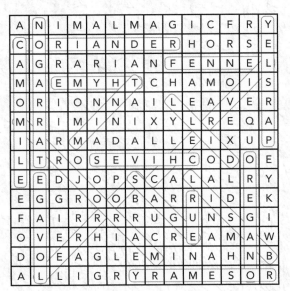

5 Scrambled words
vitamin, protein

6 Hidden foods
a. citrus; b. dates; c. plum; d. sprouts; e. sage;
f. kale; g. parsley; h. grapes; i. sardine;
j. tarragon; k. tuna; l. endive

Number and logic

1 Balancing act
One. Each knife has a value of 1, each spoon
a value of 2 and each fork a value of 4, so one
fork is needed to balance scale C.

2 Magic square

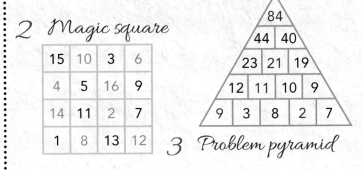

15	10	3	6
4	5	16	9
14	11	2	7
1	8	13	12

3 Problem pyramid

4 Hexagonal place mats
A (4 x 5) − 8		= 12
B (6 x 7) − 9		= 33
C (8 x 9) − 10		= 62
D (10 x 11) − 11		= 99
Therefore x		= 99

5 Orange segments
The identically placed segments in the three
slices A, B and C always add up to 28
(e.g. 11 + 2 + 15 = 28). Therefore x = 10.

6 Fruit corner
Apple (A) = 90 cents, Banana (B) = $1.10.
The trick is to multiply each equation by a
number that makes it possible to eliminate
one of the variables (Apples):

6A + 3B = $8.70   Multiply x 5
5A + 7B = $12.20 Multiply x 6
1 = 30A + 15B = $43.50 ($8.70 x 5)
2 = 30A + 42B = $73.20 ($12.20 x 6)
Subtract 1 from 2, and you are left with 27B
and no A.
27B = $29.70 ($73.20 - $43.50)
one B = $1.10 ($29.70 ÷ 27)
one A = 90 cents

7 If ... then
A. Two tuna and one chicken salad

B. National Egg Month is before National
Strawberry Month

Spatial and visual

1 Draw a line

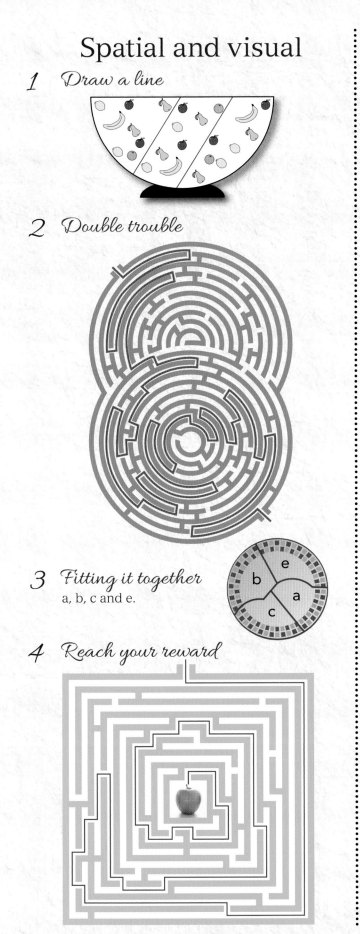

2 Double trouble

3 Fitting it together
a, b, c and e.

4 Reach your reward

Memory and concentration

1 Spot the differences

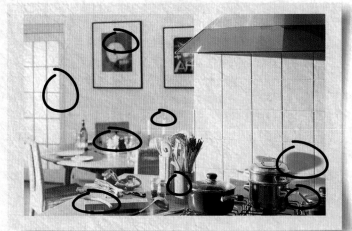

2 Time to eat
red wine
whole-grain bread
napkins
pear
pitcher of water
pepper
parsley
saucepan
cup and saucer
apples

3 The brain and food
1. False. 2. True. 3. False. 4. False. 5. False.
6. False. 7. False. 8. False. 9. True. 10. True.
11. True. 12. True. 13. True. 14. True. 15. False.

4 Odd one out
Jug c.

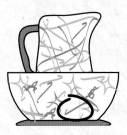

Glossary

ACETYLCHOLINE

Acetylcholine is a neurotransmitter, or brain chemical messenger, involved in many different parts of the nervous system. It is a major neurotransmitter in muscle contraction, as well as being important to attention and sensory perceptions.

ALZHEIMER'S DISEASE

Alzheimer's disease is a common type of dementia that is caused by the deterioration of the nervous system, with abnormal cells forming plaques in the brain and interfering with normal function.

ANTIOXIDANTS

When it reacts in your body, oxygen can form harmful substances called free radicals that damage cells. Since we can't live without oxygen, we have a complex system of antioxidants to protect us from this damage. Antioxidants work together to neutralize free radicals, and include some of the vitamins (such as vitamin C), minerals (such as zinc) and many other substances that are found in plant foods.

B-GROUP VITAMINS

Vitamin B_1, thiamine, is used in the body's energy generation processes and for maintaining normal neurological function.

Vitamin B_2, riboflavin, is essential for obtaining energy from food for your brain cells. It is also needed in the process that produces serotonin.

Vitamin B_3, niacin, is involved in the production of serotonin. Dementia is typically seen in niacin deficiency.

Vitamin B_5, pantothenic acid, is needed for metabolism of glucose and fat to supply energy. It is also essential for production of the most common neurotransmitter, acetyl choline.

Vitamin B_6, pyridoxine, promotes the production of mood-boosting serotonin, and some studies have found a connection between memory and vitamin B_6 status. Vitamin B_6 also helps to protect against homocysteine.

Vitamin B_9, folate, is important in maintaining myelin. It also has an important role in protecting against inflammatory homocysteine levels, which are thought to damage blood vessels and contribute to an increased risk of dementia and stroke.

Vitamin B_{12} comes only from animal foods and works with folate to maintain the myelin that protects nerve cells. As well as being important in the production of neurotransmitters, vitamin B_{12} also helps to protect against inflammatory homocysteine.

BETA-CAROTENE

Beta-carotene is the plant form of vitamin A (retinol). It acts as an antioxidant as well as being important for healthy eyesight.

BLOOD GLUCOSE

Your body uses glucose as fuel for every cell. This glucose is obtained from the carbohydrates in your diet, which are broken down and absorbed as glucose into the bloodstream. It is thought that uncontrolled high blood glucose levels could cause inflammatory damage in the body, including the brain.

CALCIUM

Apart from making your bones strong, calcium is important for helping to control blood pressure, and is also involved in producing nerve signals throughout the entire nervous system.

CARBOHYDRATES

Sugars, starchy foods such as pasta, bread and cookies, are all carbohydrates, that is, chains and clusters of sugar molecules that are broken down to produce glucose as fuel for your body.

CARDIAC DISEASE

Your heart pumps blood around your body and brain to take oxygen and nutrients to every cell. It relies on a system of blood vessels to carry the blood, but if these become narrowed, inflexible or blocked, your cells run out of fuel and can become damaged or die. Cardiac disease is usually the result of a build-up of cholesterol deposits in the blood vessel walls, other changes in the blood vessel tissue, or damage from high blood pressure.

CAROTENOIDS

Carotenoids are a family of colorful pigments in food that are similar to beta-carotene. They have antioxidant activity and are being studied for their anticancer effects (see Beta-carotene).

CEREAL GRAIN FOODS

Many of our staple foods are based on cereal grains such as wheat, rice, barley, rye, quinoa and so on. These can be very nutritious if processing is kept to a minimum, as in whole-grain bread or whole-wheat pasta, or they can be potentially harmful because highly processed starches can promote high blood glucose levels and potentially inflammation in the body.

CHOLESTEROL

Cholesterol is a fatty substance that is essential for some of the body's processes, but which can cause problems if levels are too high. Cholesterol is produced in the body from fats in the diet. LDL cholesterol ("bad" cholesterol) can be deposited in blood vessels and cause them to narrow or become blocked. HDL cholesterol ("good" cholesterol) collects damaging LDLs and transports them to the liver for disposal.

CHOLINE

Although choline is not a vitamin, it is very closely related to the B-group vitamins and is essential for the synthesis of neurotransmitters and maintaining the myelin sheath that protects the nerves, as well as being a component of cell membranes. Choline is the precursor of acetylcholine, the most common neurotransmitter, important for memory and muscle control.

DEMENTIA

Dementia refers to any brain disease that decreases brain functions such as thinking, memory and attention. Alzheimer's disease is a common form of dementia that involves abnormal tissue building up in the brain, but other causes of dementia include damage from alcohol excess, infection, changes to the cardiovascular system, and loss of the myelin that protects neurons.

DEPRESSION

Depression is a mood disorder, typically involving a low or sad mood state and a loss of interest in activities that are normally enjoyed. Since mood is strongly influenced by brain chemicals, there has been considerable research interest in how food affects mood. Foods associated with a reduced depression risk include omega-3 fats, and a Mediterranean style of eating, high in unprocessed foods, beneficial fats and plant foods.

DOPAMINE

Dopamine is a neurotransmitter, or brain chemical messenger, that activates pleasure centers in the brain and is also involved in regulating your daily sleep–wake cycle.

ESSENTIAL FATTY ACIDS

There are two particular fatty acids that are essential for health, but which our bodies can't make for us. This means we have to obtain them from food. They are linoleic acid (found in nuts and seeds, and needed for healthy skin and immune function) and alpha-linolenic acid, or ALA (found in fish and shellfish, and needed for normal brain function and immune function).

FOLATE (VITAMIN B_9)

see B-group vitamins

GLUTAMATES

Glutamate is one of the amino acids, the building blocks of protein. Glutamates in food are formed by protein breakdown (such as during the aging of cheeses or processed meats) and associated with savory "umami" flavors. Some people have undesirable food sensitivity reactions to foods that are high in glutamates.

GLYCEMIC INDEX (GI)

When you eat a carbohydrate food, it is broken down to make glucose as fuel for your body. The glucose appears in your bloodstream as the carbohydrate is digested and absorbed. The glycemic index (GI) is a measure of how quickly this happens. For example, food that is quick to digest and absorb can release a lot of glucose into the bloodstream at once, giving it a high glycemic index (or high GI) value. Low-GI carbohydrate foods, such as whole-grain breads, whole-wheat pastas, and whole-grain cereals, release glucose into the bloodstream more slowly. This can help you feel full longer and have a steadier supply of fuel for your brain.

HOMOCYSTEINE

Homocysteine is an amino acid not found in food—it is formed in the body. High levels of homocysteine seem to be a marker for cardiovascular disease risk, and may promote oxidative cell damage. B-group vitamins B_6 and B_{12} help to get rid of homocysteine.

INFLAMMATION

Your body's response to injury or infection is designed to protect you from harm, kill bacteria, remove damaged cells and promote healing. This whole process is called inflammation and is normally carefully controlled. When you aren't suffering from any injury or infection, ongoing inflammation can be harmful, causing stress in the body and damaging healthy tissue. Factors that can promote such inflammation include smoking, obesity, lack of sleep, anxiety and depression.

IRON

Your blood needs iron to help carry oxygen to your cells, to obtain energy. Iron is found in both animal foods (such as lean meat) and plant foods (such as whole grains and legumes). The form of iron contained in plant foods is harder for your body to absorb. However, eating them with a source of vitamin C, or with an animal iron source, helps your body to absorb the iron better. This means you will obtain more iron if your legume dish contains tomatoes or peppers, for example, or if you have some fruit with your breakfast cereal.

LEGUMES

Legumes or pulses include the members of the bean and pea family—peas, chickpeas, kidney beans, all types of lentils, soybeans and cannellini beans. Rich in fiber and minerals, they are a good plant source of protein.

LUTEIN

Lutein is a carotenoid, found in green leafy vegetables and in egg yolk. Along with zeaxanthin, it appears to be important in healthy eyesight and may protect against age-related macular degeneration.

LYCOPENE

Lycopene is a carotenoid pigment with a bright color responsible for the redness of tomatoes, watermelons, papaya and pink grapefruit.

MACULAR DEGENERATION

Macular degeneration is a major cause of vision loss in older people. The macula is the center of the visual field where detail is seen (for reading and face recognition), and vision is lost there when the retina is damaged. High blood pressure and saturated fat intake seem to increase risk of macular degeneration, while antioxidants such as lutein and zeaxanthin seem to be protective.

MAGNESIUM
A mineral important for the normal function of every cell in your body, magnesium is found in green leafy vegetables, nuts, seeds, spices and whole grains.

MEDITERRANEAN DIET
A diet high in plant foods and beneficial fats, and low in processed foods with small amounts of animal foods, is often referred to as a Mediterranean-style diet. This way of eating has been shown in many research studies to be good for long-term health of the brain and heart.

METABOLISM
Metabolism is the process of converting food and oxygen into the energy we need to live, and the substances that keep our bodies working normally.

MICRONUTRIENTS
Micronutrients are nutrients that we need only in tiny quantities. These include the vitamins and most of the minerals that are essential for good health.

MONOUNSATURATED FATTY ACIDS
Monounsaturated fatty acids are found in olive oil, nuts and seeds. They appear to be protective of brain function in the long term, shown in studies of the Mediterranean diet, which is high in monounsaturated fats.

MYELIN
Nerve cells, or neurons, have a long, thin tail like a communications cable, which is covered with a layer of insulation called myelin. This layer protects the neuron and helps it communicate faster and more efficiently.

NEURONAL COMMUNICATION
Nerve cells, also called neurons, each have a long tail called an axon that acts like a communications cable, carrying electrical signals by branching and linking to other neurons. At each junction point, or "synapse," chemicals called neurotransmitters take the message to receptors on the next neuron.

NEUROTRANSMITTERS
Neurotransmitters are chemicals that carry messages between nerve cells in the brain. Different neurotransmitters may activate particular areas of the brain, or be involved in specific types of messages, such as in stress or pleasure.

NIACIN (VITAMIN B_3)
see B-group vitamins

NORADRENALINE
Noradrenaline is a neurotransmitter, or brain chemical messenger, that is involved in the body's stress response. It gives you a surge of energy and keeps you alert.

OMEGA-3 FATTY ACIDS
Omega-3 fatty acids are found in fish and seafood, flaxseeds and walnuts. They seem to have an anti-inflammatory effect that may help to preserve brain function in the long term. They also seem to promote more flexible and responsive brain performance.

OXIDATIVE STRESS
Oxidative stress occurs when you don't have enough antioxidants. Although you need oxygen to live, it can react in your body to form harmful substances called free radicals that damage cells. The body's antioxidant system is supposed to protect you from this damage, but an inadequate or ultra-processed diet may mean you don't have sufficient antioxidants to meet your needs when demand is high (due to weight gain or smoking, for example, or during illness).

PANTOTHENIC ACID (VITAMIN B_5)
see B-group vitamins

PHOSPHORUS
Along with calcium, phosphorus is essential for strong bones, but it is also present in every other cell in your body as it is part of the body's energy system. It is also involved in nerve transmission, making it important for normal brain function. Phosphorus is found in all foods, but is particularly high in animal foods such as meats and dairy products.

PHYTOESTROGENS
Phytoestrogens are estrogen-like substances that come from plants such as legumes and alfalfa. These have a gentler effect than the estrogen in your body, and can be helpful during menopause by blocking the stronger undesirable effects of estrogen. This can reduce symptoms such as hot flushes.

PHYTONUTRIENTS
Phytonutrients are any nutrients that come from plants. These include vitamins but also many of the antioxidants that we obtain from plant foods.

POLYPHENOLS
The many different kinds of antioxidants include polyphenols (such as isoflavones, found in soybeans; and quercetin, found in onions and apples), which are thought to have powerful brain-protective effects, reducing the risk of cell damage from free radicals.

POTASSIUM
Potassium, found in all plant foods, is essential for every cell in your body. In particular, it maintains the electrical conductivity of your brain and nerves. It also helps to keep blood pressure under control.

PROTEIN
Your whole body is made of protein, and you need a regular intake to maintain normal healing, repair and growth. Animal flesh, eggs and milk are high in protein, while most plant protein sources are lower in protein. These include legumes, nuts and seeds.

PYRIDOXINE (VITAMIN B₆)
see B-group vitamins

RIBOFLAVIN (VITAMIN B₂)
see B-group vitamins

SALT
Table salt, or sodium chloride, enhances the flavor of our food. But excess sodium causes your blood pressure to increase as you get older. Based on the Dietary Guidelines for Americans, a publication that the Departments of Agriculture and Health and Human Services Departments release every five years, the U.S. Food and Drug Administration recommendation is to limit sodium intake to no more than 2300 mg each day— the equivalent of 1 teaspoon of salt from all sources—but many people eat double this or more, mostly in processed foods rather than salt that is added at home.

SELENIUM
Selenium is an important part of the body's antioxidant system, forming part of an enzyme that fights harmful free radicals. Selenium is found in legumes, seeds and nuts, in particular, Brazil nuts.

SEROTONIN
Serotonin is a neurotransmitter, or brain chemical messenger, that promotes a pleasant, relaxed state. Serotonin is important in getting ready for sleep.

STROKE
Stroke is a loss of brain function caused by a blockage in the blood flow to the brain, or bleeding in the brain. Increased risk is associated with high blood pressure and/or increased levels of fats in the blood.

THIAMINE (VITAMIN B₁)
see B-group vitamins

TRYPTOPHAN
One of the building blocks of protein, tryptophan is an amino acid that is used to produce serotonin, so foods high in tryptophan (such as lean meat, poultry and fish) tend to promote a pleasant, relaxed state, ready for sleep.

URIDINE
Uridine works together with choline to repair brain cell membranes, and together uridine and choline are now being investigated in research that explores how to reduce age-related loss of brain function. Foods high in uridine include tomatoes, yeast, liver and broccoli.

VITAMINS
see also B-group vitamins

Vitamin A, or retinol, is found in animal foods such as organ meats and eggs, and is essential for normal vision.

Vitamin C, also known as ascorbic acid, works as part of the body's antioxidant system as well as being essential for healthy skin and gums. Vitamin C is found in a variety of plant foods such as red peppers, tomatoes, berries and citrus fruit.

Vitamin D, essential for bone health, is made by your skin when it is exposed to sunlight. It is also found in foods such as some fish. Vitamin D deficiency seems to be associated with increased risk of depression, cognitive impairment and dementia, but it is not clear whether or not taking a vitamin D supplement can decrease this risk.

Vitamin E is part of the body's antioxidant system as well as being important for healthy skin and blood. It is found in avocado, as well as seed and cereal grain oils. Vitamin E deficiency is associated with nerve and muscle problems, making it essential for normal brain function.

Vitamin K is found in green leafy vegetables. It is an essential part of the process that helps blood to clot. Without it, serious damage to the body can result in significant blood loss.

WHOLE-GRAIN FOODS
The starch in a cereal grain is covered with layers of fibrous bran. Although this bran is rich in nutrients and fiber, beneficial to health, it is usually removed in processing. Choosing whole-grain foods, which are less processed, means you get the nutritional benefits of the bran as well as energy from the carbohydrates.

ZEAXANTHIN
Zeaxanthin is a carotenoid found in green leafy vegetables and in yellow foods such as corn and saffron. It seems to be important for healthy eyesight and may protect against age-related macular degeneration.

ZINC
Optimal brain function requires zinc in large amounts. Zinc, found in lean meats, seafood and legumes, is important in many processes of cell metabolism, and also plays a role in neurotransmission. Zinc deficiency causes problems with learning, memory and attention.

Index

A Reader's Digest Book

Consultant Suzie Ferrie, Advanced Accredited Practising
Dietitian
Designer Vivien Valk
Project Manager Deborah Nixon

Photographer Maree Homer
Stylist Louise Bickle
Food Preparation Tracy Rutherford
Recipes Suzie Ferrie, Deborah Nixon, Tracy Rutherford,
    Jody Vassallo
Copy Editor Justine Harding
Puzzle Editor Margaret McPhee
Proofreader Susan McCreery
Indexer Glenda Browne
Senior Production Controller Monique Tesoriero

Photography credits
Photographs are the copyright of Reader's Digest, except the
following:
Chapter openers pp 22–23, 50–51, 88–89, 152–153, 228–229:
Shutterstock
With thanks to Mud Australia, mudaustralia.com and
No Chintz Textiles and Soft Furnishings, www.nochintz.com

Cover Baked beets with balsamic-glazed shallots, walnuts
and feta, page 145; Tuscan-style chicken, bean and tomato
soup, page 53; Blueberry yogurt tart with ginger crust, page
256; Beef bolognese with tagliatelle, page 221
Spine Baked beets with balsamic-glazed shallots, walnuts
and feta, page 145
Back cover Chicken and vegetable curry, page 202; Blueberry
and oat breakfast muffins, page 32; Beef and broccolini salad,
page 79
Title page, clockwise from top left Oatmeal with dried
fruit compote, page 28; Spicy lentil soup with butternut
squash, tomatoes and green beans, page 64; Trout, egg and
asparagus salad, page 73; Glazed tomatoes with raisins,
almonds and garlic, page 141; Smoked paprika lamb with
whole-wheat couscous, page 222; Whole-wheat walnut and
grape focaccia, page 263; Saffron and pistachio puddings with
cardamom and honey syrup, page 235
Foreword, from left to right Berry yogurt swirl with
walnuts and pepitas, page 25; Roasted red pepper and tomato
soup, page 63; Baked beets with balsamic-glazed shallots,
walnuts and feta, page 145; Beef and vegetable skewers, page
219; Chewy nut bars, page 245

Brainpower Cookbook was first published in 2015 by
Reader's Digest (Australia) Pty Limited.

ISBN 978-1-62145-320-8

We are committed to both the quality of our products and the
service we provide to our customers. We value your
comments, so please feel free to contact us.
    Reader's Digest Adult Trade Publishing
    44 South Broadway
    White Plains, NY 10601

For more Reader's Digest products and information, visit our
website:
    www.rd.com (in the United States)
    www.readersdigest.ca (in Canada)

Printed in China

10 9 8 7 6 5 4 3 2 1

Weights and measures Sometimes conversions within a
recipe are not exact but are the closest conversion that is a
suitable measurement for each system. Use either the metric
or the imperial measurements; do not mix the two systems.

The information in this book should not be
substituted for, or used to alter, medical therapy
without your doctor's advice. For a specific
health problem or dietary concern, consult
your doctor for guidance.